This newly revised edition of a famous
household work of reference is as interesting
as a novel and as informative as its sister
volume, *Pears Cyclopaedia*. Even today,
medicine remains a subject of widespread
ignorance among civilised people. *Pears
Medical Encyclopaedia* is in no way a
substitute for a doctor's professional attention,
but it covers the wide range of Medical
Matters, relates modern medicine to its social
background and talks sheer good sense on
many controversial and taboo topics. For
example, a worried mother looking up
appendicitis will learn that this condition
cannot be caused by swallowing pips, seeds or
fruit stones, and on referring to the entry on
obesity will be told that an overweight child
is almost certainly eating too much, whatever
the state of its glands.

Pears Medical Encyclopaedia

J. A. C. BROWN

SPHERE BOOKS LIMITED
30/32 Gray's Inn Road, London WC1X 8JL

Copyright © J. A. C. Brown 1962
Revised 1963, 1965
Reprinted by arrangement with
Pelham Books Ltd
First Sphere Books edition 1967
Reprinted June 1967, January 1970, February 1974

TRADE
MARK

Set in Linotype Times

Printed in Great Britain by
Hazell Watson & Viney Ltd
Aylesbury, Bucks

ISBN 0 7221 1906 2

INTRODUCTION

THIS book assumes no medical knowledge on the part of the layman but since its aim is to be scientific and, within the limits imposed by space, reasonably detailed, it may also prove useful to nurses and others who wish to refresh their memories or refer to something outside their own immediate field. Its contents have been arranged in the following way:

(1) Symptoms are included as well as actual diseases, since it is these that are likely to attract first attention and their true significance is not always apparent (e.g. vomiting does not necessarily indicate that something is amiss in the stomach). Therefore headache, vomiting, diarrhoea, colic, breathlessness, and so on have taken their place in alphabetical order from which the reader can refer to the diseases they may indicate.

(2) The commoner diseases appear under their usual names and from these references may be made to the system affected, the anatomy and physiology of which is described together with some of the less common diseases which may attack it.

(3) Amongst other items included are certain drugs or groups of drugs, some of the most frequently used medical terms, medical and surgical procedures, etc. In certain cases the names of proprietary drugs are given when, as is often the case, these are more generally familiar than the official title.

Having made these few points about how the dictionary should be used it is necessary to say something about why it has been written at all and to give a few words of advice about the best way of handling problems of health or disease in association with the family doctor (some of whom have expressed considerable doubts about the wisdom of making more than a minimal amount of medical information available to the general public). As to the first issue the answer is simple: it has been written in the belief that so far as possible all knowledge should be available to anyone who seeks it and that, in the particular case of medical information, those who feel that too much can be harmful are barking up the wrong tree since the choice is no longer between some knowledge or none at all but between correct and incorrect information. With an increasingly

5

educated population learning daily about medical matters from newspapers, radio, and television, it is impossible to keep people in the dark and every family doctor knows perfectly well that what is not supplied openly and freely will be filled in by rumour and old wives' tales. Of course, the writer, who has had his share of general practice, can understand very well why some physicians feel that the public can have too much ill-digested medical knowledge; for it is extremely galling to find a patient scrutinising one's prescription with a jaded eye ('Oh, it's only such-and-such'!) or demanding why he has not been given the new drug he read of just yesterday in the daily paper and which seems admirably suited to his own condition. That the simple remedy may be the best and certainly the safer or that he does not suffer from the disorder for which the new drug is intended nor know of its very unpleasant side-effects may not occur to the patient. But this is not an indication for making the futile attempt to stem the flow of medical information to the public but rather for increasing the flow of accurate information. After all, so far as nonsense is concerned, there is little to choose between the patient who believes that the new 'wonder drug' will cure some illness with which he is not afflicted, that glucose will give him energy or that vitamins will stop him from feeling tired, and the old-fashioned variety who wants something to 'clean his blood' which is 'overheated' or holds that rheumatism is caused by 'impurities' or 'crystals' in some unspecified area of his body. An attempt is made here to deal with both ancient and modern types of nonsense.

The second issue is that which concerns the patient's attitude to matters of health and disease and here it is absolutely essential to insist that *no book is a substitute for a doctor's advice* even if the patient is himself a doctor. The individual who, rightly or wrongly, does not feel that he can trust his doctor implicitly should change to another (although he would be well-advised to consider first the possibility that he may be wrong and, consciously or unconsciously, is seeking someone who will give him the advice he wants to hear rather than unpleasant truths he would prefer not to hear). Confidence between doctor and patient is not only important, it is part of the treatment. Diagnosis and treatment are not purely mechanical matters but depend in part upon the doctor's estimate of his patient's total condition including his character and personal problems. Thus the fact that Mr Smith has a raised blood-pressure and that there are drugs in existence which can lower it does not lead inevitably to the conclusion that the drugs should be used because the raised pressure may be relatively harmless and the effect of drugs both harmful and unpleasant in a particular case. The 'typical' illness described in a text-book is one thing while Mr Smith's version of the same disease may well be quite another. An intelligent patient is perfectly entitled to ask his doctor's opinion of the latest tranquilliser and whether or not it would be suitable in his own case, but he would be very foolish if he tried to insist on having it prescribed or refused to accept his doctor's advice and obtained it elsewhere. What it is necessary to consider is that the report of the drug he has read in the daily papers is quite likely to have been written up from a hand-out obligingly supplied by the firm making it to a 'scientific correspondent' whose main interest is in nuclear physics, whereas what the doctor knows from actual clinical tests reported only in medical journals is that the drug in question has been shown to help some patients and in others to produce (to take just some of the effects additionally produced by certain tranquillisers) giddiness, depression to the point of suicide, or epileptiform fits. Even when the short-term results are good, the long-term ones have sometimes been serious diseases of the blood or liver. The corollary to 'never try to diagnose your own condition' is 'never try except in minor conditions to treat yourself.'

Another good rule is that one should *never believe what he hears from non-medical sources and he should never give any medical advice to others.* It is impossible to assess the amount of rubbish talked by otherwise intelligent persons or the amount of harm their well-meant advice may lead to, and doctors are all too familiar with the patient who has been kept from getting proper treatment by someone who has recommended a patent medicine which he or she has taken until it is too late and what remains of his life is to be numbered in weeks rather than months or the almost equally tragic cases who have listened to their neighbour rather than their doctor and spent years in a state of unnecessary anxiety and fear. Hardly anyone (and least of all the 'practical' man) has the slightest idea of what constitutes scientific proof of the value or otherwise of a particular form of treatment and to many it is proof enough that some carefully selected exhibitionists have given their evidence on television that 'Buxom Salts' cured their rheumatism or that Mr Jones' backache was cured by manipulation from an un-qualified practitioner – perhaps it was, but what if someone else's backache is caused by tuberculosis of the spine? How many, for example, realise that the mere observation that 90% of cases felt much better or even lost all or most of their symptoms after being treated with drug X proves just one thing: that 90% of cases *felt* better *after* being treated by drug X? It does not prove either that they are better or that, if they are, the results were produced by the drug; for, in order to prove that, it would be necessary to show (*a*) that by objective tests they were cured or relieved, and (*b*) preferably how drug X was able to produce this effect. Confidence (both on the part of the patient and the doctor), faith, and the effect of emotions on the body, can produce strange and impressive results – not that this is unworthy of consideration especially when feeling better is accompanied by actually being better and even merely feeling better is an excellent thing provided it is not confused with cure. Thus it may be recollected that cortisone when first introduced caused those suffering from long-standing rheuma-toid arthritis to leap in their hundreds from their invalid chairs and sometimes to walk for the first time in many years until it was conclusively shown that in most cases its objective effect is slightly less potent than that of aspirin in the same disease. All diseases have a large superadded psychological element of hopelessness, anxiety, and depression or fear which when re-moved by faith or renewed confidence can make an immense difference to the patient's state and, as noted elsewhere, may even be the main cause of his state as in the psychosomatic disorders. But it must also be remembered that, as the old philosophers realised centuries ago, the fact that B follows A does not prove that A caused B. The majority of diseases are self-limiting and would clear up without medical intervention and with or without a 'wonder drug,' carrying a potato in the pocket, or dieting exclusively on orange juice.

It is important, too, that *one should not be misled into believing that there is any necessary connection between the dramatic nature of a patient's symptoms and the real serious-ness of his condition*; sometimes there is, sometimes not. Thus a young child may have a high temperature or even delirium and look extremely ill yet the next morning be demanding vociferously to be allowed out of bed, whereas another who merely looks 'run-down' with a very slight temperature may well have diphtheria. The adult with 'terrible' headaches may simply have mother-in-law trouble, but the young uncomplaining woman who looks slightly anaemic may have pulmonary tuberculosis. The degree of temperature in particular bears only the slightest relation to the severity of the disease and there must be many doctors who wish fervently that some parents had never known of the existence of the clinical thermometer which can be of little value unless they know what the reading means and a considerable nuisance to both doctor and child when they don't. To be sure, a raised temperature means that *something* is wrong but the mother would not have taken the temperature in the first place unless she had already suspected as much, and even if the temperature is completely normal, it does not follow that all is well. One can be very ill with a completely normal temperature. A temperature chart in a hospital which shows how a fever rises and falls is extremely useful to the trained eye, an isolated reading tells little except that an infection is probably present.

Finally, the patient should *always be completely frank with his or her doctor about everything*, answer all his questions (including those about his intimate personal life) truthfully, and have no false modesty about any sort of examination that may be required. After all, one goes to a doctor for help and nobody can give help on inadequate information nor is any physician likely to be surprised or shocked by anything he hears – a man who is being virtually compelled to listen to the details of his patients' private lives many times a week whether he asks for them or not is unlikely to be either morbidly curious or taken aback by any individual patient's confidential disclosures. It is necessary to mention this because modern medicine is becoming more and more concerned about the relationship between the individual's way of life and his personal problems on the one hand and the illnesses he develops on the other so that it is no longer possible wholly to separate the two. Equally, one should be honest with the doctor about one's doubts and if it appears necessary (or even if it would simply add to one's confidence) then by all means ask to be referred to a specialist. But never under any circumstances should a patient go to see a specialist first about symptoms which have recently appeared as is so often done on the Continent; specialists are very clever people but not unnaturally tend to be biased in favour of their own subject and what is really needed by the individual who is confronted by an illness which is new to him is that he should first see a 'generalist' – that is, a family doctor who knows something about everything. If the trouble does not clear up under his care then a specialist's advice may be asked or even insisted on, but the doctor should be allowed to choose the specialist or at least to discuss the subject reasonably since the patient is not always the best person to decide what sort of specialist should be consulted. For instance, the fact that the most noticeable symptom relates to the eyes is not necessarily an indication to consult an eye specialist because the symptom may be caused by disease beginning in a quite different part of the body. If the patient will pay attention to these few rules he will not only spare himself much anxiety but bring about a much more satisfactory relationship between himself and his doctor.

Abdomen: the part of the trunk below the chest from which it is separated internally by a muscular partition known as the diaphragm, and above the pelvis or bony basin with which it is continuous internally. Behind it lies the spinal column and the lower ribs, but for the most part it is protected at the sides and in front only by the layers of transverse muscle running forwards from the spine and the vertical rectus abdominis muscles in the middle. Above the muscles lie the skin and a layer of fat of varying thickness whilst beneath lies another layer of fat covered with the cellophane-like membrane known as the peritoneum which covers all the internal organs as well. It is infection of this membrane which is known as peritonitis. The principal contents of the abdominal cavity are the digestive organs – i.e. the stomach and small and large intestines together with the associated glands of the liver and pancreas (*see* Digestive System), the two kindneys on either side of the spinal column with their tubes or ureters running down to the bladder in the pelvis (*see* Kidneys), and the spleen which, although lying somewhat further back, occupies much the same position on the left side as the liver does on the right. Lying at the rear alongside the spinal column are the main artery and vein of the body (the aorta and vena cava) and some important nerves (*see* Nervous System) although, of course, the spinal cord itself lies inside the bony tube within the spinal column. The pelvis below the abdomen proper contains the rectum or end of the digestive tract, the bladder with the beginning of the urethra through which the urine passes to the outside, the prostate gland beneath the bladder in the male, and in the female the ovaries, the Fallopian tubes, and the womb. Diseases of the abdomen and pelvis are dealt with under the various systems affected, or in the commoner conditions under their most usual name.

Abdominal Injuries: considering the apparent vulnerability of the abdomen which in its larger part (*see* above) is unprotected by bone, serious abdominal injuries affecting the internal organs are relatively uncommon except in the case of car accidents, crushing accidents, or falls from a considerable height. In these the liver or spleen may be ruptured but this is not necessarily fatal unless a large blood-vessel is torn when haemorrhage may be too severe for an operation to be performed in time. Rupture of the stomach or intestines may occur but this is more likely to be the result of a wound than of a blow; since the germ-laden contents of the bowels escape into the abdominal cavity immediate operation and the use of antibiotics is necessary if peritonitis is to be avoided. Rarely, a sudden and unexpected blow delivered in the region of the solar plexus when the abdominal muscles are relaxed may lead to sudden death from shock (q.v.). Straining to lift a heavy weight or even straining to pass a bowel motion may lead to a hernia or rupture in which a loop of intestine is pushed through a part of the abdominal wall (see Hernia).

Abortion: the premature expulsion of the contents of the pregnant womb prior to the seventh month of pregnancy. As used in medicine the term does not carry the usual popular significance of criminal abortion and simply refers to a miscarriage whatever its cause (see Miscarriage) or to removal of the foetus by a gynaecologist for medical reasons.

Abrasion: an abrasion is an area in which the surface layer of the skin has been rubbed off, for example by being drawn over a rough surface. When a really large area is affected it is obviously wise to consult a doctor, but small bruises should be dealt with by careful washing of the area affected to clear away any foreign matter. Suitable antiseptics are Dettol or Cetavlon in the dilutions recommended on the bottle, and the area should then be covered with a piece of surgical gauze (or a *clean* handkerchief if nothing else is available) smeared with vaseline or an antiseptic cream such as Cetavlex to prevent sticking. On the whole the less interference after this has been done the better and it is unnecessary to keep on using antiseptics on subsequent occasions since this only delays healing. Excellent dressings with antiseptic gauze attached are supplied by several firms and these may be used on small bruises but do not do away with the necessity of preliminary washing with soap and water if antiseptics are unobtainable. When an abrasion is badly contaminated with soil it may be wise to go to the local hospital for inoculation against the possibility of tetanus.

Abscess: localised area of infection anywhere in the body characterised by the fact that it is shut off from the surrounding tissues and sooner or later becomes filled with pus which ultimately causes it to burst. If the part affected is on the surface of the body the classical signs of inflammation will be observed: swelling, redness, pain, and warmth in the surrounding area. Usually, although this depends on the size and site of the abscess, there is some degree of fever which in severe cases may be high (for an account of the bodily changes occurring *see* Inflammation). Infection may be caused in one or other of three ways: (1) By the entry through a small cut or abrasion of germs which may either be foreign to the body or those normally found on the surface of the skin; in the case of boils (q.v.), which are small abscesses, entry is through the small skin lubricating glands especially when clothing constantly rubs on the part. (2) By the entry of a foreign body carrying infection, as in the case of knife or bullet wounds or some material which has been swallowed and 'gone down the wrong way' into the lungs or bronchi. (3) By the spread internally of germs already in the body as in a burst appendix or following pneumonia or the spread of middle ear infection to the brain.

The earliest sign of an abscess on the surface of the body is an area of redness which is painful and hard to the touch. Only later with the formation of pus does it become soft and may then burst by itself. The best treatment at this time is to apply a kaolin poultice covering a larger area than that actually affected; wet dressings of boric lint covered with gamgee tissue, although once popular, are less convenient, stay hot for a shorter period, and cause the skin to become sodden and devitalised. If this is done in time the abscess may resolve itself, but unless it is a very small one it is best to seek medical advice since it may need to be opened and penicillin or sulphonamide drugs given. (For abscesses in special parts *see* Bone, Breast, Lung, Appendix, Whitlow, and Gumboil.) Quite different in their origin from the above are the abscesses sometimes found in the liver following amoebic dysentery and the 'cold' abscesses of tuberculosis so-called because they produce no temperature; these are described under the diseases causing them.

Acetic acid: the essential principle of vinegar produced from the fermentation of wine or malt. Commercial acetic acid is derived from the distillation of wood with subsequent separation from tar and in its pure form is solid when it is known as glacial acetic acid, a caustic used for destroying warts. Ordinary vinegar was formerly employed as a cooling toilet preparation and, in the proportion of two or three tablespoonfuls to a quart of water, it may be used to sponge those who are suffering from the sweats of fevers from which it gives pleasant if temporary relief. Headaches are also helped in this way with a wet compress, but modern drugs have made this rather outdated as a form of treatment.

Acetone: a substance found in the urine primarily in severe cases of diabetes (in which case its sweetish smell can usually be noted in the breath during or prior to diabetic coma). However, it is also found in wasting diseases such as cancer, after prolonged vomiting, and sometimes in the acute fevers of childhood.

Acetylsalicylic Acid: (*see* Aspirin).

Achlorhydria: means an absence of the normal hydrochloric acid in the gastric juice. It is found in about 4–5% of normal people in whom it appears to lead to no ill-effects but is the rule in cancer of the stomach, pernicious anaemia, and sometimes in chronic gastritis.

Achondroplasia: a form of dwarfism in which the trunk is of normal size whilst the arms and legs are abnormally short and the head relatively large. Most of the dwarfs seen in circuses are of this type which is inherited, of unknown cause, and unalterable; the less frequently-seen dwarf of the 'Tom Thumb' type has perfectly-proportioned limbs and body and in this case defect of the pituitary gland in the base of the brain is to blame.

Acidity and Acidosis: two much misused terms, the former when employed in a general sense meaning nothing at all, the latter referring to a condition which occurs in such serious illnesses that it can hardly be what people ordinarily mean when they make use of the word. In fact, the blood is always alkaline so that even in acidosis all that is meant is that it is less alkaline than it should be; but in severe diabetes which has been inadequately treated or not treated at all, in prolonged starvation, persistent vomiting over a long period, and the final stages of kidney disease, the accumulation of acetoacetic and other acids when the body is unable to deal properly with fats leads to what may properly be described as acidosis. Obviously this is only one aspect of a generally serious condition and must be dealt with by treating the underlying disease. 'Acidity' is often used of stomach conditions where the pain is believed, sometimes wrongly, to be caused by excess acid. But the point it is necessary to make is that in the sense of a *generalised* 'acid' state of the body no such condition exists, although in former times vague symptoms were frequently ascribed to it especially in children.

Acne: a chronic skin disease affecting the sebaceous (i.e. fat or grease) glands on the face, shoulders, back and chest. It occurs mostly in people between the ages of fourteen and twenty since it is during this period that sebaceous glands become active and the typical 'blackheads' or even large pimples and small boils cause a good deal of embarrassment at an age when one tends in any case to be particularly sensitive about personal appearance. Several factors are involved, the first being a greasy skin (seborrhea q.v.) resulting from the glandular changes occurring from puberty onwards; the second, infection on the surface which by entering the sebaceous ducts causes blockage with the formation of the typical blackheads; and, thirdly, these may become infected with other germs than the acne bacillus causing pus formation and the larger sores. Treatment must initially be directed to the fundamental state which is the greasy condition of the skin and scalp; the hair should be shampooed at least twice a week, preferably with a non-soapy detergent type of hair-wash or one of the many proprietary medicated ones, and the face should be washed frequently. Greasy applications or ointments should not be used on the affected parts which should be dabbed night and morning with sulpho-calamine lotion or Crooke's 'Dermasulf.' It is also possible to obtain non-greasy creams suitably medicated and flesh-tinted for day-time use such as 'Eskamel.' The blackheads may be squeezed out either with clean hands or a special extractor obtainable at chemist's shops, but when they are inflamed, large, and have no 'head' they are best left alone since squeezing will only worsen the condition and tend to spread the infection. In more severe cases, a skin specialist may recommend ultra-violet rays, X-rays, a course of vaccine injections, or hormone treatment. Diet is probably not regarded as being so important as it once was, but it is as well to cut down on carbohydrates such as sweets, cakes, or too much white bread.

15

Acne Rosacea: more usually known as rosacea and formerly described as 'grog-blossom' is a condition of the skin of the face in which there is a red, greasy, and coarsened area with enlarged blood-vessels typically in a butterfly shape spreading across the nose and widening out over both cheeks. Associated with this, and probably its basic cause, is chronic dyspepsia or gastritis. The title 'grog-blossom' arose from the belief that rosacea was invariably associated with chronic indulgence in alcohol, but this is less than kind to the commonest type of sufferer who is the middle-aged lady of blameless habits save for an addiction to strong and frequent cups of tea. It is true that in former times such people as coachmen who were exposed both to the elements and to the temptation of frequent noggins of the steaming-hot rum so eloquently described by Dickens at stopping-points on their route tended to develop very red noses and cheeks, but the alcoholic of today rarely shows this symptom although the facial veins may be enlarged when liver disease is present and it is unfortunately the case that, if the wages of sin are sometimes unpleasant, the wages of extreme virtue are on occasion no less so. The fact would seem to be that rosacea is associated with anything that leads to frequent flushing of the blood-vessels in the face, and this includes frequent exposure to harsh weather, the menopause or change of life in women, hot foods such as curries, and hot or irritant drinks which produce gastritis when carried to excess, e.g. undiluted spirits or strong and overstewed tea taken on an empty stomach throughout the day. The treatment of rosacea should be left to the doctor, but obviously it must in part be directed to removing the basic gastritis which will involve the giving up of irritant foods and drinks with the use of appropriate medicines and in women treatment of any glandular defects. Enlarged veins can be dealt with by electrolysis and much can be done to improve the appearance.

Acriflavine: a powerful antiseptic, one of the aniline derivatives, which was, and still is, used either in liquid solution (1 in 1000 of water), in liquid paraffin, or as a cream for dressing wounds. Like iodine and other of the older antiseptics it is on the whole being replaced by more modern preparations which do not produce the unsightly yellow discoloration of the skin and interfere less with healing (*see* Antiseptics).

Acrocyanosis: a condition found especially in young women in which there is coldness and bluish discoloration of the hands and feet spreading sometimes to the nose and ears. It should be referred to a doctor who will probably be able to help with one of the new vasodilator drugs which improve the circulation (*see* Arteries, Diseases of).

Acromegaly: a state produced by overactivity of the front part of the pituitary gland at the base of the brain. When this begins in early life before the bones have stopped growing increased height or gigantism results and the general appearance (depending upon the severity of the condition) becomes somewhat gorilla-like with prominent forehead and cheekbones, a large lower jaw, long dangling arms with big hands, big feet, and a tendency to stoop. In later life an enlargement of the face bones, hands and feet, a bent back and general coarsening of the expression without gigantism results. Other symptoms such as disorders of vision and sexual impotence may be present in the more severe cases. The condition should always be referred for skilled treatment since, although some types are merely the result of an overactivity of the gland which does not progress any further, others are due to a more serious underlying cause which may require operative or X-ray therapy. Diabetes is sometimes associated with acromegaly.

A.C.T.H.: the abbreviation for adrenocorticotrophic hormone, a secretion of the pituary gland which has the function of stimulating the cortex of the suprarenal glands above the kidneys causing them, among other effects, to produce more cortisone. A.C.T.H. was first isolated in 1933 from the pituitary glands of animals which is still its only source, but was not used medically to any extent until 1949 when it appeared to be helpful in rheumatoid arthritis although its first promise in this condition has not been fulfilled. Its general action is the same as that of cortisone (*see* Cortisone, Endocrine Glands).

Actinomycosis: a disease caused by the ray fungus (actinomyces bovis) and originally noted in cattle from which the fungus was isolated by Bollinger in 1877 and shown to cause the swellings and ulcers around the mouth known by farmers as 'big jaw,' 'lumpy jaw,' or 'wooden tongue.' A year later it was found in man (although the species in this case is the slightly different streptothrix actinomyces). The name of ray fungus is derived from its appearance under the microscope

17

which shows tiny clumps of matted yellow threads from the centre of which club-shaped bodies radiate like a minute sun. These bodies are just visible to the naked eye in the pus produced by the disease. Infection ordinarily takes place through the mouth by food and it used to be thought that the human infection arose from the farmhand's habit of chewing straw or grain or directly from contact with cattle which were themselves infected. This has since been doubted, but it is noteworthy that a high proportion of those contracting the disease have been concerned in occupations dealing with cereals and chiefly with barley. Actinomycosis is a chronic disease which frequently begins with toothache and difficulty in opening the mouth; a swelling then appears at the angle of the jaw which ultimately discharges pus both into the mouth and outwardly. From there any part of the body may be affected, but most commonly the lungs and the intestines. In the former case there is chronic cough and sputum containing the fungus is expectorated, in the latter there may be no symptoms until a perforation occurs leading to peritonitis and on investigation ulcers are found in the bowels. However only a bacteriologist can make a certain diagnosis by finding the fungus in the pus or excretions. Needless to say, this is a serious disease, especially when it has spread from the mouth elsewhere, but mild cases may be cured in six to nine months. In others the outlook is less favourable. The drug generally used has been potassium iodide but penicillin and other antibiotics now give good results. However, the main treatment in most cases is surgical.

Acupuncture: a method of treatment with no known scientific basis used for the relief of various pains and diseases according to the credulity of the operator. It consists simply in inserting needles 2–3 inches long either into the parts affected or parts which, rightly or wrongly, are supposed to influence them; the procedure is relatively painless. Acupuncture is still quite widely used on the Continent where it is presumably based on some pseudo-scientific rationale, but it originated in China centuries ago where it was believed that by such an operation the harmful vapours which allegedly gave rise to certain disorders could be released from the body.

Addisonian Anaemia: a now infrequently-used term for pernicious anaemia which was named after its discoverer (*see* Pernicious Anaemia).

Addison's Disease: a disease first described by Dr Thomas Addison in 1849 the same year in which he also described pernicious anaemia. Born near Newcastle upon Tyne and educated at Edinburgh University, Addison became a famous physician at Guy's Hospital, London, and his account of this disease which he correctly attributed to destruction of the suprarenal glands (q.v.) is still valid: 'Anaemia, general languor or debility, remarkable feebleness of the heart's action, irritability of the stomach, and a peculiar change of colour in the skin.' The coloration begins first on such exposed areas as the face and hands and ranges from yellow to dark brown or even black as it spreads over the rest of the body. Extreme weakness on slight exertion, fainting attacks or giddiness and noises in the ears due to low blood-pressure, palpitation, nausea with or without actual vomiting, and sometimes diarrhoea, complete the picture. The destruction of the suprarenal glands may be due to tuberculous infection, growths, or haemorrhage but leads to loss of their essential hormones which are necessary to life, e.g. in maintaining the blood-pressure and the contractility of the muscles. Addison's disease is rare in childhood or old age being commonest during the twenties and thirties and, until recently, the only treatment was the administration of large doses of common salt which delayed its ultimately fatal conclusion although rarely longer than three or four years after the first appearance of symptoms. Today, however, the administration of the missing hormones in the form of deoxycortone and/or cortisone by injection or mouth enables most patients to lead a completely normal and healthy life. Since this is a form of substitution therapy like the use of insulin in diabetes it has to be continued permanently.

Adenitis: inflammation of the lymph glands (*see* Glands) which are situated in various strategic parts of the body to trap germs which would otherwise spread into the circulation. Each gland in a group is about the size of a small bean and, although they occur in many areas, the most obvious ones from the outside are those in the groin (which may become painful and swollen in infections of the legs), those in the armpit (similarly affected in infections of the hands and arms), and those behind the angle of the jaw (which become enlarged in throat and mouth infections). In glandular fever (q.v.) or

19

infective mononucleosis the glands of the neck become swollen, but otherwise the treatment of adenitis is the treatment of the infected part which has led to the swelling. Enlargement may also be due to non-inflammatory conditions, e.g. Hodgkins' disease (q.v.).

Adenoids: (*see* Tonsils and Adenoids).

Adenoma: a benign tumour composed of glandular tissue, for example in the thyroid gland. Benign tumours are non-malignant ones unrelated to cancer.

Adhesions: the uniting together of structures which should normally be separate by fibrous tissue resulting from acute or chronic inflammation. This usually happens in the cavities of joints or in the pleura or peritoneum covering the lungs and abdominal organs respectively. Thus in the hip-joint inflammation leads to the outpouring of fluid into the cavity (which is nature's way of lubricating irritated surfaces and so reducing pain) and from this fluid solid fibrin – the material which forms blood-clots – separates out. Ordinarily this is later absorbed, but if this does not occur it gradually turns into strong fibrous tissue which unites the normally mobile surfaces of the ball-and-socket joint causing ankylosis and making movement limited or impossible. Similarly, after an attack of pleurisy, the lung may become adherent to the chest-wall or after peritonitis and occasionally following operative interference the stomach, intestines, or other abdominal organs may become united sometimes leading to pain or even obstruction of the bowels. Adhesions may also affect the ovaries and womb in women following an infected miscarriage or similar disease. If the condition is severe enough surgical intervention may be necessary although this sometimes leads to further adhesions. It should be added that some people who complain of 'adhesions' are highly neurotic individuals who make a hobby of seeking operations and are either exaggerating the trouble produced by real adhesions or imagining the presence of non-existent ones. In this respect they resemble the victims of another fashionable condition, visceroptosis or 'dropping' of the abdominal organs which, even when it does occur, may be associated with gross exaggeration of the disability and its significance.

Adrenalin: a hormone secreted by the medulla or central part of the suprarenal glands. Its function in nature is to prepare the body functions for emergency (in animals for fight or flight) and its administration therefore leads to a rapid pulse, pallor of the skin and a reduction of blood-supply to the digestive organs so that more becomes available for the muscles, the transformation of glycogen in the liver into glucose which is an immediate source of energy, dilation of the pupils and the bronchi or breathing-tubes (*see* Endocrine Glands). First prepared by Takamine in 1901 from the glands of animals, it is now prepared synthetically, and is used in medicine in a 1/1000 solution in water, dissolved in oil, or as an ointment for external application. The injection is given for asthmatic attacks, as a heart stimulant, or in cases of diabetics suffering from an overdose of insulin; it is combined with local anaesthetic especially in dentistry to control bleeding during tooth extraction. The cream is used in the treatment of fibrositis, although whether adrenaline cream has any effect whatever in this condition is a matter of opinion. Adrenalin is ineffective when given by mouth, but substances with an adrenalin-like action such as ephedrene are used in tablet form or as ingredients of a linctus in asthma.

Aerophagy: the neurotic habit of swallowing air, usually unconsciously, which is the cause of gastric flatulence (*see* Flatulence).

Aerosol: a suspension of extremely finely-divided liquid or solid particles in a gas such as air or oxygen which is designed for various purposes so far as medicine is concerned, but generally (*a*) for detroying disease-carrying pests such as mosquitoes or lice, (*b*) for purifying the air and combating diseases carried by droplet infection in public buildings, (*c*) for inhalation by patients with diseases of the lungs. The method of delivery may be a hand-operated spray or nebulizer but the more usual appliance today (in the first two cases) is the release of the aerosol by pressing a button on a container in which the material is kept under pressure. Aerosols for pests usually contain D.D.T. and are extremely effective, those for 'purifying' the air of a room and destroying air-borne germs contain perfumes and such antiseptics as hexylresorcinol or propylene glycol. The efficacy of the latter is dubious; for, although the scent or perfume (which in some cases is more unpleasant than the smell it is designed to cover) conceals the original odours, there is no sense in which it can be said to make stale air fresh for this can only be done by ventilating the room. The antiseptics are certainly capable of killing germs in a bottle, but whether they remain suspended in the air long enough to be effectual in preventing droplet infection from people coughing and spluttering at close range is quite another matter. In a crowded cinema spraying in order to be effective would have to be carried out so frequently that many would prefer the risk of infection. The medicated aerosols used in lung disease may contain adrenaline or isoprenaline for the relief of asthmatic attacks or antibiotics such as penicillin and streptomycin when infection is present.

Afterbirth and Afterpains: (*see* Pregnancy and Labour).

Agar: sometimes known as agar-agar is a vegetable jelly obtained from seaweed and largely used in the East to make soups and jellies as gelatine is here. Before the Second World War most agar came from Japan, but it is now made in the U.S. and the Commonwealth. In medicine, agar is used by bacteriologists to make their culture media of broth or blood on which bacteria are grown more solid. It is also given either by itself or, more usually, combined with other ingredients in constipation; for, although agar itself is an inert substance with no pharmacological effects, it absorbs water into the bowel and makes the motions more fluid. Such proprietary preparations as Agarol and Petrolagar, as their names indicate, contain agar along with other substances.

Age, Problems of Old: (*see* Geriatrics).

Agglutination: the clumping together of small bodies in a fluid suspension in particular of blood corpuscles when they are brought into contact with the serum of an incompatible blood-group or of bacteria exposed to the serum of a person or animal which has developed immunity against them. The former reaction is important for testing the compatibility of blood-groups prior to blood transfusion, the latter is used in bacteriology, e.g. in the Widal reaction for typhoid fever when the addition of a patient's serum to typhoid germs in solution produces agglutination if the disease is typhoid but fails to do so if it is something else (*see* Blood, Infection).

Agoraphobia: an irrational fear or phobia of open spaces, for example of crossing a street. It is a symptom of neurosis (q.v.).

Agranulocytosis: a serious but not very common blood disease in which ulceration of the throat and mouth is accompanied by a diminution of the number of granulocytes (one type of white blood cell), initially in the bone-marrow where they are pro-duced, and subsequently in the blood-stream. The disease results either following some long-standing suppurative con-dition especially in the mouth and throat or, in some cases, from taking of such drugs as amidopyrine (which used to be used in place of, or combined with, aspirin), the antibiotic chloramphenicol, and certain sulphonamides. This cause is now infrequent because the drugs concerned are either avoided or given under careful supervision (*see* Blood).

Ague: a vague and now outdated term for malaria when it used to occur in this country, or, since diagnosis was not always accurate in those days, for other acute fevers confused with malaria.

Air-sickness: one form of travel-sickness similar in origin to car-sickness and sea-sickness. There is little necessity to suffer from this condition nowadays when so many useful proprietary pre-parations exist which can prevent it (e.g. Avomine, Drama-mine); hyoscine hydrobromide in doses of 1/60–1/120 grain may be used. These drugs can only be obtained on prescription.

Albinism: a condition of the skin, hair, and eyes in which the individual, known as an albino, shows an inherited lack of pig-ment. Albinism may be partial in which case there are irregu-larly-shaped patches of white in the skin or hair, or complete when the skin of the whole body is lacking in pigment having a pale pink colour, the hair is white, and the irises of the eyes being unpigmented are also pink owing to the bloodvessels at the back of the eye showing through the transparent iris and retina. Since too much light is able to enter the eyes of albinos they are often screwed up in bright sunlight and such people are frequently short-sighted. Curiously enough, although all the human races may show albinism (as well as animals and plants), it is commonest amongst Negroes in whom it may also be partial or complete. White rabbits with pink eyes are albinos, but some mammals living in countries which are likely to be snow-covered for part of the year show periodic albinism, the white colour of the fur serving as protective coloration during the winter months. Albinism is inherited as a Mendelian reces-sive character (*see* Heredity).

Albuminuria: albumens are proteins which enter into the com-position of all living organisms varying according to their

23

source of origin. The main ones found in food products are egg albumin in the white of egg fibrinogen and haemoglobin in blood, myosin in meat, caseinogen in milk, casein in cheese, and gluten in flour. Albumins show the following characteristics: they are colloidal and do not pass, as salts do, through parchment membranes or the membranes of normal living cells; they are coagulated by heat following which they become insoluble in water until treated with caustic alkalies or mineral acids; they are precipitated by various chemicals such as alcohol, tannin, nitric acid, and mercury perchloride. Albumin is not normally found in the urine, since as mentioned above it should not pass through the kidney cells unless they are damaged as happens in nephritis (q.v.) or inflammation of the kidneys. However, its presence in the urine does not necessarily mean that the kidneys are damaged for it also occurs in any inflammation of the lower part of the urinary tract where pus or blood is produced: e.g. pyelitis (q.v.), cystitis (q.v.), and urethritis (see Urethra). Heart diseases severe enough to produce congestion of the kidneys, many fevers, severe anaemia, and drugs or poisons, may be accompanied by albuminuria the significance of which is as serious as the disease causing it. Albumen may be found in the urine of perfectly normal people in about 4–5% of cases, usually in those between the ages of 8–18 or over, and this condition described as cyclic, functional, or orthostatic albuminuria disappears whilst the individual is lying down but reappears on his assuming the erect posture. Probably it is due to temporary congestion of the kidneys when standing up, but, in any case, it has no pathological significance. During pregnancy, the urine should be regularly tested for albumen as this may indicate approaching complications which can be arrested when discovered in time. Albumen is easily tested for owing to its properties of precipitating when various chemicals are added or coagulating when boiled; in the simplest test urine is heated to boiling point at the upper level of a test-tube to which a little acetic acid has been added. The appearance of a white turbidity in the heated area in contrast with the clear lower part indicates the presence of either albumin or phosphates, and the addition of a few drops of nitric acid increases the turbidity when albumin is present but clears it completely when it is due to phosphates which have no pathological significance.

Alcohol: A name given to a whole series of organic chemicals, the only ones relevant to medicine being methyl or wood alcohol produced by the dry distillation of wood and found in methylated spirits, and ethyl alcohol found in varying degrees in alcoholic drinks and derived in this case from the fermentation of such varied substances as grapes, barley and other cereals, apples, potatoes, and, in fact, almost any starchy or sugar-containing material. Methylated spirits contains about 10% of wood spirit, a little paraffin oil, and an aniline dye which are added to make it undrinkable; for this reason methylated spirits together with ethyl alcohol intended for commercial or scientific purposes is duty-free, whereas that intended for drinking has a heavy excise duty levied on it in the British Isles and elsewhere. Unfortunately its nauseating taste does not always stop methylated spirits from being drunk either neat or, in the form of 'red biddy,' mixed with cheap wines, and this dangerous habit amongst the vagrant class may lead to blindness, neuritis, and death. Ethyl alcohol completely free from water and other impurities is known as 'absolute alcohol.' In medicine and science, alcohol is used as a solvent since it is capable of dissolving many substances not soluble in water particularly fats, oils, and resins; in the form of 'rectified spirit', containing 90% alcohol by volume, it is used in the making of tinctures, essences, and weaker spirits of from 10–20% strength. But apart from these laboratory processes its medical uses are few. Externally, alcohol is used to remove grease from the skin and sterilise it prior to giving injections, to harden the skin of the feet prior to a long walk, or in those confined to bed for long periods in order to prevent bed sores. Rubbing alcohol to massage the body after a bath or exercise is popular in America and similar products are used on the Continent although less so here. Internally, there are virtually no indications for the use of alcohol so far as medicine is concerned; that is to say, there are no conditions for which it need be prescribed. But in those accustomed to its use, a drink before a meal, wine during a meal, or the nightcap of whisky no doubt play their part in aiding digestion or quelling nervous tension or inducing sound sleep. So-called 'tonic wines' in which a burgundy or claret-type wine is medicated with such substances as glycero-phosphates, meat extract, or some protein material which is supposed to 'build up' the nerves are entirely useless and in their effect no different from the un-medicated product – except that they taste nastier. Spirits should never be given to those who are in a fainting or col-lapsed condition, since they are more likely to choke than re-vive them. The only good reason for taking alcohol is that one likes it. Roughly speaking the alcoholic content by volume of the various types of drink is as follows: (1) Spirits such as whisky, rum, brandy, gin, which are distilled after the process of fermentation to increase the alcoholic content contain about 40%, but liqueurs may contain 50% and vodka, if 'proof' spirit, up to 57%. (2) Fortified wines such as port, sherry, and madeira are wines to which spirit has been added after fermentation and contain about 20% of alcohol. (3) Ordinary wines such as claret, hock, moselle, and champagne contain 10%, burgundy about 14%. (4) Beers and cider range from 2–5%, and strong ale to about 8%. (5) Home-made wines made from cowslips, rhubarb, raspberries, parsnips, raisins, etc., are quite as strong as ordinary table wines and may be even stronger, some con-taining as much as 20% or more of alcohol.

Alcoholism: or addiction to alcohol is a difficult subject to dis-cuss since most people are strongly prejudiced about the sub-ject one way or another. Thus on the one hand we have the obvious fact that abuse of alcohol leads to a great deal of misery, marital unhappiness and broken homes, a certain amount of crime, and produces physical and mental disease both directly and indirectly. Directly, by the physical effect of alcohol on the body and indirectly by the fact that those in a drunken state are more likely to contract venereal disease, succumb to ordinary illnesses such as pneumonia if they are chronic addicts, and, of course, to endanger the lives of them-selves and others by causing motor or other accidents. On the other hand, there can be no doubt that some people can drink very considerable quantities of alcohol throughout a long life without showing any apparent ill-effects whatever, and that in most cases alcoholism is a symptom rather than a disease in itself. Thus, although alcohol may be the immediate cause of a broken home, it is extremely likely that the home would have been broken up even if the problem of alcohol had never arisen since those with a happy home life are unlikely to take to drink in any circumstances. Similarly it could well be argued that, if the evil effects of alcohol are constantly discussed, its good effects in oiling the wheels of social inter-course and reducing tension have usually been ignored and it might be said with more than a grain of truth that moderate amounts of alcohol have kept some people going who would otherwise have found it difficult to carry on reasonably good relationships with their families or friends. Pearl in America, for example, has shown as the result of a most painstaking statistical study that, if heavy drinking considerably lowers the average expectation of life, the moderate drinker has a higher than average expectation.

The general (although by no means universally accepted) be-lief today, amongst those who have studied the problem scien-tifically is that the physical diseases brought about by the excessive consumption of alcohol are the result of its indirect effect in producing malnutrition rather than any direct toxic one. The repeated consumption of strong spirits, especially on an empty stomach, leads to a chronic gastritis of the stomach and probably inflammation of the intestines which interferes with the absorption of food substances and notably of vitamin B group; this, in turn, damages the nerve cells causing alco-holic neuritis, injury to the brain cells causing certain forms of insanity, and in some cases cirrhosis of the liver. The alco-holic is not necessarily the sort of person who becomes ob-viously drunk on frequent occasions and is more commonly the man or woman who drinks steadily throughout the day often without any immediate effect being apparent to others. Later, however, symptoms which are partly due to physical effects, partly to the underlying neurosis which is at the root of the trouble in most cases, and partly social, begin to show themselves. He (or she) eats less and drinks more, often begins the day with vomiting or nausea which necessitates taking the first drink before he can show himself in public, his appear-ance tends to become bloated and the eyes are often red and congested, his work suffers, he forgets to keep his appoint-ments and becomes indifferent to his social responsibilities, his craving for drink becomes insatiable and, when he is unable to get it he becomes shaky, irritable, and tense. Since he is ashamed of his condition, he tries to hide it and often, instead of drinking openly, hides his bottles throughout the house. His emotions are less controlled and he gets angry or tearful readily, tells facile lies, and a minor illness or cessation of the supply may lead to an attack of 'D.T.'s' (delirium tremens). In another type, there may be no craving for alcohol for quite long periods, until a sudden impulse makes it seem absolutely necessary to have a drink and the sufferer in a few hours becomes dead drunk and quite uncontrollable; this form is rather less frequent than the other and is known as 'dipsomania.' In severe cases the alcoholic may die from cirrhosis of the liver – although this is not so common a result of drinking as it used to be – or an attack of pneumonia or some other infection not ordinarily fatal to healthy people may be so to him; in other cases there may be gradual mental deterioration with loss of memory (Korsakoff's Psychosis). Nearly all cases of chronic alcoholism should be referred to a psychiatrist who is almost certain to recommend treatment in an institution or nursing-home because it is necessary to have complete control over the situation for several months and the patient cannot be relied on to abstain without supervision. The main principles of such treatment are: complete abstention, psychotherapy to find any psychological causes of the condition, and the general building-up of impaired physical health. Concentrated injections of vitamins may be given, and in some cases drug treatment designed to create repulsion against alcohol is employed. Amongst these are apomorphine treatment in which the patient is allowed to drink as much as he likes but given injections which cause severe vomiting with the idea that drink and vomiting will form unpleasant associations. Another method is the Danish drug 'Antabuse' which when taken regularly causes the patient to feel so ill after drinking that it may turn him against the habit. Unfortunately, when left to themselves, some patients are more likely to neglect taking Antabuse than alcohol. A promising development of late is the social treatment of the disease in the organisation known as Alcoholics Anonymous, an informal organisation of men and women 'for whom alcohol has become a major problem, and who, admitting it, have decided to do something about it.' Those who wish to join the group should write to BM/AAL, London, W.C.1.

Aldosterone: a hormone secreted by the cortex of the adrenal glands which plays a major part in maintaining the balance of salts in the body (*see* Endocrine Glands).

Alkalies: are substances, usually oxides, hydroxides, or carbonates and bicarbonates of metals, which neutralise acids to produce salts. The commonest are those of potassium, sodium, calcium, aluminium, and magnesium. Strong ammonia, caustic soda or potash, and washing soda are caustic poisons which have no place in medicine except in the case of caustic soda which is sometimes used for removing warts; weak solutions of ammonia or washing soda may be used to apply to insect bites or stings. But the main use of the alkalies is in hyperacidity of the stomach for which the chief products are: sodium bicarbonate, calcium carbonate (common chalk), magnesium carbonate, magnesium trisilicate, and aluminium hydroxide. These may be used alone or in mixtures. Although there is no harm in using sodium bicarbonate (baking soda) from time to time when nothing else is available its regular use is unwise (a) because it produces gas in the stomach and leads to flatulence, (b) because it is the most strongly alkaline and has therefore the greatest tendency to upset the acid–alkali balance of the body. Magnesium trisilicate and aluminium hydroxide are the safest in this respect, although it is important to emphasise that prolonged dyspepsia should be medically investigated and not self-treated.

Alkaloids: are extremely potent substances found mostly in plants and widely used in medicine. Their general properties are that (as the name indicates) they are alkaline in reaction and, if used therapeutically, mostly extremely poisonous when taken beyond the correct dosage, they are insoluble to a greater or less extent in water but soluble in alcohol (hence those given by mouth are usually either in the form of tablets or tinctures – i.e. alcoholic solution); and most have a bitter taste. Alkaloids have names ending in -ine, and certain drugs with similar properties but non-alkaline in reaction have names ending in -in – e.g. digitalin, aloin. Common alkaloids are atropine from the belladonna plant, cocaine from coca leaves, caffeine from tea and coffee, morphine with codeine and other drugs from opium in poppy-juice, nicotine from tobacco, quinine and quinidine from Peruvian bark, strychnine from nux vomica seeds. The only common alkaloid from animal sources is adrenaline from the medulla of the suprarenal glands. Digitalin is one of the principles of digitalis from the fox-glove leaf.

Allergy: an exaggerated reaction to various foreign substances usually of a protein nature that are harmless in similar amounts to ordinary people. The substance responsible ordinarily produces a reaction which is the same in a given individual for a specific substance and bears no relationship to that which it might lead to in normal people to whom it is given in large amounts, i.e. a material to which a person is allergic produces typically *allergic* symptoms such as an asthmatic attack, hay-fever, nettle-rash, or dermatitis when given in even small doses, but large enough amounts of the same material would produce typically *toxic* symptoms in the normal person. Broadly speaking allergic symptoms are typical of the person, toxic symptoms are typical of the drug given. The reason for this is that the basis of the allergic reaction is the same in all cases and the particular reaction it produces depends upon the part of the body mainly affected which is related (*a*) to the individual and his past history, and (*b*) to the mode of entry of the allergen. Thus allergens in foods tend to cause dermatitis, pollens hay-fever, and dust and animal danders asthma.

As is well-known, infectious diseases (q.v.) are accompanied by the production in the blood-stream of substances known as antibodies resulting from the reaction of the body to the invading germs and these antibodies help both to destroy the invaders and to produce varying degrees of immunity against subsequent infection by the same germs. It is believed that the same effect takes place with allergens, but in this case for some unknown reason the antibodies are formed either within or on the surface of the body cells instead of in the blood-stream. The allergen–antibody reaction damages the cell walls and liberates a substance known as histamine which is the cause of the actual allergic response. Histamine produces two main effects, (*a*) it increases the permeability of the small blood-vessels causing the fluid part of the blood or serum to leak into the tissues, (*b*) it brings about spasm of certain groups of muscle, notably in the bronchial tubes. The former effect leads to the swelling (oedema), the blisters, and the irritation of the skin, nose, and eyes, the latter to the asthmatic attacks in allergic subjects. It is not known with any degree of certainty what makes a person allergic. In some cases heredity may play a part, but there can be little doubt that in many, if not all, the psychological element certainly does. Thus it is known that allergic-type symptoms can arise from purely psychological causes as in the well-known instance of a person allergic to roses developing asthmatic attack in the presence of artificial flowers which she thought were real, and nettle-rash or blisters often arise when there is a history of psychological shock but none of exposure to allergens. Blisters, indeed, can be produced under hypnosis. Treatment of allergic diseases depends on the individual case, but includes: (1) removal of or from the source of trouble as when feather-stuffed pillows, animals in the house, flower or grass pollen, or dusts at work are responsible; (2) a course of desensitisation by giving increasing doses of the allergen over a long period which is more likely to be successful in hay-fever than in other cases; (3) psychotherapy in a very few selected cases; (4) the use of the new anti-histamine drugs which, by antagonising the effects of histamine, relieve or even remove the symptoms without permanently curing the condition. Since there are a considerable number of these drugs it may be necessary to try out a number before finding the most suitable one. Cortisone or hydrocortisone creams or sprays give considerable relief when applied locally to allergic skin conditions. Asthma of allergic origin is by far the most difficult of these conditions to treat, perhaps because of its larger psychological element.

Aloin: an extract from aloes, the dried juice of a plant found in the West Indies and East Africa. It is used as a purgative but because its powerful action tends to cause griping aloin is usually given in a pill containing other substances to counteract this effect (e.g. aloin, belladonna, strychnine, and cascara). One of the best-known proprietary preparations of this sort is 'Alophen' pills produced by Parke Davis & Co. Ltd., the usual dose being 1–2 pills at night. However, although effective, such pills are for occasional rather than regular use and the regular use of any purgative is bad in principle (*see* Constipation).

Alopecia Areata: a form of baldness brought about by nervous disturbances such as shock or worry. Since the hair grows back again in 99% of cases with or without treatment, there can be little doubt that most of the letters written to makers of 'hair-restorer' by grateful customers were written by those suffering from this condition (*see* Baldness).

Amidopyrine: a drug, also known as 'Pyramidon,' which has the same effects in reducing pain and lowering temperature as aspirin. Its use is unjustified in view of the fact that it is no more potent than aspirin and considerably more dangerous as it occasionally leads to the serious blood-disease of agranulocytosis (q.v.).

Aminophylline: a combination of theophylline and ethylene diamine which produces an increased flow of urine, dilates the breathing-tubes, and improves the blood-supply to the heart. It is therefore used in the form of injection, suppositories, tablets, and capsules (sometimes in combination with a sedative) in the treatment of bronchial asthma, angina pectoris, or in order to reduce the amount of fluid in the body as in the oedema of heart disease.

Amnesia: partial or complete loss of memory, although the latter is almost inconceivable since without memory no intellectual functions would be possible. The commonest form is verbal amnesia where words or names are forgotten, but varying types and degrees of amnesia are found in old age and other organic conditions in which the brain cells are impaired by disease directly affecting them or, indirectly, through a poor blood-supply due, e.g. to arteriosclerosis. However, most cases of poor memory or loss of memory are largely psychological in origin, the poor memory of anxiety neurosis being caused by lack of attention in one obsessed with his own troubles, the genuine amnesia of hysteria being a mechanism of retreat from some intolerable situation (*see* Neurosis, Arteriosclerosis, Psychosis).

Amoeba: a group of single-celled microscopic animals belonging to the group of protozoans. The common amoeba found in pond-water is just visible to the naked eye and, of course, harmless as are also certain species normally found in the human intestinal canal. However other types are capable of causing disease such as the Entamoeba histolytica which is the cause of amoebic dysentery (*see* Infectious Diseases, Dysentery).

Amphetamine: amphetamine sulphate or its related form dexamphetamine is a drug closely related to adrenaline and therefore capable of stimulating the sympathetic nervous system. It is also known under the trade names of 'Benzedrene,' 'Dexedrene,' and in combination with a sedative as 'Drinamyl' or 'Daprisal' which also contains an analgesic or pain-killing drug. It was formerly used in inhalers for colds because of its ability to reduce congestion by shrinking the nasal lining, but has now been discontinued for this purpose because of its other dangerous properties and its tendency to cause insomnia. Amphetamine stimulates the brain and usually produces a feeling of well-being and an increased capacity for work by reducing fatigue and depression; for this purpose it has a place in the treatment of minor neuroses and depressive states with or without a sedative. Since, especially in the form of dexamphetamine, it tends to reduce the appetite, it has been used in the treatment of obesity. On the other hand, amphetamine is one of the 'pep pills' which can cause addiction and in some may increase rather than reduce nervous tension. So far as weight reduction is concerned there are many safer and more effective substances available. Amphetamine, although commonly peddled illegally, should only be obtainable on a doctor's prescription and taken under medical supervision.

Amyl Nitrate: an oily liquid which evaporates readily and has the effect of relieving spasms and dilating the blood-vessels. Hence it is used as an inhalation in capsule form for relieving the pains of angina pectoris.

Amyotrophic Lateral Sclerosis: a degenerative disease of the nervous system which leads to wasting of the muscles primarily in the hand but later in the arm and shoulder or face with weakness in the affected areas. The legs, on the other hand, become stiff and spastic and are not wasted but their spasticity causes difficulty in walking. The disease affects men more often than women and usually those over the age of forty. Diagnosis and treatment are a matter for the neurologist.

Anaemia: there are many types of anaemia, references to which are given under the heading of Blood Diseases (q.v.), but the simplest classification is that between ordinary anaemias described as microcytic hypochromic anaemia (i.e. characterised by a reduced number of red cells in the blood, each cell being smaller than normal and containing less haemoglobin or red colouring matter), and those such as pernicious anaemia (q.v.) which are described as megaloblastic hyperchromic anaemias (i.e. characterised by a reduced number of red cells, each of which is larger than normal and contains relatively more pigment, many being immature forms). The present entry concerns only the former type, that is to say, common or secondery anaemia so called because it is secondary to some other condition which has resulted in loss of blood, defective formation of blood, inadequate intake of iron

33

in the food or defective absorption of iron from the intestines and stomach. At this point it is necessary to make it clear that although 'anaemia' is often used as an explanation for feeling generally run-down, nervousness, poor appetite, and so on it leads to these symptoms much less frequently than is often believed and can only be diagnosed with certainty by actually testing the blood. The mere fact that somebody looks pale is no proof that anaemia exists and is no indication for self-treatment with an 'iron tonic' because iron is quite useless to those who are not lacking it. In the apparent absence of other illness the most usual cause of anaemia is excessive menstrual loss in women which forms the greater bulk of mild cases. Nor is it correct to speak of a 'tendency to anaemia' or to continue for years or months taking iron mixtures or pills which can only have the effect of wasting money and upsetting the digestion. One either has anaemia to a measurable degree or one has not and in this type of case it is unnecessary to take iron beyond the point at which the blood has been returned to normal which should be a matter of a few weeks. It is also a mistake to think that capsules or pills containing other substances such as liver or stomach extract, vitamins, etc., are of any advantage over the simple iron preparations in the Pharmacopoeia. Some forms of iron are more elegant or disturb the digestion less than others, but additional ingredients are useless and even harmful since if the case happens to be pernicious anaemia the real state of affairs is likely to be concealed if pills containing these substances have been taken. Simple secondary anaemia is therefore caused by (1) loss of blood as in heavy menstruation, after childbirth or an operation, or bleeding from the intestinal tract as in gastric or duodenal ulcer or haemorrhoids. (2) Defective blood formation after or during infections particularly chronic ones, and more rarely in chronic kidney disease. (3) Lack of sufficient iron in the diet is a rare cause of anaemia since the sufficient daily intake of 12 mgm or 15–20 mgm in pregnancy is found in most diets, but it does become important if blood is being lost which the intake is inadequate to replace. (4) Inadequate absorption of iron occurs in such intestinal diseases as ulcerative colitis where the diseased intestinal canal is unable to make use of the iron supplied in the diet. The treatment of secondary anaemia is the treatment of the condition causing it, preceded in most cases by a blood-examination to confirm the diagnosis, and the subsequent giving of one or other of the many iron preparations (*see* Blood, Pernicious Anaemia).

Anaesthesia: means in the first place a loss of feeling particularly for the senses of touch or pain which occurs in certain psychological states and in organic disease where damage to the sensory nerves or their centres has occurred; more generally it is applied to the deliberate induction of total or partial insensibility for the purpose of performing surgical operations. It is in the latter sense that anaesthesia is dealt with here.

In ancient times the use of such drugs as 'nepenthe' (probably opium) is described by Homer and hemp (cannabis indica, marihuana) was used to produce near-insensibility prior to surgical procedures by the Scythians and the ancient Chinese. Mandrake, mentioned by Shakespeare, was used during medieval times. None of these, however, was capable of doing more than reducing pain. In 1785, a Dr Pearson of Birmingham suggested the use of ether for asthmatic attacks and in 1800 Sir Humphrey Davy observed the anaesthetic effects of nitrous oxide or laughing gas, proposing its use in surgical operations; in 1818 Faraday and several American physicians noted the anaesthetic effects of ether. But the first practical application of nitrous oxide in this way was in 1844 by an American dentist Dr Horace Wells of Hartford, Connecticut, and it was another American dentist Dr Morton of Boston who first used ether. In the same year (1846) the first operation in Britain under ether anaesthesia was carried out by Lister and in the following year J. Y. Simpson of Edinburgh initiated its use in childbirth, discovering the use of chloroform a few months later. Ethyl chloride was tried and abandoned for the time being and until recent times gas, ether, and chloroform held the field. Today the chief anaesthetics used for general anaesthesia are nitrous oxide either alone or in combination with oxygen, ether, chloroform, ethyl chloride, chloroform-ether mixture, or trichlorethylene, all of which are given by inhalation; thiopentone (trade name 'Pentothal') is a barbiturate drug administered intravenously. For local anaesthesia eucaine, novocaine, and in operations on the eye cocaine are used, and for spinal anaesthesia stovaine, tropocaine, and novocaine.

Nitrous oxide is used alone only for brief operations as in

35

dentistry but combined with oxygen can be employed for longer ones when it is accompanied by the administration of analgesic drugs such as morphine and muscle relaxants such as curare. It has the advantage of being safe and relatively free from after-effects, whilst ethyl chloride which is also used for short operations such as the removal of adenoids tends to produce sickness and headache as after-effects; sometimes ethyl chloride is used to induce anaesthesia being then followed up by ether or nitrous oxide. Ether is for longer operations and does not act so rapidly as the other two. It may either be given by the open method of dropping on a gauze mask held over the patient's face or with a bag and facepiece. Chloroform is less frequently used nowadays in the pure form as it can be dangerous, but in a mixture with ether it is both safe and convenient. Thiopentone (Pentothal) and hexabarbitone given intravenously are very quick-acting barbiturates used either for short operations or for inducing rapid anaesthesia to be followed by something else in longer operations. Local anaesthesia for very minor operations can be briefly produced by 'freezing' with a spray of ethyl chloride which evaporates quickly covering the area with a thin layer of frost and thus deadening pain, but for other procedures the synthetic cocaine products eucaine and novocaine are injected either directly into the area or further up into a nerve which supplies the area producing nerve block. Cocaine itself, although used as drops of watery solution for pain in the eyes and sometimes in a cream for local irritation is little used in any other field of medicine since it leads to addiction more readily than almost any other drug and can be dangerous if absorbed into the system. Spinal anaesthia is used more on the continent than here and its principle uses are for operations on the lower part of the body especially when the patient's general condition makes general anaesthesia inadvisable. Some anaesthetics are injected by the rectum. Trichlorethylene or 'trilene' has recently been found to have the valuable property in the form of a pocket inhaler of deadening pain in cases of emergency or in childbirth; it can be administered either by the patient himself or by someone else. When self-administered the patient need only breathe enough to keep the pain under control and since it is both safe and effective it forms a useful substitute for morphia.

Modern techniques make the production of anaesthesia relatively safe even when the patient is dangerously ill or debilitated or when the operation lasts for prolonged periods. With the use of supportive drugs, analgesics, and the relaxant curare it is possible to keep him unconscious for many hours with a minimum amount of anaesthetic. The new methods of hypothermia and 'artificial hibernation' in which the temperature of the body is so lowered by packing in ice that its metabolic processes are reduced to a minimum so that they are, as it were, just 'ticking over' makes long and extensive operations possible with small quantities of anaesthetic and consequent advantage to the patient. Operations carried out under modern conditions are extremely safe and the patient is unlikely to know of anything that occurs between the moment when he gets his first injection in bed and the time when he wakes up in bed once more. Sickness is the exception rather than the rule, and those who (as frequently happens) worry lest they should give away important secrets under an anaesthetic need not trouble themselves. Nobody ever does.

Analgesics: are drugs which deaden pain without loss of consciousness, some (e.g. aspirin, mixtures of aspirin with other substances such as phenacetin and codeine, and some of the more recent proprietary preparations such as Panadol) being taken by mouth to act on the central nervous system, others being applied locally as lozenges containing benzocaine for sore throat or creams applied to the skin for itching or muscular pain to act on the nerve-endings. Creams used for itching are more correctly called 'antipruritics' and those for muscular pains which act by producing a sense of heat 'counter-irritants.' Adrenalin cream is not a counter-irritant, but is supposed to act by relaxing muscular spasm. Local anaesthetics could, strictly speaking, be described as coming under the above definition but the word 'analgesic' is more generally used for aspirin and the opium derivatives such as morphine which act on the pain centres of the brain. The latter are only available to doctors who may prescribe them for severe pain. Colic due to spasm of the intestines or biliary and renal tracts are treated by 'antispasmodics' which relax the spasm (e.g. belladonna) with or without central analgesics.

Anaphylaxis: is virtually synonymous with allergy (q.v.) but is usually applied to the symptoms which may develop following the injection of serum such as diphtheria or anti-tetanus inoculations ('serum sickness'). In rare cases a second injection given at a certain interval after a first to which the patient has become allergic may cause sudden death by 'anaphylactic shock.'

Androgen: the only hormone secreted by the testes, the male sexual glands, is testosterone which is partially responsible for sexual development in a masculine direction. Androgens are adrenal hormones which have a testosterone-like action, testosterone itself, or any other hormones which have a virilising effect (*see* Endocrine Glands).

Aneurine: Vitamin B1 (*see* Vitamins).

Aneurism: a localised bulging in the wall of an artery usually caused by a degeneration of the inner lining which may occur in almost any part of the body. A *true* aneurism is of this type, whereas in a *false* one all the coats have given way and the bulge is only supported by the thickened fibrous tissues of the structures surrounding the artery. In a *dissecting* aneurism blood has got through a weakness in the inner wall and passed between the outer walls of the artery for a varying distance. *Miliary* aneurisms are tiny bulges (like a millet seed) usually found on the vessels in the brain. Classification is also according to the area in which they occur, e.g. abdominal, thoracic (in the chest), popliteal (behind the knee), axillary (in the armpit), etc. The cause of aneurisms varies: in former times it was commonly chronic syphilis which usually affected the aorta in the chest but today this is rather rare owing to early treatment of the disease, atheroma in which an excessive amount of cholesterol in the blood-stream has led to the formation of localised deposits on the arterial walls may cause aneurism in the abdominal aorta (*see* Arteries, diseases of) and elsewhere, tuberculosis of the lungs may lead to aneurism in the pulmonary artery mainly through weakening the supporting tissues, and small aneurisms may occur where there is localised sepsis or in many areas simultaneously in generalised infection. The immediate cause of an aneurism may be strain but this can only be effective when the arterial coat has already been weakened; this was notably the case in popliteal aneurisms behind the knee which were common in the days when horse-riding was more frequent than it is now. The only really common aneurisms today are in the brain due either to arteriosclerosis or to weak areas in the circle of blood-vessels surrounding the base of the brain present from birth.

There are no specific symptoms of aneurism; for, except when they are on the surface where a swelling which pulsates with the heartbeat can be seen or when sudden haemorrhage arises, what symptoms are present are those brought about by pressure on the surrounding structures and therefore vary from one area to another. The blood inside an aneurism may clot thus bringing about spontaneous cure, or, if it is discovered in time, the clotting process may be induced artificially by surgical means. Where an alternative circulation is present the artery may be tied, but of course it is necessary to treat the underlying cause medically. Advances in modern surgery have now made it possible to treat large aneurisms, for example in the abdominal aorta, by completely removing the affected part and replacing it by a plastic tube. Occasionally aneurisms result from bullet or knife wounds, and very rarely such an injury may cause an artery and its vein to join together.

Angina: in its less modern usage is a term applied to any disease which brings about a sense of suffocating or choking as in swellings of the throat (e.g. quinsy or Vincent's angina, q.v.). Today it is almost entirely applied to Vincent's angina and angina pectoris, a heart disease described below which gives rise to similar sensations.

Angina Pectoris: a heart disease the main symptom of which is the occurrence of paroxysmal attacks of severe pain or a sense of oppression sometimes mistaken for indigestion in the heart region but spreading over the chest and left shoulder region and characteristically down the left arm. The attacks are brought about by exertion or emotional stress and their immediate cause is spasm of the coronary blood-vessels which supply the heart muscle. Typically, the sufferer from chronic attacks develops pain whilst walking or emotionally distressed which ceases when he sits down or relaxes, differing in this way from the sufferer from coronary thrombosis where the vessels become actually blocked by clotting, producing identical symptoms with the exception that the pain may occur at any time, often in bed and unrelated to exercise or emotional stress, and does not disappear on resting but may remain for some days. Although the pain in angina is brought about by spasm it is seldom the case that spasm alone is the cause and the arteries are usually narrowed through arteriosclerosis or atheroma long before the attack occurs. Sometimes a single attack may be fatal, but more usually there is a series of attacks which may either increase in intensity or simply cease especially if the patient adheres carefully to medical instructions. In severe pain there is often an accompanying sense of impending death, shallow breathing, a generally shocked appearance with cold sweats, and restlessness with a feeling of extreme anxiety. Treatment is a matter for the doctor but involves rest, instruction about exercise when the patient is able to get about, sedatives and vasodilator drugs which relieve the spasm (these may be given either for use in emergency or taken over a prolonged period of time). Surgery has been employed in such techniques as putting sterile talc into the pericardial sac surrounding the heart to increase the blood-supply by the irritation induced, transplantation of the internal mammary artery from the inside of the breast-bone to the heart, and, more recently the use of a free vein graft whereby a piece of vein taken from elsewhere in the body is used to connect the aorta (the main artery of the body) with the coronary veins, thus reversing the flow of blood through vessels which do not develop arteriosclerosis. These operations are in the experimental stage and are rarely performed, medical treatment usually being adequate. It is worth noting that the vast majority of people who have pain in the heart region are not suffering from heart disease of any sort, but when in doubt the doctor should be consulted (*see* Coronary Thrombosis).

Angiography: the injection of radio-opaque substances into the blood-vessels in order to make them visible on X-ray plates. This demonstrates whether they are narrow or not, the presence of aneurisms (q.v.), and vascular tumours such as angiomata.

Angioma: a simple tumour or cluster of large or small blood-vessels which is sometimes found in the internal organs (where in the brain it may occasionally give rise to haemorrhage) and fairly frequently in the form of naevi or 'birth-marks' on the skin which may be unsightly but not dangerous. Treatment is only indicated when they are giving rise to inconvenience or appear unsightly and this will depend on the size, small ones being cauterised with an electric needle, larger ones being removed surgically under local anaesthesia. Also known as Haemangiomas, these tumours do not become malignant.

Angioneurotic Oedema: a condition usually found in young adults of either sex in which there is varying degrees of swelling particularly about the face and hands, although sometimes elsewhere. It appears in attacks either after eating foods to which the individual is allergic or after emotional stress. The eyelids and lips especially become tight and uncomfortable from the swelling and the face looks puffy so that it may be impossible to open the eyes. Occasionally diarrhoea and vomiting are present. The patient is usually of a sensitive and nervous disposition and the attacks sometimes run in families; danger only arises if the glottis or throat is affected when he runs the risk of choking. Angioneurotic oedema as the name indicates has a large neurotic element in its causation, but the exciting cause is ordinarily allergy (q.v.) to certain substances, usually foods. The immediate treatment of an attack is to give an injection of adrenaline as is done in most acute allergic conditions; the later treatment is dependent upon finding and avoiding or desensitising against the allergen, the use of antihistamine drugs, and perhaps psychotherapy. Usually the patient 'grows out of' the attacks.

Ankylosis: the condition of a joint which has become fixed so that the ordinarily movable parts become capable of only a limited degree of movement. The causes are inflammation which has died down leaving the bones attached by scar-tissue, joint deformities, or actual union of the bones, and these may be brought about by a fracture, tubercular infections, rheumatoid arthritis, or long immobilisation as when fractures are being treated or amongst the Indian fakirs who as part of their religious devotions hold a limb for years in the same position. Sometimes ankylosis is brought about deliberately by surgical operation (e.g. in prolonged pain) this operation being known as arthrodesis.

Ankylostoma: the hook-worm, a parasite causing the disease of ankylostomiasis found mainly in tropical countries but also in Western Europe and the Southern States of America. In temperate lands it is usually found amongst workers in damp and insanitary conditions such as mines and sewers or underground tunnels. The eggs of the parasite are expelled in the motions of an infected person and hatch in warm damp soil

41

into larvae or immature forms which burrow through the skin of the feet, enter the blood-stream and pass to the lungs, where being coughed up they are swallowed into the stomach and intestines, there as adult worms 1–2 cm. long to attach themselves by their hooks to the lining of the bowels where they may cause fatal haemorrhage. Milder attacks cause nausea and vomiting with the development of anaemia which results in millions of individuals throughout the world being unable to lead a normal active existence. Treatment is by purgatives and vermifuges (drugs for driving out worms) such as carbon tetrachloride which is extremely effective. But the main effort has to be directed against bad sanitation, the use of human faeces for manure, and the habit of going about barefoot in surroundings where infection may occur.

Anopheles: the name given to a group of mosquitoes widely distributed throughout the world some species of which transmit to man the malaria parasite. Two types both found in England, Anopheles maculipennis and A. bifurcatus, are capable of doing this although malaria is now rarely contracted here (*see* Malaria).

Anorexia Nervosa: a nervous condition confined mainly to young women who refuse to eat, sleep very little, and yet remain very active. Sometimes the state begins with an obsession that the person concerned is becoming overweight, appetite being at first restricted by deliberate intent and then being genuinely lost. Emaciation may become severe and even result in death, the patient often deceiving her attendants as to the amount of food she has taken. Treatment is psychological but, of course, in severe cases the first thing to do is to ensure adequate intake of food by compulsion if necessary. Psychiatric advice should always be sought.

Antabuse: a proprietary name for disulfiram (*see* Alcoholism).

Antacids: medicines for treating gastric acidity (*see* Alkalies).

Antihelminthics: drugs for causing the expulsion of parasite worms, also 'vermifuges.'

Anthracosis: the greyish-pink or black changes in colour in the lungs of miners, but found in varying degrees in most city-dwellers due to the inhalation of coal-dust or soot. There is no evidence that it leads to any harmful results.

Anthrax: a serious disease caused by a bacillus which affects cattle and sheep chiefly in Australia, Russia, and S. America, and is spread to man either by direct contact or by contact with the hides, fleeces, or diseased meat. It is also known as woolsorter's disease, malignant pustule, rag-picker's disease, and, in animals, splenic fever or murrain. In both man and animals it takes two forms: external and internal. The external type can occur by infection through cracks or cuts even from hides long-removed from the animal; a 'boil' appears on the area, often the face or arm, and the inflamed area spreads until a small area of pus appears at the centre which bursts to produce a black scab about half-an-inch in diameter. There is a high fever and great prostration which disappear within about ten days in cases which recover. The internal form is caused either by breathing in the spores which the bacillus gives rise to and which may persist for very long periods in the hides, or by eating infected flesh or drinking infected water. In this case pneumonia with haemorrhages from the lungs or bleeding from ulcers in the intestines with gangrene of the spleen occurs and is almost always fatal without treatment by anti-serum, penicillin, or aureomycin which has reduced deaths to one tenth of their former incidence. Preventive measures include destruction by burning of all infected hides and bodies, disinfection of premises, and forbidding of grazing in an infected area. Anthrax is uncommon in Britain, although a minor epidemic occurred in Bradford in 1880.

Antibiotic: a collective name for any substance derived from micro-organisms or fungi which is capable of destroying infections, e.g. penicillin, aureomycin, chloromycetin, streptomycin (*see* Penicillin, *et al.*).

Anticoagulants: drugs which reduce the clotting-power of the blood and are therefore useful in diseases such as coronary thrombosis brought about by clotting leading to interference with blood-supply, in this case to the heart muscle. They include heparin obtained first from liver tissue but only effective by injection, dicoumarol from spoiled sweet clover which produces a bleeding disease in cattle through its anti-clotting activity and is cheaper and capable of being given by mouth, and the slower-acting phenindione, a synthetic. Proprietary preparations are: 'Tromexan,' 'Sinthrome,' 'Pularin,' 'Marevan,' 'Marcoumar,' etc. Their use requires periodic checks to make sure that the coagulating power of the blood is not too greatly reduced.

Antigen: a substance which causes the formation of antibodies in the blood which act in opposition to material (*see* Allergy) or infections introduced from without (*see* Infection).

Antihistamine Drugs: drugs which antagonise the action of histamine liberated from the body cells in cases of allergy (q.v.) thus leading to the symptoms of the various allergic diseases. They are extremely effective in many cases, possibly least so in asthma and most in skin conditions and hay-fever. Of the thirty or forty drugs available it is worth noting (*a*) that their effects in individuals vary so that one may help whilst others may not and it is therefore sometimes necessary to try several, (*b*) that, whilst most have some sedative effect and tend to make the patient drowsy, some have this effect in a greater degree than others, e.g. 'Benadryl,' 'Phenergan,' and Promezathine' are more sedative in effect than 'Thephorin,' 'Piriton,' and 'Antistin.' This is important in those who have to drive, climb heights, or keep a clear mind generally.

Antimony: a metal similar in its effects to arsenic and formerly much used in the treatment of fever and bronchitis, or in the form of 'tartar emetic' as an emetic (for which it is not to be recommended), antimony is now used only in the treatment of certain tropical diseases. Since it is very poisonous to protozoa, tartar emetic is sometimes given in 2% solution for Kala-Azar (Leishmaniasis) and in sleeping sickness (trypanosomiasis) as twice-weekly intravenous injections. Filariasis, yaws, oriental sore, and relapsing fever are also treated in this way. Stibophen or Fouadin is used in bilharzia and Stibosan and Neo-Stibosan in Kala-Azar.

Antiphlogistin. substances used as plasters in the treatment of inflammation on the surface of the body, the most familiar being the cataplasma kaolin. This is much the best form of applying heat to infected areas as it does not make the skin wet and sodden like boric lint but rather absorbs liquid and retains heat for longer periods. The plaster may be applied by placing the tin in a little water and boiling (taking care not to let the water into the kaolin), then spreading the kaolin on lint and carefully applying it to the skin as hot as possible without burning or causing discomfort. An alternative method is to apply the plaster cold to the lint and heat it under a toasting grill.

Antipyretics: drugs or methods which reduce fever, e.g. cold-sponging, wet-packs, aspirin, phenacetin, quinine.

Antiseptics: strictly speaking the term refers to substances which prevent putrefaction by destroying or arresting the development of the germs which are the cause of the process as distinct from disinfectants which destroy the germs causing disease. However, the two words are so often confused that they have become virtually synonymous and it is in this sense that they will be used here. It was Louis Pasteur (1822–95) who first discovered the function played by germs in causing disease although initially in non-medical fields such as fermentation and diseases of the grape-vine, and Semmelweiss, an Austrian, who first showed their influence in wound infections leading to sepsis in 1847. Lord Lister (1827–1912) first used antiseptics during surgical operations and in the treatment of wounds by his introduction of carbolic acid. Various processes have the effect of destroying the germs of putrefaction (e.g. extreme heat or cold, drying, etc.), thus surgical instruments are sterilised by boiling, and canned foods which are boiled and then hermetically sealed can be kept almost indefinitely; refrigeration by arresting the development of germs can keep food safe from putrefaction during transport or in the home refrigerator; drying has been used for centuries as in dried fruits, meat, and fish. In jam, the high concentration of sugar prevents the development of bacteria by withdrawing moisture from them. Some food preservatives (e.g. sulphur dioxide) are still used, but to nothing like the same extent as formerly.

Most authorities today (even when they practice it in order to impress others or to protect themselves from charges of negligence) think very little of the necessity for disinfecting houses after ordinary infectious diseases (*a*) because it is unlikely to have any effect, and (*b*) because it is usually thought that the majority of childhood fevers are best contracted and got over with since they are much more dangerous in adult life. Houses, of course, may be *disinfested* to get rid of parasites such as bed-bugs and clothing to get rid of lice or scabies mites. Many proprietary disinfectants are available for disinfecting drains, lavatory pans, and sinks; nearly all are highly effective but most are poisonous and some corrosive if they get on to the skin. There is really little necessity nowadays to

45

use carbolic acid or the older and more crude products with strong odours. The majority of household disinfectants contain coal-tar products such as cresol, products of chlorine, or formaldehyde but in a more sophisticated form which is equally effective and smells clean and pleasant.

Amongst the most common antiseptics which have been used on the body are boric acid dissolved in water or as an ointment, a weak but non-poisonous or irritant antiseptic; hydrogen peroxide, strong but non-poisonous and useful for removing wax from the ears, dirt from wounds, or as a gargle; iodine and iodoform, now rarely used; potassium permanganate as a gargle, douche or hand-wash; acriflavine, brilliant green, gentian violet, and other aniline dyes for the skin; eusol, like the proprietary 'Milton,' a chlorine product. But the use of antiseptics on the body has been greatly reduced in recent years. In surgery the aseptic method which ensures that everything touching the body is sterilised has replaced the antiseptic method long ago; antiseptics are used for the initial cleaning of wounds but since nearly all hinder the process of healing we are much less prone to use continuous applications, and antibiotics have greatly reduced the dangers of infection. When they are necessary the modern proprietary antiseptics such as Dettol or Cetavlon are used in preference to the older ones. Gargles are pleasant when one has a bad taste in the mouth, but nobody believes that they have any significant healing effect, and antiseptics in the bath unless required for some definite purpose, are unnecessary and a bad idea since soap in itself is quite antiseptic enough. In short, the best use for antiseptics is on drains, surgical instruments, and in cleaning wounds. The less they are used otherwise without medical advice the better.

Antitoxins: (*see* Blood, Infection).

Antivenine: a serum produced by the injection of increasing doses of snake venom into animals which leads to the production of antitoxins in the serum which is effective against the bite of the specific snake if given within an hour of the injury.

Antrum: a natural space within a bone, especially the maxillary sinuses in the upper jaw-bone between the eye and the mouth and the mastoid antrum behind the ear (*see* Sinusitis, Mastoiditis).

Anus: the two sphincters or rings of muscle at the end of the bowel where the rectum opens to the exterior (*see* Haemorrhoids, Fissure, Constipation, Rectum, Diseases of).

Anxiety Neurosis: (*see* Neurosis).

Aorta: the main artery of the body (*see* Circulatory System).

Aperients: (*see* Constipation).

Aphasia: means a defect of the power of speech or its complete absence caused by damage to the centres in the brain connected with the function. Usually this is caused by a stroke or apoplectic attack in which haemorrhage, clotting (thrombosis), or a displaced clot which has arisen elsewhere (embolism) causes their destruction, but in some cases disease of the nerve tracts is responsible. Aphasia takes various forms because the various functions connected with reading, writing, understanding, and hearing are found in different parts of the cerebrum on the surface of the brain whilst the lower centres which directly bring the muscles of speech into action under control of the cerebrum are found in the brain-stem or medulla. Thus damage to the inferior frontal area on the left side in right-handed people (and vice versa) brings about an inability to speak although intelligence and silent reading or writing are unimpaired, whilst damage to the area just above this leads to agraphia or the inability to write rationally without any defect of the hand movements being present. These two are together known as motor aphasia, whereas loss of power of taking in and understanding words seen or heard are known as word blindness or word deafness respectively and as sensory aphasia collectively. In the latter case the damage is further back in the temporal region of the cerebrum and in word blindness there is a failure to understand the written word although there is no defect of vision, in word deafness a failure to understand the spoken word although hearing is unimpaired. An attack of aphasia may be temporary and last for only a few hours, but more frequently it is permanent and there is also some intellectual defect. Treatment is that of the cause.

Aphonia: or loss of voice may be partial or complete and is caused by disease of the nerves supplying the throat muscles, such infections as laryngitis, or neurosis. In the latter case aphonia is brought about by the unconscious desire not to speak, or to be unable to speak in a particular situation (*see* Laryngitis).

Apomorphine: an emetic, related to morphine, which given hypodermically produces vomiting (*see* Alcoholism).

Apoplexy: stroke brought about by cerebral haemorrhage, embolism, or thrombosis, and leading to unconsciousness and varying degrees of paralysis. In embolism a clot may form in a diseased heart and, becoming dislodged, pass to the brain and block a blood-vessel leading to sudden loss of consciousness and the other symptoms of apoplexy; the outlook of recovery of function is better in this case than in the other two types. Thrombosis may come on more gradually in elderly people with diseased blood-vessels and poor circulation leading to gradual formation of a clot within the brain arteries, but haemorrhage (the commonest type of apoplexy to which the word is usually applied) is generally sudden in its onset although the processes leading to it may have been occurring for some time previously. Ordinarily those who have an apoplectic attack are between the ages of forty to sixty and the commonest predisposing causes are atheroma (i.e. one form of arteriosclerosis with degeneration of the lining of the arteries leading to weakness), and chronic kidney disease leading also to changes in the heart and arteries together with a high blood-pressure. However the condition may occur in younger people and even in children usually as the result of congenital aneurism (*see* Aneurism) in the arteries surrounding the base of the brain. Recent evidence seems to suggest that in many cases of stroke the blockage is in the arteries of the neck rather than inside the head. The symptoms are more or less sudden loss of consciousness with flushed face, heavy breathing, and blowing out of the cheeks with each breath. The paralysis is not immediately apparent at this stage but is usually noticeable when one lifts the limbs and finds them much more flaccid on one side of the body than the other. Sometimes apoplexy is mistaken for narcotic or alcoholic poisoning but can usually be distinguished by this flaccidity on one side which causes the limbs to flop down powerlessly when lifted and the contracted pupils in contrast with the usually dilated pupils of poisoning by narcotics or alcohol. (The smell of alcohol on the breath is not a safe guide since apoplexy may occur after taking alcohol and, especially in the case of haemorrhage from the middle meningeal artery which may result from injury through a fall after drinking too much, people have frequently died through being locked up in the cells as cases of simple drunkenness). Sometimes sudden paralysis of one side may occur without the onset of unconsciousness. The immediate cause of the attack may be exertion or straining, emotional outbursts, drinking bouts or too much food, fits of severe coughing, etc.

The immediate treatment is to loosen the patient's clothing, particularly about the neck, move him as little as possible, keep him warm, and send for the doctor. *Stimulants, whether alcoholic or not must never be given,* nor, for the matter of that, should any food or drink so long as the patient is unconscious or semiconscious. The most dangerous period is the first twenty-four hours after the attack and even the first two or three days; after three weeks, however, some degree of improvement should be seen and may by this time have reached its full extent so far as paralysis is concerned.

Appendicectomy: (American, Appendectomy) removal of the vermiform appendix.

Appendicitis: it is a strange fact that appendicitis was almost unknown prior to 1886 although how far this is due to more careful diagnosis and how far to modern habits in eating and living nobody can say. The condition is caused by bacterial infection of the appendix, a useless relic of our primitive past located in the right lower part of the abdomen and attached to the caecum at the point where the small intestine enters the large intestine or colon; it is never caused by the swallowing of fruit stones or pips as is so commonly believed. In a typical case the patient is young (80% occur under the age of 30) and begins to have discomfort in the stomach region or the upper part of the abdomen; this becomes more severe and is accompanied by vomiting and slight fever and gradually localises itself in the right lower part of the abdomen. Sometimes constipation has been present for several days prior to the attack. But appendicitis is not always easy to diagnose and pain may occur in other parts since the organ is extremely mobile. If untreated the appendix may burst leading to an appendix abscess or peritonitis, therefore it is a general rule for the surgeon to operate when any doubt exists. For the average uncomplicated case the usual period in hospital is one week. Medical treatment with antibiotics alone is never used unless there are very good reasons for it or the patient is out of reach of surgical attention. Other types of appendicitis have been described as 'chronic' or 'recurrent' and these are characterised by periodic attacks of pain over the appendix area, loss of appetite, nausea, and constipation lasting for a period of months or years. A considerable number of surgeons doubt whether these cases really exist, but the only sensible procedure is to be advised by one's own surgeon who is best qualified to know in a particular case whether operation is, or is not, necessary.

Apraxia: the loss of power to carry out regulated and co-ordinated movements caused by disease of the nervous system.

Argyrol: a mild antiseptic of silver in combination with protein used in 5–25% solution in water to treat conjunctivitis or to wash out the bladder. The fact that it is the same colour as tincture of iodine has sometimes led to serious accidents to the eye when the latter has been used in mistake, and that it is also inconvenient by reason of the staining it is liable to produce on the skin or clothes has led to it being much less used than formerly.

Arsenic: a metallic poison which, like antimony, produces irritation of the stomach and intestines in sufficient amounts, leading to symptoms of gastro-enteritis. It is now rarely used in medicine save in certain skin diseases and, of course, in the form of salvarsan or neosalvarsan (arsphenamine) Ehrlich's great discovery for the treatment of syphilis, yaws, and relapsing fever. As a poison it has the disadvantage for the criminal that it is perhaps the most easily identifiable of all such substances, but its relative availability in sheep-dips, fly-papers, and in dyeing has endeared it to the hearts of the unimaginative.

Arteries: (*see* Circulatory System).

Arteries, Diseases of: arteries, particularly the larger ones, are very elastic and pulsate with every beat of the heart; when an artery is cut this quality causes the cut end to shrink and draw itself within the outer fibrous coat leaving a smaller opening to be closed by blood-clot. The layer within the fibrous coat is composed of muscle tissue supported by elastic fibres, and the innermost layer is further elastic tissue covered with smooth flat cells like paving-stones. From within the layers are known as intima, media and adventitia. In disease it is the two innermost layers with which we are most concerned since it is there that the trouble usually begins. As people grow older the media or middle coat of their arteries tends to become less elastic and more rigid especially in the middle-sized vessels, but when this change is pronounced or comes on too early in life it is known as arteriosclerosis or hardening of the arteries. Such a condition seems to be partly hereditary, is sometimes (but by no means always) associated with high blood-pressure, and more often with diabetes or a tendency to gout. It need not necessarily produce symptoms, but obviously this depends on how early the condition starts, what other diseases may be present, and which arteries are affected and how badly. Thus in the brain it is conducive to cerebral haemorrhage, in the coronary vessels of the heart to angina or coronary thrombosis, in the kidneys to a form of chronic nephritis, and in the legs to circulatory disturbances. Mentally some of the changes normally found in old age may occur: the patient tends to be forgetful especially of recent events, less so of the more distant past; he is emotionally unstable and easily moved to tears or anger; he becomes self-centred and irritable. In atheroma there is localised thickening of the intima or inner coat with the formation of yellowish plates and a degeneration which may gradually spread to the other layers leading to swellings which in the case of the smaller vessels interferes with the blood-supply to the parts surrounding them and in larger ones may cause aneurisms (q.v.). The plaques are composed of cholesterol and the condition is believed by some to be in part due to too much cholesterol in the blood from a diet too rich in animal fats; in time they may become calcified and chalky so that the arteries instead of being elastic become like pipe-stems. Atheroma leads to much the same changes as arteriosclerosis with risk of thrombosis especially in the heart and brain. Another disease in which the thrombosis is mainly in the vessels of the legs is *thromboangiitis obliterans* which is found in comparatively young people between the ages of 25–50. Mostly they are males who smoke too many cigarettes and, allegedly, more commonly Jews; possibly the condition is a form of allergy to tobacco. The legs become red and swollen when hanging down, but pale when lifted up, pulsation is absent in the arteries behind the knee and at the side of the ankle, and blisters or gangrene of the toes may occur. The treatment is a matter for the specialist,

51

but may consist of various medical measures including the giving up of smoking and sometimes surgical removal of the 2nd to the 4th lumbar ganglia of the sympathetic nervous system, which ordinarily causes constriction of the arteries concerned, may be advised. Thromboangiitis obliterans is also known as Buerger's disease, and often the first sign is pain on walking which is relieved by rest. Similar pains, although more often burning in nature than cramp-like, are found in *erythromelalgia* a disease found in women between the ages of 30–50. Here, however, the pain is most usually on the soles of the feet and may be brought on by heat as when lying in bed or in summer-time. There is no swelling or gangrene and the disease is primarily a nervous one which may be treated by drugs or occasionally by operation to divide the pain-producing nerves. Spasm is also the cause of *Raynaud's disease* which is commoner in the hands although the feet, nose, and ears may be affected. Here again, the patient is usually a woman between the ages of 30–50 who notices that her fingers or toes suddenly become pale at the tips and on warming ache or throb. In more severe cases one or more fingers may become blue or black and very occasionally this may lead to localised gangrene. Various forms of treatment may help, either medical or surgical or both, but the condition has a tendency to disappear after several years. Often modern vasodilator drugs are sufficient to bring about a cure. In *acrocyanosis* the hands and feet of young girls are cold and blueish-red owing to poor circulation but they develop no other symptoms and the condition clears up in time with vasodilator drugs or spontaneously.

Arthritis: inflammation of a joint or joints due to rheumatoid arthritis, osteoarthritis, gout, tuberculosis, injury, or occasionally gonorrhoea and other infections (*see* Joints, Diseases of, Gout, Rheumatism).

Artificial Insemination: is the introduction of semen into the vagina by artificial means which, although long used in animal breeding, has only comparatively recently been used in human beings in cases where a married woman is unable to have children in the ordinary way either owing to her husband's sexual impotence or actual sterility. Where the husband's semen is normal and impregnation does not take place because of some impediment to intercourse as in impotence the method known as A.I.H. (artificial insemination by the husband) is used in which the husband's semen is injected by a syringe into the womb. In A.I.D. where the husband is sterile semen is obtained from a donor other than the woman's husband and unknown to her but known, of course, to the doctor. In both cases several attempts may have to be made. Religious bodies hold varying views on the subject but most seem to regard A.I.D. as morally wrong. It is specifically forbidden by the Roman Catholic Church.

Artificial Respiration: former methods of artificial respiration such as Schafer's and Sylvester's are being replaced by the Holger Nielsen method now adopted by the Royal Life-Saving Society and the St John and British Red Cross organisations. In this the patient is laid flat on the ground face downwards with false teeth and anything obstructing the mouth and throat removed. The arms are placed forwards on each side of the head and the elbows bent outwards so that the hands lying palm downwards, one on top of the other, are beneath the forehead. The back is then smacked hard to bring the tongue forward. The operator kneels on the right knee in line with the patient's head and facing his back, the left leg being placed with the heel near the patient's right elbow. The hands are placed on the patient's shoulderblades and the operator leans forward until his straight arms are vertical, causing the patient to force air out of his chest. This takes $2\frac{1}{2}$ seconds and the hands are then moved along the arms until the patient's elbows are reached; done slowly and deliberately this should take 1 second. The arms and shoulders of the patient are then lifted upwards until the weight of the chest is felt but without moving either chest or head and this causes inspiration lasting a further $2\frac{1}{2}$ seconds. The elbows are then lowered and the operator's hands move back to the shoulder-blades to repeat the cycle.

Another valuable method is Eve's rocking method in which the patient is rocked up and down whilst lying tied to a stretcher, the tilt of the rocker extending 45 degrees from the horizontal. This is carried out 10 times per minute and has the advantage of stimulating the circulation as well as the respiration. The mouth-to-mouth method may also be used.

Asbestosis: a special form of pneumoconiosis caused by the inhalation of asbestos dust i.e. mainly magnesium silicate.

53

Unlike the pneumoconiosis of miners the damage does not occur in nodules and patches but consists in a diffuse fibrosis or scarring throughout the lungs accompanied by emphysema (q.v.) and thickening of the pleural lining. The symptoms are breathlessness, bluish discoloration of the skin due to cyanosis and cough with sputum containing asbestos bodies; there may be clubbing of the fingers. Treatment is a matter for the doctor, but prevention is the main point and this consists primarily in dust suppression by wet drilling as in Canada where asbestos mining is carried out. Similar precautions are taken in Britain in the manufacture of asbestos textiles.

Ascaris: the roundworm, in appearance very similar to a large earthworm (up to a foot long), which is parasitic in human and horse intestines (*see* Worms).

Ascites: swelling of the abdomen due to fluid exuded from the blood-vessels in such conditions as heart, kidney, and liver diseases.

Ascorbic Acid: the chemical name of synthetic or natural vitamin C (*see* Vitamins).

Asepsis: the procedure in surgical operations in almost universal use today whereby, instead of the use of antiseptics, all instruments, materials, surgeon's gowns and gloves, etc., are sterilised by steaming, boiling or dry heat prior to operating. Antiseptic is used only to clean the skin area where the incision is to be made and masks are worn to exclude germs from the operators' noses or throats (*see* Antiseptics).

Aspiration: the withdrawal of fluid localised in some area of the body. Formerly used for swelling of the legs or abdomen in chronic heart or liver disease this is now rarely necessary since it is more efficiently done with modern diuretic drugs. However, it is still frequently in use as in lumbar puncture to draw fluid from the spinal canal for diagnosis or treatment, in pleurisy with effusion, and in the case, e.g. of fluid in the pre-patellar bursa of the knee.

Aspirin: the proprietary name given by the firm of Bayer's to acetylsalycylic acid now commonly used in many such preparations. Aspirin relieves pain of moderate degree and reduces the temperature; it has no effect upon 'nerves', sleep (unless insomnia is due to pain), or being generally miserable. In other words, aspirin is neither a tonic nor a sedative. There is no evidence that it is any more effective when mixed with phenacetin, codeine, or caffeine nor that soluble aspirin or aspirin combined with alkali is any less irritant to the stomach. There is no point in taking more than two tablets at a time (i.e. 10 grains) since beyond this point its pain-killing power is not increased. Gastric sufferers should not use aspirin.

Asthenia: loss of strength or debility.

Asthma: a condition in which there are attacks of severe breathlessness when the patient is unable to get air in, and particularly out, of his lungs owing to spasm of the smaller bronchi which leads to swelling of the mucous membrane lining. Asthma may be truly allergic (*see* Allergy) and caused by the inhalation of foreign proteins in the form of dust to which the indivdual is hypersensitive, nevertheless in the vast majority of cases no such hypersensitivity can be found, nor when it begins for the first time is bronchitis present as invariably happens later. The condition may begin in childhood when it is often grown out of, or in early adult life when it becomes very difficult to eradicate, and there can be little doubt that the cause is in most cases primarily emotional and the first attack often follows an incident or period of emotional stress. At this stage the treatment lies, not in drugs, so much as in the right handling of the patient's emotional life which in a child is usually influenced by over-anxious parents. But the usual progress of the disease is initial emotional stress followed by a vicious circle in which fear of another attack actually leads to one, these attacks lead to bronchial infection causing the bronchi to become more sensitive to emotional stimulation and even stimulation by chemical agents such as fog, dust, etc., and bronchitis leads to emphysema (q.v.) which predisposes to further bronchitis. By this time the disease is well-established and medical treatment gives best hope of relief although the emotional origins should never be neglected at any stage. For an attack the doctor may give an injection of adrenaline, and there are various sprays inhaled from a nebuliser and usually containing ephedrene which has an adrenaline-like affect when given by inhalation or mouth. When infection is present antibiotics such as penicillin or terramycin may be given or courses of the sulpha drugs. It must be repeated that true bronchial asthma depends initially upon emotional stress in a person predisposed to react in that way rather than others. Breathing exercises carried out by a trained therapist may be helpful and sedatives sometimes help in combination with the other drugs.

Astigmatism: a defect of vision caused by distortion of the cornea (the clear membrane in front of the eye) which is cylindrical instead of globular, one axis being longer than the other. Hence objects are seen distorted so that a circle looks like an oval. The condition is remedied by the use of glasses with suitably curved lenses of which one surface forms part of a cylinder.

Astringents: are substances which cause contraction of mucous surfaces and therefore stop bleeding or discharge of moderate degree, e.g. alum (aluminium and potassium sulphate or aluminium and ammonium sulphate) used as a styptic for shaving cuts, tannic acid, or witch-hazel (hamamelis) in the form of an extract, liquor, or ointment.

Ataxia: loss of the power to control movements so that, although no muscular weakness is present, fine movements become impossible, the legs for example being thrown about as in locomotor ataxia and other diseases or the hands incapable of small movements which require careful coordination. This is due to a defect of the sensory nerves which, being damaged in some part of their course, fail to send messages to the brain giving the position of the limbs in space upon which fine movements depend.

Atebrin: the trade name of mepacrine hydrochloride given in malaria.

Atelectasis: collapse of part of the lung or failure to expand at birth.

Atheroma: (*see* Arteries, Disease of).

Atomic Radiation: nuclear weapons produce the ordinary results of any explosion by the effects of blast and burning but their specific contribution lies in the effects of radiation. The rays produced are similar in nature to those of light but shorter in wave-length and much more penetrating. Such rays do not necessarily arise from the explosion of weapons for they are also characteristic of X-rays and the radiation produced by radioactive elements as they spontaneously disintegrate or are disintegrated artifically in a cyclotron; in addition they include the cosmic rays which enter the Earth's atmosphere from outer space. Radiation of this type is dangerous to the human body in a selective way, damaging in particular the skin, the bone marrow, and the sex glands. Exposure to X-rays for measured periods leads to reddening of the skin after a latent period of a few days or as much as two weeks and a still longer exposure to destruction of the hair-follicles leading to baldness; the early workers learned to their cost that long periods of intermittent exposure can lead to chronic skin ulcers which tend to become cancerous. The effects of ionising radiation on the bone-marrow leads to its destruction and hence to aplastic anaemia from damage to the blood-producing cells in this tissue and there is considerable evidence that leukaemia in which the white blood cells proliferate is on the increase and may be related to radiation. Both these two forms of blood disease terminate fatally. Acting on the sex-cells, fertility is decreased and those children who are born are liable to be abnormal; large doses cause complete sterility. So far it would appear that actual atomic explosions have not increased the total radiation to which we are exposed by more than 1% and the greater risk is from industrial, medical, and other sources since ordinary X-rays as used in medicine increase the danger to the sex-cells by 20% and even the watch with a luminous dial produces an appreciable amount of radiation. The explosion of H-bombs produces radioactive strontium which, by replacing the calcium in bone, can lead to serious disease. Radioactive iodine and caesium also produce harmful effects.

Atophan: trade name for cinchophen used in the treatment of gout.

Atropine: an alkaloid obtained from the Deadly Nightshade plant and purified from belladonna in the leaves and roots. It is a local anaesthetic acting on nerve endings, hence is used in belladonna plaster. Internally it paralyses certain groups of nerves (esp. the vagus) and therefore leads to dry mouth (for which reason it may be given before administering an anaesthetic) and dry skin; dilated pupils (therefore given as eye-drops to simplify examination of the back of the eye or retina); relaxation of the muscles of the bronchi and other tubes such as the intestines and stomach, the bile duct, and the ureters (hence its use in colic in the bile or kidney ducts, in stomach and duodenal ulcer and pyloric stenosis in infants or bronchial asthma); and increased rate of the heart. The drug is only to be given under medical supervision except in the case of belladonna plaster which, in spite of the faith many people still have in it, is almost completely useless and much better replaced by kaolin plaster.

Aureomycin: trade name of chlortetracycline hydrochloride, a broad range antibiotic obtained by B. M. Dugger of Lederle Laboratories from a mould discovered in a spoonful of earth from a grain-field in Missouri. It is active in many bacterial infections, in some virus infections, cholera, and conditions which do not respond to penicillin.

Auscultation: the method of examination used by doctors to discover by the sense of hearing the condition of certain internal organs. It was probably used in early Greek days by application of the ear to the body when abnormal sounds in the chest could be heard, but the method of *percussion* (i.e. thumping with the fingers on the body to hear whether the sounds are dull or resonant and therefore whether the underlying organ is solid – as the lung in pneumonia – or hollow) was invented in 1761 by Auenbrugger of Vienna. The use of the stethoscope was discovered by Laennec of Paris who first used a rolled up piece of paper and later a wooden cylinder, but nowadays the binaural stethoscope with two ear-pieces is generally used and electrical stethoscopes which greatly amplify the heart and lung sounds are also available. In this way damage to the valves of the heart or in the lungs can be discovered after the student has been trained to recognise them.

Autogenous: applied usually to vaccines prepared from germs found in the patient's own body (e.g. in boils or bronchitis) and used in treating the disease they have produced in the individual concerned.

Autoimmune Diseases: a comparatively-recently discovered factor in the causation of a number of fairly common diseases is the possibility that they may result from the individual developing antibodies to certain organs in his own body thus causing them to be treated as alien and to be dealt with in the same way as other foreign agents. Antibodies (*see* Infection) are part of the defence system of the body normally used to destroy invading germs and this, of course, is their only proper and useful function, but we now know that their action can be turned to dangerous ends. Thus (*see* Allergy) foreign proteins such as pollen or house dust can lead to the formation of antibodies which are not only ineffective but damage the cell walls resulting in the liberation of histamine and the development of allergic diseases such as asthma and hay fever. More serious is the case of the baby who is born with severe jaundice because the mother has developed antibodies against her own child (*see* Icterus Neonatorum Gravis). Certain diseases appear to occur in the same person more often than might be expected by chance. For instance, diseases of the thyroid gland such as toxic goitre seem to be associated with pernicious anaemia, Addison's disease, and myasthenia gravis. All are not uncommonly associated with chronic gastritis. Examination of the blood shows the presence of autoantibodies (i.e. antibodies produced by the body against itself) and gastric and thyroid autoantibodies often appear together. However, it must be made clear that this work is at an early stage and we may summarise what is so far known as follows: (1) people with thyrotoxicosis usually show areas of inflammation in the gland which are certainly due to the development of autoimmunity; (2) this does not prove that the toxic goitre is *caused* by autoimmunity although there is a strong suspicion that this may be so; (3) a group of diseases, apparently unrelated, is commonly associated and autoantibodies are found in the blood; the only illnesses absolutely known to be caused by autoimmunity are certain serious blood diseases, but it seems that the heart damage which is the real danger in rheumatic fever results from the body mistaking part of its own heart muscle for an invading germ. It appears likely that this mechanism will be found in the near future to be important in many other illnesses.

Autointoxication: self-poisoning brought about by areas of sepsis anywhere in the body. Thus arthritis is believed by some to be caused by sepsis in tooth sockets or in the sinuses. As a term for the alleged consequences of constipation the word is now outdated since nobody who is qualified to know believes that constipation leads to 'poisoning of the bloodstream' as the manufacturers of aperients and purgatives put it, nor, for the matter of that, is there much evidence that septic foci are a cause of disease generally (*see* Constipation, Rheumatism).

Autonomic Nervous System: the part of the nervous system which regulates those aspects of body function which are not under conscious control, e.g. the heart-beat, the movements

59

of the intestines, the size of the pupils, and the blood chemistry to some extent. It has two divisions: sympathetic and parasympathetic, whose actions are opposed to each other, the former preparing the body for emergency the latter for relaxation (*see* Nervous System).

Avitaminosis: the condition of being deprived of one or more vitamins.

Avomine: the trade-name for promezathine-8-chlorotheophyllinate used successfully in the prevention of travel sickness (q.v.).

Babinski Reflex: an abnormal response to the planter reflex in which, when the finger or some other pointed object is drawn across the sole of the foot, the toes ordinarily bend downwards. In the Babinski response the great toe turns upwards and the others spread out. Such a response is normal in the first two years of life but later indicates that something is wrong with the nervous system.

Bacilli: rod-shaped bacteria, e.g. the bacillus coli (*see* Bacteria, Infection).

Bacitracin: an antibiotic prepared from the organism known as bacillus subtilis and originally isolated from a culture taken from a leg-infection in a little girl of seven years old called Margaret Tracey when she was a patient at the Presbyterian Hospital, New York. The name 'bacitracin' is derived from the surname of the child. Bacitracin is usually applied locally in mixed wound infections, boils, carbuncles, etc., but can also be given internally under careful supervision (because of possible toxic reactions) in penicillin-resistant cases.

Backache: is a symptom of many conditions some of which are localised in the muscles or bones in the neighbourhood of the spinal column whilst others are due to disease of the internal organs which shows itself in this area. Amongst localised conditions are the pains produced by *lumbago* in the loins, those resulting anywhere in the back after *strain*, sudden twisting movements, or *exercise* involving muscles not ordinarily used; in older people pain and stiffness is often present in *osteoarthritis* of the spine and at any age disease of the bones or joints can cause pain of varying severity. On the other hand, pain in the loins usually associated with urinary symptoms is typical of *kidney disease* or *pyelitis* affecting the pelvis of the kidney or the ureters leading down to the bladder and it is a common sign of pelvic disease in women with *menstrual disorders*, displacement of the *womb*, or *ovarian disease* in which case there will usually be other symptoms and the pain is dragging-down in nature. In *gall-bladder disease* pain is typically felt under the right shoulder-blade and in *gastric ulcer* or *gastritis* pain may occur at the level of the last rib on the left side of the back. Lastly, aching in the back is a sign of some infections such as *influenza* and in *psychological conditions* associated with emotional stress which brings about spasm of the muscles (*see* under the separate disorders).

Bacteria: a general term for those micro-organisms smaller than the yeasts but larger than the viruses, some of which are disease-producing, other harmless, and many useful, e.g. the nitrogenous bacteria of the soil. They are classified (*a*) in terms of their reaction to Gram's stain as Gram-positive or negative, or (*b*) by their shape. Thus cocci are round, staphylococci like small bunches of grapes, streptococci form chains and diplococci pairs, bacilli are rod-shaped, and yet others are curved or wavy (spirilla), comma-shaped (vibrio), or corkscrew-shaped (spirochaete). (For further details *see* Infection).

Bacteriophage: an entity, which may be a virus or an enzyme, first described by d'Herelle in the early years of this century. It has the property of attacking colonies of bacteria, causing them to disintegrate and die and was used in the treatment of some bacterial diseases before the discovery of antibiotics.

Bagassosis: an acute or chronic lung disease similar to silicosis caused by the inhalation of dust from 'bagasse' which is broken sugar-cane after the extraction of sugar. Bagasse, used in the making of artificial boards, contains 6% silica.

B.A.L.: contraction of British Anti-Lewisite or dimercaprol discovered during the last war by Professor R. A. Peters of Oxford originally as an antidote to lewisite poisoning. Subsequently it was found to be a useful treatment for poisoning with some of the heavy metals such as lead, arsenic, antimony, and gold or mercury.

Balanitis: inflammation of the parts beneath the foreskin.

Baldness: a very common condition occuring mainly in men and much less frequently in women in one or other of three conditions: (1) during acute fevers, myxodema (q.v.), syphilis and tuberculosis when, with the exception of myxodema, the loss is usually slight and recovers when the disease is cured; (2) in nervous illness such as following an emotional shock where the baldness may be partial or total but nearly always recovers with or without treatment, although the new hair is often of a lighter colour or even white; (3) hereditary baldness which is by far the commonest type. There is no treatment for baldness for, with the exception of hereditary forms, the hair grows back by itself, and it may safely be assumed that any hair-restorer that works has been used in cases of alopecia areata which, being of the second type, recovers in any case spontaneously. Hereditary baldness is inevitable although it is possible that in the future when more is discovered about controlling hormones it may be prevented or at least delayed. Probably it is related to the male hormone in the blood-stream and this, at least in part, is why baldness is relatively rare in women. Hair 'foods,' like nerve-foods, do not exist, but the hair should be shampooed at least once a week (preferably with a non-soapy shampoo) or when excessively greasy two or three times a week.

Banti's Disease: (*see* Splenic Anaemia).

Barber's Itch: (*see* Sycosis).

Barbiturates: a group of drugs, derived from barbituric acid or malonylurea, which are used for their sedative or sleep-inducing (hypnotic) properties. They are divided into groups according to their period of action, the long-lasting ones being phenobarbitone (Gardenal or Luminal), barbitone (Veronal), and barbitone sodium (Medinal); medium-acting are allo-barbitone (Dial), butobarbitone (Soneryl), amylo-barbitone (Amytal), and pentobarbitone (Nembutal); short-action barbiturates are cyclobarbitone (Phanodorm), quinal-barbitone (Seconal) and hexobarbitone (Cyclonal or Evipan). The first group acts from 12–24 hours, the second 6–10, and the third 3–6. Barbiturates are dangerous drugs which are only obtainable on a doctor's prescription. They should always be kept locked up and, when taken at night, the exact dose should be taken and the rest put out of reach since poisoning has occurred in cases where the individual has forgotten during the night how many he has taken and in a semicomatose condition swallowed more. Nikethamide, beme-gride, and picrotoxin are specific antidotes to barbiturate poisoning, but in these days unless the doctor advises otherwise there exist much safer and equally potent sedatives for general use. In some tablets barbiturates are combined with an emetic to combat the effects of overdosage.

Barium Meal: a dose of barium sulphate in water used to outline the stomach and intestines or sinuses in X-ray work since these parts would not be visible in an ordinary X-ray and are made opaque by barium.

Basedow's Disease: the continental name for Grave's disease or exophthalmic goitre (*see* Goitre).

Basilicon Ointment: an old-fashioned but innocuous ointment made of resin, lard, wax, and almond oil.

B.C.G. Vaccine: the Bacillus Calmette-Guérin vaccine introduced by these two men in France about 1908 which is used for immunising against tuberculosis infection. It is used either in the case of infants or children who are exposed to special risks of infection (as when the mother or another relation has T.B.) or in young adults such as nurses who have been shown by tests to have no natural immunity and are proposing to work with tuberculous patients.

Beat Elbow, Hand or Knee: a term applied by miners to swelling and inflammation of the joints concerned usually arising from constant pressure and ingrained particles of dirt whilst at work. It is found also in other occupations and usually subsides with treatment by poultices although it sometimes goes on to suppuration with the formation of pus.

Bed Bugs: a wingless blood-sucking insect known scientifically as *cimex lectularius* which hides by day in cracks in walls or floors or in grooves in beds. The eggs hatch out into larvae in 6–10 days which become adult in about six weeks and cause small itching sores on the human body. Bed-bugs are best dealt with by a D.D.T. spray.

Bed Sores: are areas of inflamed skin which may break down and ulcerate, usually arising upon the pressure-points in patients confined to bed over long periods with chronic illness, especially in those who are old, thin, debilitated, or suffering from diseases or damage to the nervous system. The sores are commonest on the shoulders, elbows, heels, buttocks, ankles, and other parts which press upon the bed and are at first blue, subsequently becoming ulcerated with the formation of a black slough which coming off leaves an open sore likely to extend in area. The most important measure is prevention and the skin of these parts should be washed daily, dried carefully, then rubbed with spirit and finally dusted with zinc oxide or boric acid powder. When an area becomes red or bluish it should be padded with cotton-wool and an airring or air bed used; ulcers should be treated by the doctor who may recommend cetrimide (Cetavlon) as liquid or as a water-soluble cream, sulphonamide powder or sulphonamide and penicillin. More recently barrier creams and sprays containing silicones have been used twice daily to prevent bedsores, e.g. 'Rikospray Silicone' which is in aerosol form.

Belladonna: (*see* Atropine).

Bell's Palsy or Paralysis: paralysis of the facial nerve which enters the face immediately below the ear and supplies the muscles connected with facial expression. There may be no apparent cause for the paralysis or it may be due to draughts as in driving a car with the window open in cold weather, to an injury in front of the ear, a fractured base of the skull, or as part of the paralysis in a cerebral haemorrhage. Its presence is made obvious by the patient's inability to shut the eye on the affected side, to smile, or blow out his cheeks. It is doubtful whether treatment makes any difference to a condition which usually clears up by itself when due to the first two causes. Obviously, if the nerve is divided by injury or affected by a stroke or fracture healing is likely to be slow or may not occur at all.

Bemegride: or its proprietary form Megimide is a drug used in the treatment of barbiturate poisoning (*see* Barbiturates).

Benadryl: is an anti-histamine drug otherwise known as diphenhydramine used in the treatment of allergic conditions. In the form of Benylin it is combined with other drugs for use as a cough linctus (*see* Antihistamines).

Benzedrene: (*see* Amphetamine).

Benzocaine: a cocaine substitute used as 2% in olive oil in nasal disease or hay fever and in 10% ointment form for haemorrhoids and other conditions of the skin associated with itching.

Benzyl Benzoate: is used as a lotion in the treatment of scabies.

Berger Rhythm: the normal rhythmical changes in electrical potential passing as waves over the brain in electroencephalograms. Also known as alpha waves they merely indicate that the brain cells are undisturbed and discharging simultaneously; for they appear only in the absence of mental activity when the eyes are shut and disappear when the eyes are fixed on some object or when a difficult mental problem is being considered. Abnormal waves are found in pathological conditions of the brain. (*See* Electro-encephalography).

Beri-beri: a vitamin difficiency disease at one time prevalent in the East but never very common in European countries. There are two main types, the wet in which the heart-muscle becomes flabby and the patient weak and oedematous (i.e. with swelling of the legs and abdomen due to excess fluid leakage into the tissues) and the dry, in which the main damage is to the nerves in the limbs so that the patient is unable to walk properly. It is caused by lack of vitamin B1 or aneurine and is only likely to occur in those who live exclusively on diets of polished rice from which the vitamin-containing embryo has been removed, or in infants fed on tinned foods where heating has destroyed the aneurine. Alcoholics suffer from neuritis of this type due to the gastritis produced by strong spirits interfering with the absorption of the vitamin but beer drinkers are not affected since beer is rich in it. British prisoners of the Japanese during the last war suffered from Beri-beri and the treatment is to supply the missing substance in large amounts by injection or oral concentrates.

Bicarbonate of Soda: baking soda (*see* Alkali).

Bile: a thick, bitter-tasting, golden-brown greenish-yellow fluid secreted by the liver and stored in the gall-bladder. It contains mucus, water, bile pigments which are brown (bilirubin) and green (biliverdin), bile salts (of glycocholic and taurocholic acids) and is discharged into the intestine through the bile duct a few inches below the stomach. Bile is particularly an excretion from the liver resulting from the destruction of red blood cells when they have become old and partly a secretion which aids the process of digestion especially of fats and destroys some of the germs in the bowels. In jaundice (q.v.) either the bile ducts are blocked or there is too great a destruction of blood cells as in the hereditary disease of alcho|uric jaundice and when this happens, the bile circulates in the bloodstream giving rise to the yellow or brown coloration of the skin. Normally from 1–2 pints of bile are excreted daily, but most of this goes back into circulation and only a small amount is expelled in the faeces. 'Biliousness' or 'liverish' troubles are largely imaginary diseases popular in those who have been in the East and amongst men and women on the Continent; they are polite names for gastritis brought on by dietary indiscretions or drinking too much and have no particular connection with the liver or bile. The vomiting of bile is another condition usually considered to have sinister significance, but any attacks of repeated vomiting may show discoloration of the vomit with bile whether the cause be trivial or serious.

Bilharzia: a tropical disease found in Egypt, Africa, Arabia, and Iraq which in areas where it is endemic may affect 90–100% of the inhabitants. The parasite's life-history begins when a man bathes in or drinks infected water when the small swimming forms enter the body by penetrating the skin from which they pass to the portal vein below the liver where they pair and remain for six weeks until, as adults, they swim against the blood-stream to the pelvis where the female lays eggs which have a sharp spine that penetrates into the bladder in the case of schistosomum haematobium or into the rectum when the parasite is s. mansoni and pass out in the urine or faeces depending on the type. If they enter water they hatch out into small moving larvae which seek out a water-snail within which they develop into cercariae ready to find a new human victim. The female is slender, round, and about 1 in. in length, the male about ¾ in. in length, flat and leaf-shaped and their courting takes place, as we have seen, in the portal vein.

Infection results in fever and in the urinary type there is blood in the urine, in the intestinal type blood in the faeces and diarrhoea. In both cases treatment is by injections of antimony tartrate which have proved very successful. Needless to say, bathing in or drinking of infected water should be prohibited and the water supply should be cut off from time to time in order to kill the snails. Without treatment the disease may go on for years when it may recover of itself or lead to slow death. A third type of schistosomiasis (s. japonicum) is found in the Far East and is similar to the intestinal type already described. Bilharzia is one of the greatest plagues of the world.

Binet-Simon Test: the earliest form of intelligence test devised in 1904 by the Frenchman Alfred Binet in collaboration with Théophile Simon. Items such as 'point to nose, eyes, and mouth' (for age 3) to 'repeat months of the year' (one of the questions at age 10) were standardised for children of various age-groups according to the average performance of the group in the population as a whole. When a child of 7 passed all the tests for age 7 his mental age was said to be 7 and his Intelligence Quotient (mental age divided by chronological age × 100) was said to be 100; if his real age was 8 years 6 months and he could only pass a test for 88 months his I.Q. would be 88/102 or 86. In the form revised by Terman this test is still in use for the younger age-groups. An I.Q. of at least 120 is necessary before an individual would have much chance of passing into a university.

Biotin: one of the dozen or so vitamins of the vitamin B complex; deficiencies lead to skin diseases and a smooth tongue.

Birth: the average child weighs 7 lb. at birth. A *still-born* child is 'any child which has issued from its mother after the twenty-eighth week of pregnancy and which did not at any time after being completely expelled from its mother breath or show any other signs of life.' *Premature birth* is one which takes place before the natural time but in which the child is capable of surviving. A birth which takes place so prematurely that the child must necessarily die is known as an abortion or miscarriage (*see* Miscarriage, Labour).

Birth-marks: are of various kinds the most common being the 'port-wine' type (*see* Naevus). Pigment spots are often raised above the surface of the skin and may be more or less hairy (*see* Moles).

Bismuth: a metal used either as such or as a salt in medicine. As a powder for dusting on wounds, sores, and moist conditions of the skin bismuth subnitrate has been used as a mild antiseptic and astringent either alone or with zinc oxide and starch. Internally, bismuth subnitrate and carbonate is used for gastric or duodenal ulcers or for diarrhoea – it must be remembered that such preparations turn the motions black, hence they may mask bleeding from the bowel which has the same effect. In X-ray work for making the intestines opaque to the rays bismuth has now been replaced by barium (q.v.). Bismuth metal in a state of fine subdivision is used with

67

arsenic or penicillin in the treatment of chronic syphilis. Compounds of bismuth with arsenic are Bismarsen and Bistovol used for the same purpose.

Bites, Stings, and Poisoned Wounds: in general people treat *dog-bites* with a great deal more care than is justified especially when they occur in this country. Ordinarily they need only be treated with an antiseptic as any other wound of comparable degree unless the risk of rabies or hydrophobia exists when more active measures require to be taken (*see* Rabies). *Snake bites*, too, are ordinarily insignificant in Europe where only two or three deaths occur every year in contrast with the world total of about 25,000–30,000 yearly of which at least 20,000 occur in India. In Asia the poisonous snakes include the cobra, king-cobra, krait, and others; in America, the rattlesnake, copperhead, and moccasin; in South America, the fer-de-lance and the coral snake; and in Australia, the death-adder, tiger snake, copperhead, brown snake, and black snake. The sea snakes of the Indian and Pacific oceans are almost all poisonous. But in Britain the only poisonous snake is the adder or viper which rarely does any great harm to human beings by its bite. Symptoms of severe snake-bite are swelling and paralysis of the bitten part, with general depression, palpitation, difficulty in breathing, followed by collapse, total paralysis, and convulsions ending sometimes in death. Treatment consists in sucking the wound after applying a tourniquet in the area between the bite and the heart and the injection, if available of antivenine (q.v.) which is given both intravenously and in the skin about the bitten area. The general treatment is for shock (q.v.). *Poisonous fishes* are limited to the Indian and Pacific oceans (although of course any wound from a fish's spines may turn septic), the poisons may cause heart-failure in a few cases. *Tropical centipedes, scorpions, and tarantulas* may cause painful, put rarely fatal bites and anti-scorpion serum is available. Bites from *fleas, lice, and mosquitoes* are irritating but in this country extremely unlikely to spread any diseases. Lice may be got rid of by a D.D.T. spray and, if on the hair, a 2% emulsion of D.D.T. will remove them. Stings from *bees* or *wasps* are painful but may be alleviated by the use of a mild alkali such as baking soda or weak ammonia in the former and a weak acid such as vinegar or lemon juice in the latter; better than either for both types (or indeed any type) of sting is anti-histamine cream. If the sting remains in the wound it should first be removed.

Blackheads: (*see* Acne).

Black Motions: the most important cause of black motions is bleeding from the intestinal tract either in the stomach or bowels. Both bismuth (contained in some proprietary medicines for the stomach) and iron taken for anaemia cause black motions but in the absence of these causes the opinion of a doctor should always be sought whether other symptoms be present or not. Medically, black motions are known as Melaena.

Blackwater Fever: a condition associated with malaria of the malignant tertian type and brought on by the administration of quinine, the name is derived from the colour of the urine which is dark red or almost black owing to the presence of haemoglobin resulting from the breakdown of the red blood cells within the blood-vessels. The onset is sudden with headache, vomiting, severe backache, and prostration, the patient is restless and anxious with difficulty in breathing. Both liver and spleen are enlarged and tender and jaundice appears a few hours after the illness has begun. The urine may actually be suppressed with the results that uraemia and death occurs from the retention of substances which should normally be excreted. Mild cases recover in a day or so, but in more severe cases there may be a succession of attacks leaving the patient in a weak state from extreme anaemia and weakness of the heart. Treatment consists in absolute rest with intravenous transfusions of glucose, saline, and plasma. Antimalarial drugs may have to be given, but quinine and pamaquin should be avoided.

Bladder: *Gall-bladder* (*see* Liver, Gall-bladder Diseases). *Urinary Bladder* lies in the pelvis in front of the rectum and can hold, when fully distended, about a pint of urine. The two ureters passing down from the kidneys enter the bladder (which is roughly pear-shaped with the narrow part pointing downwards and backwards) at the rear of the base and from the same area the urethra leaves it to pass to the exterior. The inside of the bladder is lined with flat irregularly-shaped epithelial cells over a fibrous layer in which there lie many blood-vessels and above this is a coat of muscle fibres running in all directions which make it able to contract and increases its strength. Covering all in the upper but not the lower part is a coat of the general peritoneal lining of the abdomen. The condition of the bladder, when necessary, is investigated by a number of techniques. Thus the urine (q.v.) may be tested for abnormal chemical substances such as sugar or albumen or for germs, blood-cells, or pus under the microscope; the specimen may either be passed in the ordinary way or (especially in the case of women) drawn off by a *catheter* which is a thin rubber, metal, or guttapercha tube sterilised, of course, beforehand. Catheterisation is done for the medical examination of a specimen uncontaminated from outside sources, for washing out of the bladder, or in cases where the urine cannot be expelled voluntarily. The inside of the bladder may be investigated by a *cystoscope* which is a long thin metal tube arranged as a telescope with a tiny electric bulb at the end through which the inside of the bladder can be clearly seen and tumours, ulcers, and blood coming from the bladder wall or the ureters observed.

Cystitis: is known in mild cases as a 'chill' or 'cold' in the bladder and its symptoms are pain of a dull, aching kind over the region of the lower abdomen or in the small of the back, usually fever, and the desire to pass frequent small quantities of urine which may have an unpleasant smell. It results in those who are generally run-down so that germs which ordinarily live in the urine or pass through from the bowel but do not multiply in the normal state create an infection. The usual type is bacillus coli normally present in the bowels, and in this case the reaction of the urine is acid. Bilharzia and tuberculosis of the bladder wall are rarer causes, the former occurring only in those who have contracted the condition in the Middle or Far East. Similarly, anything which irritates the lining of the bladder or slows down the flow of urine can lead to cystitis, hence prolapse of the womb in women and enlargement of the prostrate gland (at the base of the bladder surrounding the urethra) in elderly men may cause cystitis or a stone in the bladder and disease of the nearby rectum lead to the same result. But the first is much the commonest cause and in this case the giving of potassium citrate with mandelic acid, sulphonamides, or antibiotics will rapidly clear it up. In other cases the primary underlying cause will have to be dealt with first, although these drugs will give relief in the meantime. A *stone or calculus in the bladder* may be of any size from tiny crystals that sometimes arise after eating rhubarb or strawberries which contain oxalates, to stones the size of a hen's egg or even larger. The former may cause brief irritation but need no further treatment, the latter composed of urates in those subject to gout or phosphates in those with chronic infections of the bladder may have to be treated by litholapaxy (i.e. crushing the stone with a lithotrite, an instrument passed up the urethra) or lithotomy (i.e. surgical operation through an opening in the abdomen or perineum). It is impossible to remove a stone by any other means although there is a popular belief that they can be dissolved by something taken by mouth. No such drug exists. *Tumours*, both malignant and benign, are found in the bladder and are often discovered for the first time by the passage of large amounts of bright red blood; the usual cause is a papilloma which resembles a varicose vein and can be dealt with by cauterisation through the cystoscope. Occasionally the badder is ruptured either by a crushing injury or spontaneously in old men with a history of bladder or prostate trouble. Naturally this requires surgical treatment.

Blaud's Pills: pills used in the treatment of anaemia containing iron carbonate (*see* Anaemia).

Blepharitis: inflammation of the eyelids due to infection is extremely common, especially in children, the commonest form being a stye (hordeolum) usually caused by staphylococci, the organisms commonly responsible for boils. Another type resembles dandruff with loose scales and in this case ulceration may occur. Styes require hot bathing frequently carried out and sometimes need to be opened or the hair whose follicle is infected pulled out to let the pus escape. In both types of blepharitis an ointment containing sulpha drugs can be applied; penicillin is also in use but can give rise in sensitised people to severe reactions. Drops or creams containing cortisone in combination with an antibiotic are very soothing, as cortisone reduces the inflammation.

Blindness: may be caused by injury either to the eyes or to the back of the brain (occipital region) where messages of sight are received and the tracts and nerves connecting them. The injury may be physical as in a war wound or brought

71

about by a tumour or haemorrhage within the brain. Other causes are senile degeneration of the macula (the most sensitive part of the retina at the back of the eye), cataract, glaucoma, and general diseases such as diabetes and syphilis from birth which accounts for less than 1% of all cases. A 'blind person' is defined by the National Assistance Act of 1948 as one 'so blind as to be unable to perform any work for which eyesight is essential.' In the case of children the term includes not only the totally blind but those who cannot be taught by visual methods, even by the use of large print, blackboard writing, or lenses for magnifying ordinary print. At the end of 1956 the number of registered blind people in England and Wales was 96,019. Of these 3·6% were totally blind, 11·1% were able to perceive light only, and 57·3% could perceive hand movements (*see* Cataract, Corneal graft, Glaucoma).

Blisters and Counter-Irritants: counter-irritants, as the name implies, are used in order (*a*) to distract attention from an already existing pain by the production of irritation in the area, and (*b*) to increase the flow of blood, thus improving the local circulation. In former days a *cautery* like a small branding-iron was employed and *vesicants* were used to produce actual blistering of the skin or even the formation of pus by the use of *pustulants*, but none of these are employed now, although *rubifacients* which make the skin red may produce blisters on a sensitive skin. The usual use for counter-irritants is in rheumatic pains for which they are still popular, and in strains or muscle injuries, but they are still employed by a few for application to the chest in bronchitis and pneumonia or pleurisy, in sciatica and lumbago, etc. It is doubtful whether counter-irritants are of much use in chest complaints and they have the disadvantage of being messy. However those who gain relief from plasters, rubs, and medicated wool will certainly come to no harm by applying them. Most rubifacients are varying mixtures of such irritants as mustard, turpentine, cajuput oil, capsicum, tincture of iodine, and so on which are applied either in the form of liniments such as methyl salicylate, camphorated oil, or terebinth, or ointments such as capsicum or eucalyptus. Most people use proprietary preparations for rubbing into the skin such as Algipan, Capsolin, Cremalgin, Finalgon, Iodised Oil with Methyl Salicylate, Rubriment, or Transvasin. Adrenaline cream and aconite ointment are not rubifacients; the former, which may or may not be of any use, is alleged to relax muscular spasm, the latter which numbs the nerve endings is dangerous.

Blood: the blood-stream is the canal system of the body which carries substances essential to life from one part to the other and takes to the refuse disposal units its waste-products. Thus it carries, partly in the red blood cells and partly in solution in the liquid part of the blood, the oxygen breathed into the lungs and returns to the lungs to be breathed out the waste gas known as carbon dioxide which results from the combustion of food in the cells. From the intestines it carries the digested foods through a large system of veins (the portal system) to the liver where they are changed to make them suitable for absorption. Blood also carries those defence materials which help to destroy infection in any part of the body: the antitoxins and antibodies and the white cells which destroy the bacteria when they have been dealt with by antibodies. And, just as it transports food materials around the body, so it carries away waste in liquid form to be disposed of by the kidneys. Blood consists of a liquid part known as plasma and floating about in it the red cells or erythrocytes and the white cells known variously as leucocytes, lymphocytes, and eosinophils each of which is subdivided into sub-types. In one cubic millimetre (i.e. an area about the size of a pin-head) there should normally be about 5 million red cells and 5 thousand white cells. From examination of the blood the physician can tell a great deal about the patient's health, e.g. too few red cells means anaemia, too many, polycythaemia, and if the red cells are not only reduced in number but large in size and of primitive type the condition may be pernicious anaemia. In acute septic conditions the leucocyte count may be increased to 30,000 or more, and in some chronic diseases or in whooping cough or glandular fever the number of lymphocytes may be increased. Eosinophils are increased in many allergic conditions. Doctors also consider such factors as the number of platelets (which are very tiny cells connected with clotting), the fragility of the red cells, and the sedimentation rate which is the length of time it takes for red cells to sink to the bottom of a tube. The coagulation time is also important.

The main blood centres are in the liver, spleen and bone-marrow; the former destroys poisons circulating in the blood and makes prothrombin which is necessary to clotting, it also stores blood as does the spleen which manufactures both red and white cells before birth but hands the task over to the bone-marrow where all the red cells and most of the white ones are made thereafter. However, all through life the spleen creates certain types of white cells and has the further function of destroying the old red and white cells and storing their iron to make new ones. It also kills bacteria which have not been dealt with in other ways but the body, although it can well manage without the spleen, cannot live without the liver or the bone-marrow.

Blood groups: all human beings of whatever race, belong, in respect of their blood, to one of four groups which depend upon the capacity of the serum of one person's blood to agglutinate the blood cells of another's. The reaction depends on antigens known as agglutinogens in the red cells and others known as agglutinins in the serum. There are two of each, the agglutinogens being known as A and B and it follows that anyone's blood cells may have (1) no agglutinogens, (2) agglutinogen A, (3) agglutinogen B, and (4) agglutinogens A and B. These are the four groups and the practical consequence is that, in a blood-transfusion, the person giving and the person receiving the blood should belong to the same group.

Blood, Diseases of: simple *anaemia* of the secondary type and *pernicious anaemia* are dealt with elsewhere as are also the *leukaemias, Hodgkin's disease,* the *purpuras,* and *haemophilia.*

Blood-poisoning: or septicaemia is a serious condition divided into septicaemia proper in which the bacterial toxins are circulating in the blood-stream, and pyaemia in which bacteria are circulating and cause thereby abcesses in various parts of the body where they settle down. The cause may be an infected wound or sore in which the body defences have broken down and are unable to limit the spread of the infection; this is especially the case in infection of the womb after childbirth. Such bodily conditions as diabetes and alcoholism may predispose to septicaemia when infection is present. There is a very high temperature with profuse sweating and shivering attacks (rigors), pains in the joints and muscles, and in pyaemia signs of localised abscesses may also be present. Death used to be inevitable until the discovery of the sulpha drugs and antibiotics.

Blood-Pressure: the blood-pressure is highest (systolic pressure) at each heart-beat and goes down to a minimum (diastolic pressure) as the heart relaxes. In young adults the blood-pressure is usually about 120/80 and it tends to increase, although this is by no means always the case, with age. In certain diseases, e.g. nephritis, in disorders of the ductless glands, or in the condition known as essential hypertension the pressure is raised and it is lowered in some cases of anaemia or Addison's disease. Blood-pressure is something everybody 'has' and it is not correct to use the word for high blood-pressure or hypertension (q.v.) as is frequently done.

Blood-spitting: or haemoptysis is a symptom of a great many diseases or none at all, but first it is necessary to know whether the blood was vomited or coughed up. Vomited blood from the stomach is usually brown in colour and has a 'coffee-grounds' appearance, unless it comes from the oesophagus as in oesophageal varices where there is usually a history of chronic alcoholism. Blood from the lungs is usually bright red and frothy and may be caused by pulmonary tuberculosis, mitral stenosis (a disease of the mitral valve of the heart), an infarct of the lungs (i.e. an area which has been shut off by a blood-clot in a small artery), pneumonia, chronic bronchitis or bronchiectasis, a tumour, various other lung infections such as actinomycosis or hydatid disease (tape-worm infection), pneumoconiosis, such blood disorders as purpura, leukaemia, pernicious anaemia, an aneurism, or vitamin deficiency as in scurvy. On the other hand blood coughed up may simply have come from the nose or back of the throat as in sinusitis and tonsillitis, nose-bleeding, or nose-picking, and it may also come from bleeding gums. In these cases it is likely to be non-frothy and dark red. Often the cause is trivial but a doctor should always be consulted even when the cause is believed to be known.

Boils: or furuncles are caused by three separate factors in each case: (1) the presence of germs (usually staphylococci) on the surface of the skin, (2) lowered bodily resistance to these particular germs, (3) the existence of pressure or rubbing causing the infecting organisms to be pushed through the skin or into a hair follicle. Hence boils usually occur in the nose or the shaving area of the face in men when dirty handkerchiefs and towels have rubbed them in, or where the clothes cause friction, e.g. the back of the neck, the arm-pit, the wrists, on the back under a belt, and in the groin or buttocks. Quite often there is a whole series of boils occurring one after the other or simultaneously and in this case it is usually advisable to have the urine tested for sugar as boils are common in diabetes. The short-term treatment is to apply a boil dressing which may be obtained ready-made from the chemist's or a kaolin poultice if the boil is a large one and the area permits. Boils on the face and particularly in the nose may be smeared with Cetavlex cream and *must on no account be squeezed or interfered with,* otherwise the infection may spread inside the skull with serious or even fatal consequences. The long-term treatment if many boils are present is to keep the skin clean by frequent washing with soap and water and hot baths with Dettol added according to the instructions on the bottle when the boils are on the trunk. In some cases a course of vaccine injections may be given which may be either a stock or an autogenous vaccine (q.v.), but in the vast majority of cases the sulpha drugs or antibiotics suffice.

Bones: the skeleton is made up of both bone and cartilage the latter being found where the ribs join the breast-bone and in the larynx, hyoid bone and windpipe. Bone is built up of varying amounts of fibrous tissue and mineral salts, mainly calcium phosphate and carbonate, and as a child's bones contain nearly two-thirds fibrous tissues whereas those of an old man or woman contain two-thirds of mineral it is easy to see that fractures will have different results in each case the former being supple, the latter brittle. The shafts of long bones are composed of dense bone in tubular form whilst their ends are composed of cancellous bone which is hard but spongy in texture and forms the other bones of the body as well. The thin outer covering of bones is known as periosteum and the inner cavity is filled with marrow which in the smaller ones is red and the site of origin of the red blood cells. All bones are pierced by tiny canals for the entry and exit of blood-vessels and nerves and the long ones grow from a plate of cartilage about half an inch from either end until growth ceases at the age of about 16–18. Bone is kept in repair by cells known as osteoblasts which lay down fibrous tissue between the strands of which the calcium salts are deposited and other cells known as osteoclasts break up dead or damaged bone. When a fracture has occurred and the ends are brought into contact a mass of blood surrounds them which is organised by these cells into fibrous tissue and then into bone which at first is a thickened mass known as 'callus' and can be felt as a slight bulge in the bone, but later this is smoothed out except in those cases where union has not been accurate. The main bones of the body come into the four categories of long bones, short bones like those of the wrist and ankle, irregular bones like those of the face or vertebrae, and flat bones like those of the skull.

Bone, Diseases of: all three parts of a bone may be infected: the outer membrane in *periostitis*, the bone itself as in *osteitis*, and the marrow and bone together in the only important one of these three conditions known as *osteomyelitis*. Osteomyelitis is primarily a disease of children although it may become chronic and last for many years. It arises (1) where there has been a direct injury even if a quite trifling one, (2) where the infection has been carried from elsewhere in the body as in tonsillitis, a boil, or some of the fevers especially scarlet fever and typhoid. Any bone may be affected, e.g. the lower jaw in early life, but the femur (or thigh-bone) and the tibia (the inner and thicker of the two bones of the leg) are most commonly involved. Typically the origin is sudden with high fever and great pain over the site where the abscess is under tension within the bone; the patient is prostrated and cannot bear to have the limb moved. X-rays and blood-counts may have to be taken to distinguish the disease from similar-appearing ones such as rheumatism and cellulitis (q.v.), the painful stage of poliomyelitis, and the bleeding under the periosteum sometimes found in scurvy. Occasionally pain is mild or absent and it is then necessary to distinguish osteomyelitis from fever due to other causes. The sulpha drugs and antibiotics are used in treatment and, if these do not work, a surgical operation may be necessary or may in any case be necessary in later stages to remove portions of dead bone known as sequestra. Staphylococci are the usual cause of the infection, and before penicillin it was common to have a discharging sinus from the bone communicating with the skin which might continue for years. This, however, is now much less common. *Abscesses* in bone are usually tuberculous in origin and are likely to be in the bones of the leg, commonly on one or other side of the knee. There is a painful swelling, the pain being worse at night;

abscess is most frequent in boys of 14–15 and the treatment is surgical. *Exostosis* is an outgrowth of bone sometimes produced by constant irritation as in the inner side of the knee of those who ride a good deal, but it may occur in other conditions such as syphilis which tends when untreated to produce swellings of bone. In *tuberculosis* which also occurs mainly in young people the disease occurs (*a*) in the small bones of the hand or foot, (b) in the long bones, especially at the ends where it is liable to spread to a joint, (c) in the vertebrae where it may lead to curvature of the spine or a chronic abscess. There is a history of poor health, pain and swelling in the affected area, and later the skin may get red and pus forms which discharges through a sinus for many months or even years. The treatment depends on the state of the condition but consists of rest, drugs, and sometimes surgical intervention. The *tumours* of bone are chondroma, a small and harmless swelling of cartilage and bone which sometimes develops under a finger or toe-nail and is easily removed. Carcinoma (*see* cancer) never begins in bones but may spread there from elsewhere and sarcoma, if it occasionally occurs causing the bone to swell or even fracture spontaneously, is more often than not secondary to one in the adrenal glands or kidneys. *Osteitis* is a general term used of inflammatory conditions of bone and includes *osteitis deformans* in which the long bones become curved and the skull thickened in older people (40–60) presenting an appearance not unlike acromegaly (q.v.) and *osteitis fibrosa* (*see* Fibrocystic Disease) caused by overaction of the parathyroid glands in which the bones become thickened and softened. The cause of the former (also known as Paget's disease) is unknown although it seems to be inherited, the latter is cured by removing the swelling of the parathyroids which brings it about by removing calcium from the blood-stream. *Rickets* and *osteomalacia* are vitamin deficiency diseases resulting from lack of vitamin D, the former usually beginning in childhood and leading to bone deformities, such as pigeon-chest and bow legs, the latter in women who have had a number of children in quick succession thus depleting the system of calcium. Both are rare in Britain and Europe generally and are cured by the administration of the vitamin.

Boracic or Boric Acid: a mild antiseptic prepared from borax and used in dusting-powders, eye-lotions, or on lint as a fomentation. Borax (sodium biborate) has much the same effects but is mainly used in the treatment of thrush (q.v.) when it is dissolved in glycerine for use as a paint.

Bornholm Disease: named after the Danish island of Bornholm in the Baltic and also known as 'devil's grippe' is an acute infective disease in which there is fever, pain around the base of the ribs, and headache. It is due to a Coxsackie virus (q.v.) and occurs in epidemics during the summer months most commonly in younger people; lasting from a week to ten days it is never fatal.

Botulism: a rare type of food-poisoning caused by the toxin of the Clostridium botulinum found in faultily-tinned foods. The earliest symptoms which come on a few hours after the food has been taken are vomiting, abdominal colic, and blurring of vision. The later symptoms are mainly due to the action of the toxin on the nerves and include drooping of the eyelids, double vision, dilation of the pupils and weakness of the face muscles with dryness of the mouth. More than 50% of cases are fatal and, since the disease is essentially a poisoning brought about by bacterial toxins rather than a direct infection, antibiotics are useless and the main treatment is the giving of emetics and the antitoxin if available.

Brachial: connected with the arm, e.g. brachial artery and brachial plexus of nerves.

Brachycephalic: means short-headed and is a term applied by anthropologists to those races with skulls the breadth of which is at least four-fifths of the length, e.g. the so-called 'Alpine' race and the Bronze Age people of Britain. Long-headed races are known as dolichocephalic, i.e. those in whose skulls the breadth is less than four-fifths of the length such as the Neolithic peoples of Britain.

Brachydactyly: a term applied to conditions in which the fingers and toes are abnormally short as in achondroplasia (q.v.)

Bradycardia: a slow heart-beat (i.e. below 60 beats per minute) found normally in athletes, adolescents, and the aged. Bradycardia is found as a pathological symptom in convalescence, brain tumour, haemorrhage or abscess, uraemia and jaundice, and in meningitis.

Brain: (*see* Nervous System).

Bread: (*see* Diet)

Breasts: or mammary glands are typical of the most highly-developed group of animals who suckle their young and are therefore known as mammals. In the human female they begin to grow at puberty and there are usually two although additional breasts of a rudimentary type may develop anywhere in a diagonal line across the body from the armpit to the lower abdomen on the opposite side. If unsightly or embarrassing these can easily be removed. Each breast is divided into 12–20 compartments containing systems of branching tubes lined by cells that form the material composing the milk and in each compartment the tubes join together to form a single duct which opens on the surface of the nipple. There are therefore 12–20 openings and the intervening tissue between the tubes is filled with muscle fibres, fibrous strands, and fat. The efficiency of the breasts in supplying milk has nothing to do with their size, small breasts being often more productive than large ones, nor, indeed, do 'vital statistics' convey much information, depending as they do to some extent on the breadth of the back. As the breast is primarily responsive to the oestrogenic hormones of the ovary, it may vary in size or firmness with the fluctuation of hormones in the blood during the menstrual cycle and, of course, enlargement of the breast is often one of the early signs of pregnancy. Newly-born babies sometimes produce a milk-like substance from their breasts resulting from the hormones absorbed from the mother and in former times this was known as 'witches' milk.' But if the oestrogens are the main stimulus it is nevertheless the case that the cooperative effort of the whole endocrine system (q.v.) is necessary for normal growth and function so that breasts which are underdeveloped do not always respond to the administration of oestrogens (it must be remembered that the *feeling* that the breasts are too small may often obsess a woman much beyond any real need for worry and correspond very little with the true state of affairs). In some circumstances men may develop gynaecomastia or enlargement of the glands which is sometimes one-sided due to local sensitivity to hormones since oestrogens are normally present in the male as well as in the female; it is rarely caused by any deficiency of testicular development and most commonly arises in those who are being given oestrogens for medical reasons (as in enlargement of the prostate, acne, etc.) or in those who work with them. Cirrhosis of the liver or malnutrition in prisoners of war may lead to gynaecomastia which also occurs in acromegaly and other glandular disorders.

Breast, Diseases of: *acute inflammation and abscess* is most common during the suckling of a child, especially during the first two months, but slight painful swelling which does not go on to abscess formation may occur in both boys and girls at puberty. Infection usually enters through the ducts of the nipple and leads to pain, increased hardness and fullness of the breast, followed by redness of the skin in the affected area (usually the lower part) which may later burst. In the early stages kaolin poultices, regular emptying of the breast by the baby or a breast-pump, and the giving of sulpha drugs or penicillin will bring the process to a stop, but if an abscess does form the only treatment in the later stages is to open it under an anaesthetic. It may subsequently become necessary to stop the flow of milk by the giving of oestrogens such as stilboestrol. *Chronic mastitis* may take the form of a persistent abscess but most usually the term is applied to one or more lumpy areas in the breast which tend to develop in women who have had children and after the age of 30. Mastitis is not caused by infection but by some glandular disturbance of the ovaries or the pituitary gland at the base of the brain. Pain may be present which is worse before or during the first days of the menstrual period. Treatment is a matter for the doctor although mastitis, if painful, is not serious, but it cannot be too often repeated that *all lumps in the breast must be seen at once by a doctor* since they may be due to cancer which can be cured if treated immediately. Other swellings may be caused by abscesses, cysts, or adenoma which is a simple non-malignant growth and it is foolish to worry unnecessarily about something which expert examination may show not to have been cancer but even more so to delay seeking advice for what may be malignant. *Cracked nipples* are caused by lack of attention to hygiene or large strongly-sucking babies, sometimes to no discoverable reason at all. They are extremely painful and should be treated by stopping feeding for 1-2 days, squeezing out the milk by hand, and the use of stilboestrol ointment or whatever application may be advised.

Breath, Bad: or halitosis is common in many people at all times and in all people some of the time, and if it is often the case that the sufferer is unaware of the discomfort he (or she) causes to others it is equally often possible to find those who worry unnecessarily about more or less imaginary halitosis which upsets nobody. The common causes of halitosis are any condition of the nose, mouth, respiratory tract, or stomach which are associated with chronic infection or local upsets of one sort or another, e.g. bad teeth in which decaying food may lodge, infections of the gums (as in Vincent's angina or chronic pyorrhoea), chronic tonsillitis, lung diseases such as chronic bronchitis and bronchiectasis (in the latter the breath may be exceedingly foul), chronic gastritis, and diseases of the nose or sinuses which cause a discharge at the back of the throat. Constipation, except insofar as it is associated with chronic gastritis, is not in itself a cause of halitosis whatever the patent medicine advertisements may say. The treatment depends upon the cause, but in the absence of any symptoms relating to the chest or stomach the first thing to do is to see a dentist who will treat the tooth or gum infection which is the most usual cause of the trouble; if nothing abnormal is found, the tonsils and nose and throat generally may need attention. The bad breath of a hangover is caused by gastritis from strong spirits taken the night before but there are very few people who do not have bad breath in the morning which is simply the result of the relatively reduced amount of saliva produced during the night, saliva being nature's mouth-wash. Assuming that no disease is found to account for the condition, antiseptic toothpastes or mouth-washes may be used and it seems probable that chlorophyll tablets reduce the odour in local conditions although it is most unlikely that they have any effect on general ones. In some instances those who are unduly concerned about halitosis are suffering basically from a sense of inferiority and guilt which causes them to haunt the doctor's surgery in the conviction that their breath or urine and other bodily excretions smell foul and being unduly sensitive refuse to be convinced to the contrary.

Breathlessness: is caused by any condition which brings about a deficiency of oxygen in the blood and therefore may result from (a) interference in the air-passages and lungs, (b) disease of the heart which prevents efficient circulation of the blood carrying the oxygen, (c) diseases of the blood in which its oxygen-carrying capacity is reduced. Hence diphtheria, laryngismus, asthma, pneumonia, lung infections generally, emphysema, bronchitis (which leads sooner or later to emphysema), pressure from fluid or tumours in the chest cavity, pleurisy (which reduces respiratory effort because of the pain it produces), all either reduce the intake of air or reduce the lung surface available for its absorption. Most heart diseases produce breathlessness on exertion and, in serious cases, even without exertion and in anaemia of any sort the lack of red cells reduces the amount of oxygen brought to the tissues. Two other causes of breathlessness are obesity in which there is too much flesh to be adequately supplied with oxygen and the body has too much work to do to transport itself around, and fevers in which case the respirations are increased because of the extra demand made on the tissues for oxygen. Adenoids interfere with breathing, but this is usually made good by the substitution of mouth-breathing for breathing through the nose. (Individual causes of breathlessness mentioned here can be referred to in the appropriate entries).

Bright's Disease: (*see* Nephritis).

Bromides: are salts of bromine used as sedatives, the commonest being sodium, ammonium, and potassium bromide. There is really very little place for bromides in modern medicine although, when introduced well over a century ago, they were a decided advance in the production of a sedative which was effective, fairly safe, and less habit-forming than opium. But today other equally safe and potent sedatives are available which lack their objectionable features. These are: rashes which frequently develop in those who are sensitive, and a dulling of mental capacity which occurs in cases which necessitate the taking of bromides over a long period of time, e.g. epilepsy. However, in the form of a mixture of bromide and strychnine, they are still occasionally prescribed for nervous people as a 'tonic.' The mental dullness and confusion resulting from the prolonged use of bromides is known as 'bromism.'

Bromidrosis: is the secretion of bad-smelling sweat (*see* Perspiration).

Bronchial Tubes: (*see* Lungs, the Respiratory System).

Bronchiectasis: is a dilation of the bronchi or breathing-tubes which may be secondary to the inhalation of a foreign body, lung infections such as pneumonia, bronchopneumonia, and chronic bronchitis, or the pressure of an aneurism or tumour.

In the vast majority of cases it follows on chronic bronchitis whether tubercular or otherwise; for in this condition pus or discharge tends to accumulate and damage the linings of the bronchi so that a vicious circle develops in which pus accumulates, bronchitis results, and more pus accumulates with the development of a further attack of bronchitis. All the signs of chronic bronchitis are present – cough, breathlessness, occasional attacks of fever – but in this case the typical feature is the large amounts of foul-smelling pus which are brought up. Bronchiectasis is a serious disease, but the antibiotics and sulpha drugs have changed the outlook considerably and lung surgery in the form of removal of a lobe or the temporary collapse of a lung may aid in clearing it up. Ordinarily, however, treatment in the milder cases will take the form of expectorant cough medicines, courses of antibiotic, and 'postural coughing' which means that the patient spends a few minutes each morning lying face down with his head hanging over the edge of the bed at a lower level than the rest of the body coughing in order to bring up the sputum which collects during the night. In this way the vicious circle by which pus retention leads to further infection may be broken or at any rate alleviated.

Bronchitis, Acute: is primarily a disease of the very young or the rather old and is characterised by acute or chronic attacks of fever, cough with purulent sputum, and sometimes pain in the chest and breathlessness of varying degrees. Sometimes it occurs as a complication of other diseases such as measles or influenza and, although streptococci and staphylocci are usually present in the sputum, it cannot be said to be produced by any one type of germ since in general the infecting organisms are mixed types. Acute bronchitis is rarely serious in itself, but it can spread downwards to the smaller tubes and finally to the lung tissue causing bronchopneumonia where there are patches of solid infected areas scattered throughout the lungs in place of the picture found in lobar pneumonia which (a) is caused by a single type of germ, the pneumococcus, and (b) affects a whole lobe of a lung at one time and may happen at any age or time or place. Chronic bronchitis is typically a British disease (although not exclusively so) and has a direct connection with bad weather, foggy atmospheres, and city life; but there can be no doubt that much depends on the person affected. The young children who develop acute bronchitis are debilitated ones either suffering from some other disease or generally 'run-down,' the older people with chronic bronchitis who periodically develop acute attacks usually in the winter and autumn are city dwellers, more often than not those with outdoor rather than indoor jobs, and constitutionally they are likely to have a long history of childhood infections of the ear and throat, to be narrow-chested and have frequent colds, and to come from poorer rather than well-to-do homes. The treatment of bronchitis depends greatly on the doctor's skill because there are few fixed rules and what one does will be related to the acute or chronic nature of the infection, the age of the patient, his main symptoms, and his personality. Thus one would not treat in the same way a patient with a short history and one who has had many attacks with complicating symptoms of emphysema or bronchiectasis. Cough mixtures will depend upon the type of cough, the degree of breathlessness and fever; the use of antibiotics or sulpha drugs will vary with the patient; and the presence of other symptoms will determine what advice one gives about smoking, breathing exercises, and inhalations or nebulisers. Hardly any other condition taxes the ingenuity and experience of the family doctor to the same degree as bronchitis, but this we can say: that it is an infection which occurs more often in damp and temperate climates than hot and dry or even cold and dry ones; that it occurs more often in town than country dwellers; that it is related to social class and the type of work; and that (with exceptions) it is essentially a disease of the underprivileged. The annual death-rate in Britain is 25,000.

Bronchopneumonia: is basically a continuation of the above process – that is to say, it is not a disease that comes on suddenly but rather one that is either a gradual worsening of bronchitis over a period of days or a complication of another disease. Although, like lobar pneumonia, it may be associated with the pneumococcus it does not spontaneously attack otherwise healthy people and, especially in children, the primary impression given is *distress*, an anxious look, a bluish appearance of the face, breathlessness and cough. Initially the cough is dry, but later there may be a copious production of sputum, except in infants where it tends to be swallowed.

Bacterial toxins may lead to drowsiness and a rapid heart-beat. Primary bronchopneumonia is a disease of infants and young children and is not to be confused with the acute attacks of chronic bronchitis in older people or the broncho-pneumonia which comes at the end of serous illness. Treatment is with antibiotics or sulpha drugs but attention to general health is even more important after the illness than in other cases since this is not a disease of otherwise healthy people (*see* Pneumonia).

Bronchoscope: an instrument based on the principle of the telescope which is passed down the windpipe and used, by the illumination provided by a small electric bulb at the end, to examine the larger bronchial tubes.

Brucellosis: (*see* Malta Fever).

Bruise: more or less extensive areas of damage to the underlying tissues without necessarily being attended by an open wound, the bleeding having occurred beneath the skin. The general appearance is that of being 'black and blue.' Bruises are usually the result of a blow with a blunt instrument or the human fist, but may happen after a fall, especially in older people whose blood-vessels are more brittle; they are the subject of numerous superstitions, e.g. that a bruise has to 'come out,' that it has necessarily some serious significance, that it can be relieved (in the case of a black eye) by a piece of beefsteak or, if Dickens is right, by pressure against a cold lamppost. In fact, a bruise is a slight haemorrhage beneath the skin caused by a blow and may occur in the area of the actual injury or further down the body as a blow on the shoulder may lead to a black and blue patch in the region of the loins or a blow in the buttocks or thigh region to a black and blue calf of the leg; there is no meaning in saying that a bruise must come out, for it simply stays where it is until, in the course of days or even weeks, it fades away by changing from black to bluish and then to brown and yellow. The treatment is to ignore it completely except (*a*) when it causes pain or discomfort in which case a kaolin poultice is required together with some aspirin, or (*b*) when, as may happen, it is feared that further injury may be present such as a fracture which is an indication for obtaining a doctor's advice. Here it may be added that these are the only good reasons for seeing a doctor after injury. After all, if one has fallen downstairs then all that can be said is that one is likely to feel uncomfortable for some time afterwards and attention is required or would be useful only if it is felt that the pain is excessive or another injury than the visible one is thought to be likely. Apart from kaolin poultice, a cold compress of lead may help or if the application of a poultice is difficult or impossible in view of the area affected ice may be applied or a rub with liniment substituted.

Buerger's Disease: (*see* Arteries, Diseases of; Thromboangiitis obliterans).

Bunions: (*see* Corns).

Burns and Scalds: burns are caused by dry heat, scalds by wet heat, but similar effects may be produced by corrosive liquids such as strong acids or alkalis. Various degrees of burn are described, but here it will be adequate to mention three: (1) first degree burns produce simply redness of the skin as in a mild scald; (2) second degree burns damage all but the deepest layers of the skin; (3) third degree burns cause damage right down to the tissues below. Generally speaking, burns are not unduly dangerous if they involve less than one-third of the body's surface, but second or third-degree burns involving more than one-third of the body are a serious danger to life. It is necessary to consider, therefore, both the extent and the depth of a burn, and the former is usually more important than the latter so any burns which are more than trivial should be treated initially by general means such as warmth, the administration of liquids when the patient is conscious, and disturbing him as little as possible. The clothes should not be removed and *absolutely nothing* in the way of dressings should be applied – least of all ointments or fatty substances. If help is likely to be delayed the patient should be placed in a warm (not hot or cold) bath with one teaspoonful of salt or baking soda to a pint of water. Ordinary burns are best treated by the application of non-greasy Cetavlex cream and plain gauze or a clean handkerchief; blisters should not be touched except by a doctor.

Bursae: these are natural spaces in the fibrous tissues containing a little fluid and situated at points where there is constant pressure or friction. Sometimes they develop in areas where unnatural pressure is frequently applied as over corns and bunions when the footwear is too tight. The so-called 'housemaid's knee' develops excess fluid in a natural bursa in front of the knee-cap although it is often mistaken for a disease of the knee-joint itself. Treatment in general consists of poulticing, but when the fluid does not disperse it may be necessary to draw it off.

Busulphan: trade name 'Myleran,' is a preparation related to the nitrogen mustard group which has an action on dividing cells similar to that of radiation from X-rays. It is used in the treatment of selected cases of chronic myeloid leukaemia.

Byssinosis: a form of pneumoconiosis found in workers in the cotton industry who have been employed for many years in cotton rooms, blowing rooms, or carding rooms where the spinning of raw cotton is carried on. The workers are exposed to the dust inhaled during these processes but it seems probable that there is a large element of allergy. As in other forms of pneumoconiosis, the main symptoms are chronic bronchitis and emphysema (q.v.) with cough and progressive breathlessness. Typical is the 'Monday fever' which occurs when the individual has been away from work for some days and then returns.

Cachexia: means the extreme debility produced by a serious chronic illness.

Caecum: from a word meaning 'blind' refers to the dilated beginning of the large intestine lying in the appendix area of the right lower abdomen. It is, in effect, the blind alley at the end of the small intestine to which the appendix is attached.

Caesarean Section: the delivery of a child by an incision through the abdomen and womb from in front, named after Julius Caesar who, according to tradition, was delivered in this way. Previously a serious operation employed only when natural childbirth was impossible or the mother was dead, it is now done for a number of different conditions, e.g. small pelvis, disease or swellings in the womb which would make delivery difficult, cases where the placenta is placed right over the opening of the womb (placenta praevia), haemorrhage in the womb, some cases of heart disease or abnormal (breech) presentations in older women, toxaemia of pregnancy, inertia of the womb, or repeated difficult pregnancies. Thus today it does not necessarily signify any very grave condition: nor (subject to the general state of the patient) is it a particularly serious operation.

Caffeine: the alkaloid (q.v.) present in coffee and tea which gives them their stimulating properties, although freshly-made tea is unlikely to contain very much caffeine. The drug is a brain stimulant, a diuretic which increases the flow of urine, a heart stimulant (hence the palpitation some people get after drinking too much strong coffee), and a mild respiratory stimulant. It plays very little part in medicine today except as a constituent of aspirin, phenacetin, and caffeine tablets which go under an immense number of trade names, although there is no evidence that they are more effective than aspirin alone, where it is supposed to counteract the dulling effects of aspirin. Once popular in the form of caffeine citrate tablets with students prior to university examinations it has now (stupidly) been replaced by amphetamine amongst those who are unable to see that no drug will counteract the serious effects of not knowing enough. Since it increases nervous tension its use is inadvisable in these circumstances.

Caisson Disease: work in compressed air chambers is a common feature of civil engineering excavations in water-bearing strata or under water as well as in diving. Caissons or diving-bells consist of a compressed air chamber at a pressure of 1 atmosphere for each 10 metres of depth but rarely exceeding $3\frac{1}{2}$ atmospheres or 40 lb. per square inch, an air-lock in the shaft, and a communication with the open air. When returned too rapidly to normal air pressure the worker may develop caisson disease which is brought about by the fact that the nitrogen of the air is five times more soluble in the body fats than in fluids and is therefore released more slowly than oxygen and carbon dioxide so that bubbles remain in the tissues for up to twelve hours and their presence produces the symptoms. These are severe pain in the muscles of the limbs known as 'the bends,' redness of the skin with itching known as 'the itch' or 'prickles,' giddiness or 'the staggers,' and rarely a type of asphyxia known as 'the chokes.' Paraplegia (i.e. paralysis from the waist down) used to be described as 'diver's palsy' and nitrogen emboli in the blood-vessels of the brain, lungs, or heart sometimes proved fatal. Aseptic necrosis of bone used also to occur, but both these conditions are rare today. Since caisson disease never occurs at pressures of less than

18 lb. to the square inch (i.e. 40 feet of water) the *preventive* treatment is not to exceed this depth, but when symptoms have appeared the patient must be returned to the chamber to be gradually decompressed.

Calamine: in the form of impure zinc carbonate lotion is used as a mild astringent for itching skin disease. Combined with sulphur as sulphocalamine lotion it is used in the treatment of acne and seborrhea to keep the skin clear of grease.

Calcaneum: the heel-bone or os calcis.

Calciferol: or vitamin D2 is produced from ergosterol when exposed to the action of sunlight; since ergosterol occurs naturally in the skin sunbathing produces the substance which has the same action as vitamin D.

Calcification: the formation of chalky deposits in tissues as in the scars of healed tuberculosis.

Calculi: are hard stony concretions formed in the bladder, the kidney, or the gall-bladder (q.v.) usually described as 'stones.'

Callouses or Callosities: are thickenings of the outer skin layers or cuticle (*see* Corns).

Callus: the new tissue formed around the site of a fractured bone.

Calomel: is mercurous chloride formerly used as a purgative and cholagogue (i.e. a drug which stimulates the flow of bile). When used for the latter purpose it is generally taken by those whose livers are already damaged and, as mercury is a poison which accumulates especially in the liver, its use in this or indeed any other condition makes it even less desirable than the other purgatives.

Calorie: a unit of energy used in physics and dietetics. For the former purpose the small, gramme, or standard, calorie is used which is defined as the amount of heat required to raise one gram of water one degree centigrade in temperature; the large or kilogram-calorie used in dietetics is the amount of heat required to raise one kilogram of water one degree centigrade in temperature (*see* Diet).

Cancer: the general name given to the type of tumour to which the term 'malignant' is applied. These are characterised by the facts that (1) they are not surrounded by a capsule and therefore invade and destroy the tissues in which they arise, (2) they reproduce their cells in a disorderly and uncontrolled way, (3) the cells tend to be of a more primitive type than those of the tissue in which they arose, and (4) they are capable of producing metastases or secondary growths in other areas. There are two main types of cancer which are defined by the nature of the tissues in which they arose: carcinoma which develops from the cells on the surface of the body or its internal linings (epithelium and endothelium), and cancer which develops from the connective tissues of bone, muscle, tendons, etc. and is known as sarcoma. (In the terms used by embryology, carcinoma arises in the tissues developing from the outer and inner layers of the embryo, the ectoderm and endoderm, sarcoma from the tissues developing from the middle layer or mesoderm). Carcinoma is twenty times more common than sarcoma. Cancers are also subdivided more specifically according to the parent tissues from which they take their origin: thus epithelioma is cancer of the skin, adenocarcinoma cancer of the substance of a gland, glioma is cancer of one kind of nerve tissue, and meningioma cancer of the meninges lining the brain. The cause of cancer is not known but it is fairly accurate to say, (a) that in the modern view cancer is not so much a specific disease entity as a type of reaction of the body to various stimuli, i.e. it is a *category* much in the same sense that 'inflammation' is a category and not a particular illness, (b) that, consequently, it is probably incorrect to speak of 'finding the cause of cancer' since it is doubtful if there is any single cause. Thus some forms of cancer are hereditary but the vast majority are not, some are caused by chronic irritation others apparently not, some are caused by a virus whilst most are non-infective, some are associated with glandular maladjustment since they can be controlled by glandular extracts, others with the application of certain chemical substances. We do not know the *cause* of cancer, but we certainly know many *causes*, although, of course, it is entirely possible that all these different causes may finally be grouped under a single heading depending upon one immediate cause which all the various intermediate ones merely bring into action. Cancer is found amongst nearly all animals and plants and therefore there is no reason to think that it is a disease of civilisation as some are prone to suggest; it is only a disease of civilisation in the respect that civilisation enables people to live longer and, as cancer is more frequently found in older people, more live to develop it. It must be remembered, too, that civilisation brings people into contact with many substances that they would not otherwise come across, and that some of these may be carcinogenic, i.e. giving rise to cancer; e.g. cancer can be started in animals by repeatedly painting the ears with coal-tar and British scientists have isolated the actual substance in coal-tar that causes this result. It evidently plays some part in the cancers due to smoking and probably did in those of former days developed by chimney-sweeps by the rubbing of soot into the groin. The virus discovered by the French bacteriologist Rous in fowls produces cancer and can be handed on from one generation to another. Some of the factors which seem to be relevant are *injury* about which it is fair to state that there is no evidence that single injuries (although often the factor which brings a cancer, e.g. of the breast, to notice) have any effect but repeated irritation, e.g. from a dirty broken clay-pipe which inflicts injuries on the tongue and then pours tobacco and tar-laden smoke on them, from a chronic ulcer in cancer of the stomach, and in the cancer of those who work with paraffin or soot, obviously does. *Locality* is relevant but appears to be related mainly to city life versus country life which one may assume to be connected with the first factor in that the inhabitants are more frequently exposed to carcinogens. *Age*, although sarcoma occurs in younger persons, the vast majority of cases of carcinoma belong to the age-group, 50–60. *Sex* does not very greatly influence the incidence of cancer but it *does* influence where it occurs. Thus, in 1956, 48,935 men died of malignant disease as contrasted with 43,775 women; but in men the cancer was mainly in the intestines, the prostate, and the lungs, in women the site was the breasts and uterus and rarely the tongue or lungs. This fits in with the observations that stomach disease is in general commoner in men than women, that men smoke more than women, and that the sexual organs are particularly related to cancer. (We know, for example, that giving female sex-hormones causes a slowing-down in the development of cancer of the prostate in men, whereas cancer of the breast in women is slowed down by giving male sex-hormones). Cancer has apparently increased more than six times in the past seventy years, but it must be recognised that during this period people have begun to live longer, that diagnosis has become much more accurate, that people have been in contact with many more new substances, and that smoking has become much more common. It is now second in importance as a cause of death to diseases of the circulatory system – a fact which is not very impressive in view of the obvious relationship between death and the stopping of the heart-beat and the natural tendency of doctors to notify the immediate cause of death as being due to the latter when other conditions have not been diagnosed. It is only those cases which have come to autopsy where the cause of death can with more or less certainty be revealed.

A great deal of important work, both in the field of prevention and research, has been carried out in 1964. Since the early discovery of Rous that one form of chicken cancer resembling leukaemia could be passed from one fowl to another, many types of cancer have been experimentally transmitted by viruses from one species of animal to another and also to laboratory cultures of human cells. It would now appear almost certain that leukaemia is caused by viruses and, indeed, these have actually been seen; for the Imperial Cancer Research Fund has isolated an unknown virus from human bone-marrow and cultured it in large amounts whilst workers in Texas found virus-like particles in the majority of a group of children suffering from leukaemia. This raises the possibility of an anti-leukaemia vaccine and a report from America describes the case of a man on the point of death from the disease who no longer responded to the usual drugs yet made a remarkable response to the injection of six different virus preparations. This action was almost certainly due to that sort of interference between different viruses caused by the substance known as interferon (q.v.). It would appear that many types of cancer, in addition to the factors mentioned above, may be caused by *non-cancer producing viruses* which, however, produce changes in the cells of various parts of the body leaving them open to carcinogenic substances which then act as a 'trigger' setting off the process. The number of known carcinogenic substances is multiplying and extends even to the most ordinary household goods, but since many of these are dubious inferences it would be foolish to scare the reader by making statements about specific substances which may very well not be true. What it is important to realise is (1) that whatever part viruses may play in certain forms of cancer it is *not* in any ordinary sense an infectious disease, and (2) the immense importance of prevention. It has been calculated that of the nearly two and three-quarter million people who die of cancer every year at least half need not have died. Education is needed here in addition to specific methods such as cervical smears (compulsory in Russia) which detect cancer of the neck of the womb at an early stage.

Symptoms, the symptoms of cancer naturally vary according to the part affected and these are dealt with under the appropriate headings, but it is a good general rule to see a doctor when any of the following circumstances (which may or may not be cancerous) arise: pain in the stomach or indigestion arising for the first time in later life or a history of intermittent pains which become constant; any persistent swelling on the surface of the body or any generalised swelling of a single limb; a mole which may have been present for many years and changes in any way; any sore which takes a long time to heal; a persistent dry cough; changes in the menstrual periods especially when flooding develops or bleeding in between the periods; any ulcer or lump anywhere, severe constant headache with vomiting; blood in the sputum, motions, or urine. The treatment of cancer depends on the site and is always a specialist problem; in some cases (e.g. rodent ulcer of the face) the condition has no tendency to spread throughout the body and is almost always cured by X-ray or radium therapy, in others drastic surgery may be necessary. But nearly all cases can be cured if taken in time and therefore it is essential that the patient should co-operate with the doctor in reporting any of the above signs if they present themselves.

Cancrum Oris: or noma is a now rare condition of ulceration of the mouth or face on the outside occurring in weak children often after some other disease. It is caused by an infection and requires immediate treatment.

Cannabis Indica: Indian hemp, hashish, bhang or gunjah, marihuana, is derived from the flowers or leaves of this plant which is widespread in both Asia and America. Together with opium, hashish is one of the oldest known drugs and was formerly used because of the drowsiness and relative insensitivity it produces in the treatment of neuralgia and pain generally or prior to surgical operations. It has no medical uses today. Hashish or marihuana (as the American form of the drug is called) is most commonly taken in the form of cigarettes when it leads to a gay and cheerful mood with a sense of exhilaration but without delirium or excessive excitement. Visual hallucinations may also occur, but the most typical results of marihuana are the prolongation of the senses of space and time; because of the latter effect it is used by the players of jazz music when it appears to improve the sense of rhythm. The limbs may feel heavy and the eyes are bright, but there is no hangover effect although a sense of unreality may persist for some hours. Like any form of narcotic hashish is best avoided, although it comparatively rarely leads to either addiction or any other ill-effects except in those predisposed and possibly its worst effect is the sort of company its use is likely to be accompanied by.

Cantharides: or Spanish fly is a powder made of the bodies of the crushed-up and dried beetle known as Cantharis vesicatoria found in the Mediterranean countries. It is an irritant and hence used at one time as blisters to the skin in counter-irritant therapy. Together with bay-rum it is still used as a hair-tonic, but its main unofficial use is as an aphrodisiac since when taken internally it causes amongst other effects irritation of the urinary tract with erection of the penis. Since the irritability of the urethra produced by Spanish fly greatly exceeds any advantages gained in the sexual field and the kidneys may be permanently damaged it is perhaps safest for the impotent to see a psychiatrist and this would also have the advantage of dealing with the symptom's basic cause which lies in the head rather than the sexual organs in the majority of cases.

Carbohydrate: the sugars and starchy elements of a diet (*see* Diet).

Carbolic Acid: one of the first deliberately-used antiseptics introduced by Lord Lister in 1867, carbolic acid is the one still used as a standard by which to test other germicides. Apart from this use and its employment on drains and bed-pans it has no modern applications in medicine.

Carbon Dioxide Snow: or 'dry ice,' since it melts by evoporating into thin air instead of liquefying, is sometimes used as a caustic for warts. It can cause severe burns of the skin in those who use it commercially, e.g. in the preservation of ice-cream.

As a gas, carbon dioxide is used to stimulate breathing in artificial respiration.

Carbon Monoxide: a very deadly gas which is one of the components of coal-gas (q.v.).

Carbromal: a sedative and hypnotic derived from urea, carbromal is relatively safe. The proprietary form is 'Adalin' and in 'Carbrital' capsules carbromal is combined with pentobarbitone sodium; used to excess these products may lead to nausea and giddiness.

Carbuncle: a large boil with several openings and a tendency to spread (*see* Boils).

Carbutamide: a sulphonamide derivative (sulphonyl-n-butyl urea) which lowers the blood-sugar in diabetes. It is not known whether it stimulates the production of insulin by the pancreas or potentiates its activity in the body. The related drug tolbutamide or 'Rastinon' is used, like carbutamide, in the treatment of mild cases of diabetes in older people.

Carcinoma: (*see* Cancer).

Cardiac: to do with the heart. This is one of those adjectives which is often excruciatingly misused because its meaning is not understood as in 'cardiac heart' which is almost as common as 'gastric stomach'; the literal meaning of these illsounding compounds would be 'hearty heart' and 'stomachy stomach.' Cardiology is the study of heart diseases and the specialist is a cardiologist.

Cardiospasm: spasm of the muscle surrounding the opening of the oesophagus into the stomach, i.e. the cardiac sphincter because it lies at the heart end of the stomach. The condition is not common but is associated with difficulty in swallowing and later the vomiting of solid food over a period of many years. There may be wasting and, although this condition is curable, its main significance is that it may be mistaken for cancer.

Caries: decay of bones or teeth.

Carminatives: drugs (usually the essential oils and spices) which allegedly aid digestion, relieve spasm or colic, and expel flatulence. Amongst these are: cloves, nutmeg, cinnamon, lemon, pepper, ginger, cardamons, oil of lavender, peppermint, aniseed, coriander, dill, and gentian. There is no evidence that anything 'aids' digestion unless something is lacking in the first place, e.g. hydrochloric acid, enzymes; there is little evidence that these particular substances relieve to any significant extent colic or spasm; nor, since flatulence of the stomach is a neurosis, is there much likelihood that carminatives can help it. However, it is quite likely that the pleasant taste or smell of most of these condiments makes one feel hungry (as in the case of curry) and, of course, the flatulent neurotic can 'burp' at any time with or without medicine.

Carotene: the yellow colouring-matter in butter, egg-yolk, carrots and other vegetables which is built up into vitamin A in the liver.

Cartilage: the tissue forming the rib-junctions with the breast-bone, the thyroid and hyoid cartilages, the rings of the wind-pipe, and part of the external ear. It is made up of a glassy background material like semi-transparent plastic with cells arranged in rows or groups of two, and forms also the growing points of bones (q.v.) in the shape of a plate lying about $\frac{1}{2}-\frac{3}{4}$ of an inch from the ends of the long bones before they set. Fish bones are mainly cartilagenous. A tumour of cartilage is known as a chondroma; it is non-malignant.

Cascara: cascara sagrada or 'sacred bark' is the bark of the California buckthorn, used in liquid or solid form as a purgative. The more elegant forms are the proprietary 'Cascara Evacuant' and sugar-coated pills; they have the virtues and vices attached to all purgatives (*see* Constipation).

Caseation: a process found in tuberculosis and other chronic diseases in which the central part of the affected area instead of turning into pus to form an abscess develops into a cheesy mass which may later become absorbed by fibrous tissue or changed into chalk by calcification.

Castor Oil: the oil squeezed from the seeds of the castor-oil plant of India, Ricinus communis; but it should be noted that the seeds themselves (in case any herbalist wishes to use the 'natural' product) are deadly poison. In itself, castor oil is bland but it is hydrolysed in the small intestine into ricinoleic acid which by its irritant action acts as a purgative taking effect because of its site of action within 3–4 hours with more or less violence – hence its popularity with the Italian Fascists who used it in large amounts as a punishment. It has been given medicinally when, as before an operation or X-ray examination, a single rapid purgation is required but it is difficult to see why anyone else should want to use it. Locally the oil is soothing when applied to the skin as in zinc and castor oil paste or as drops to the eyes to protect them during operation. As its action on the intestines is followed by constipation it used to be given for diarrhoea caused by indiscretions of diet, etc.

Castration: the removal of the testicles (sometimes applied also to removal of the ovaries in women). This is generally done for local disease of the organs, but occasionally for cancer of the prostate gland which is less quick to develop in the absence of the secretion of the testis known as testosterone. Castration leads to results which vary with the age at which it is done. Thus before puberty the operation leads to a failure of development of the male sexual characteristics: the voice remains high-pitched, the figure becomes feminine in shape, and the beard does not grow. After puberty there are few physiological changes and such as they are these are likely to be very gradual, but, of course, complete sterility develops although not necessarily impotence as occurs in pre-pubertal cases. Pharmacological castration can be produced by the administration of stilboestrol, the synthetic female sex-hormones and leads to the same results. Amongst the other reasons for castration are (1) in animals it is done in order to make the beast more placid and put on more flesh; (2) in the sexual perversions and homosexuality (q.v.) either surgical or pharmacological castration (depending upon the law of the land) is sometimes performed to reduce the sexual impulse and keep the individual out of trouble; (3) in some states the mentally defective or seriously mentally-ill are castrated in order to prevent procreation and the handing on of an hereditary defect; (4) in women the ovaries are removed either for local disease or to prevent conception where this would be dangerous to the individual or bad for the community; (5) in the Roman Catholic Church during the 17th century the Sistine Chapel in Rome substituted 'castrati' for the imported male sopranos or 'falsettists' of Spain and such singers were much in favour during the 17th and 18th centuries in Europe, the most celebrated of all castrati being Farinelli. The voice is not quite the same as a boy's treble or a woman's soprano but has a quality most closely resembling a contralto; (6) in the East castration was performed upon male slaves whose function it was to guard the harem or seraglio for obvious reasons (*see* Endocrine Glands).

Catalepsy: a somewhat archaic word used to describe any form of suspended animation characterised by immobility and lack of movement. It is a symptom of gross hysteria and somewhat rare since hysteria became unfashionable in the more technically advanced countries.

Cataplasm: (*see* Blisters and Counter-irritants); the word refers to any type of plaster.

Cataract: an opacity in the lens of the eye more or less completely obscuring vision and occurring at different ages and from a number of causes. The commonest type is senile cataract which may occur in previously healthy eyes after the age of fifty and is largely an exaggeration of the ageing process whereby most people develop hardening of the lenses and difficulty in focusing on near objects as the years go by. In the cataract case more pronounced hardening and consequent shrinking occurring near the centre leads to 'splintering' of the lenses and shortly to opacity such as develops on unbreakable windscreens when hit by a stone. Cataract of this type has nothing to do with the general health or even with the health of the rest of the eye. Unlike this is the cataract found in children which may result from abnormalities in the mother such as defects of calcium metabolism associated with parathyroid disease or an attack of German measles during pregnancy; it is quite frequently associated with other defects both in the eye and elsewhere and therefore the outlook is not so good as in the first case. Diabetic patients are prone to develop cataract and amongst other causes are: direct injury to the lens or even a blow on the eye, prolonged exposure to heat as in glass-workers, radiation cataract caused by X-rays, radium, or atomic radiation, cataract following an electric shock. The symptoms are (1) an appearance of spots before the eyes which, unlike those seen by perfectly normal people when they pay attention to them, are immobile, (2) bright lights are sometimes seen double (e.g. street lamps seen at a distance in the dark), and there is a moderate degree of short-sightedness aided for a time by glasses, (3) gradually increasing blindness in which initially vision in twilight may be better than in full daylight since light is admitted around the more widely dilated pupil in the dark, (4) in the final stage the defect becomes apparent to others as a greyish-white mass filling up the pupil. Cataract is never treatable by drugs or applications of any sort although unscrupulous individuals have sold salves alleged to act by 'dissolving the cataract away' and since most of these contain atropine which does indeed temporarily improve vision by dilating the pupil with the effect mentioned above they often impress the sufferer although the improvement lasts only a few hours. The only treatment is an operation to remove the lens from its capsule through the opening of the pupil usually under a local anaesthetic and with perfect safety even with very old and frail patients. Ordinarily they will be allowed out of bed one week after the operation and will have to have both eyes bandaged for the first forty-eight hours after which the good eye is left uncovered whilst the affected one is dressed daily. The necessity for rest is to reduce the chance of haemorrhage into the eye or tearing of the very delicate stitches in the tiny wound. Results are excellent in more than 90% of cases and patients are able to use both their eyes within a month. Complete vision is, of course, obtained only after suitable glasses have been prescribed which take over the function of the removed lens. Cataract is not hereditary, not caused by eyestrain, not preventable by any method known to us (except in the case of the occupational cataracts), and must be operated upon as soon as discovered since if this is not done the eye will be damaged beyond repair resulting in total and permanent blindness. In about 10% of cases the cataract is in one eye only and never develops in the other. After operation and healing is completed glasses must continue to be worn, but otherwise no special care need be taken of the eyes nor is there any visible scar.

Catarrh: is one of those emotional words like 'constipation' and 'acidity' which means very little to the scientifically-minded doctor and yet refers to a real or presumed state of affairs which seems to drive otherwise sensible people to furious argument when the subject is mentioned as if one were attacking their religious or political beliefs and sends them on fruitless visits to quacks or to writing letters to advertisers of herbal or other remedies in the small announcements columns of the weekly journals. A leading dictionary defines catarrh as 'a state of irritation of the mucous membranes, particularly those of the air passages, associated with a copious secretion of mucus,' but one sometimes hears of 'catarrh of the stomach' and cannot help wondering what its symptoms are and how on earth people get to know that their stomach exhibits 'a copious secretion of mucus.' The word is rarely found in the index of modern textbooks of medicine but on looking up one of thirty years ago we find that an alternative name for acute bronchitis used to be 'suffocative catarrh.' In short, it may be concluded that 'catarrh' is an out-of-date word; that it has been applied to so many different conditions as to be almost meaningless; that it has to do with the excess secretion of mucus and therefore, in so far as it has a meaning, it is not a disease entity but a symptom found in many diseases due to quite unrelated causes. Thus a cold which is due to a virus infection is called by some 'nasal catarrh,' bronchitis is presumably 'bronchial catarrh,' chronic sinus infection which causes a drip of pus down the back of the throat may be what people mean by 'chronic catarrh,' and the older text-books say that in chronic gastritis (which is not at all common) the stomach secretes mucus – one has never seen such a case but it may well be so – yet why of all the symptoms which must additionally be present does the sufferer pick on this magically significant one? For the undoubted fact is that if chronic gastritis is really present the other symptoms are so unpleasant that the presence of a little mucus in vomit might seem to be a relatively trivial matter, and the main difference would seem to be between the people who notice it and those who do not. This observation would seem to be confirmed by the fact that there is no direct correlation between the amount of mucus present and the amount of suffering it seems to give the individual: some have a copious secretion of foul-smelling mucus and notice nothing at all, whereas in other cases one finds bitter complaints in the almost total absence of any secretion. It is not a neurosis to have a mucous discharge coming from somewhere or other any more than it is necessarily a neurosis to have constipation, but it is a neurosis to be obsessed by either to the exclusion of all else. In both cases one finds that the neurotic sufferer (*a*) has a theory of his own about how his complaint arises, his pet medicines, and fixed beliefs about what it does to him (e.g. in both cases it is alleged to 'poison the system,' to give rise to foul odours, to cause immense suffering); (*b*) is unhealthily

101

obsessed with the minute details of his excretions, whether mucus or faeces, how they smell, how they look, how they alter with each new drug; (c) is incredibly persevering in visiting his doctor, but equally persevering in rejecting any advice he may give so that one has a feeling that depriving the patient of his symptom could cause him to have nothing further to live for. Tell the sufferer from either of these complaints that his system is not being poisoned and he will demand to know why he feels as he does if this is not so, tell him that the medicines he takes on his own or demands from the doctor are far more dangerous than any effects his disease might have and that their constant use may well have serious consequences and he will ignore you, show him the latest text-book by the greatest authority and he will ignore that too because he, after all, has 'studied himself' – which of course is all too true and lies at the root of all his troubles. To conclude: 'catarrh' is a symptom of many different conditions and its treatment is the treatment of these conditions some of which are curable (e.g. sinusitis) and others not (bronchitis with emphysemo of many years standing); it may be altogether overshadowed by the patient's obsession with it, his false beliefs about it, and what amounts to his refusal to accept expert advice; the word is obsolete and should cease to be used.

Catatonia: a state in which the patient remains for hours or days in the same position and when moved tends to remain in the new position. It is symptomatic of one type of schizophrenia.

Cathartics: are purgatives (see Constipation).

Catheter: (*see* Bladder, Urinary).

Cat-scratch Fever: a mild virus infection characterised by fever and enlargement of the lymph glands. Although it appears to be introduced by a scratch, in only about half the number of cases does a cat seem to be involved and the initial injury may equally well come from a splinter or thorn. Occasionally the swollen glands may go on to abscess-formation and require surgical treatment but in most patients the disability is slight and self-limiting. Antibiotics do not seem to help.

Cellulitis: inflammation of the superficial tissues.

Cellulose: a carbohydrate substance which forms the skeleton of most plants. It is not capable of being digested by human beings and its only significance to diet is the increase in bulk which it causes, bulk being a relevant factor in some types of constipation. In the form of methyl cellulose it is used as a treatment for obesity under many proprietary names ('Cellucon,' 'Celapose,' 'Celevac' etc.) where its action is to absorb fluid taken with the tablets and by swelling in the stomach still the pangs of hunger. Its advantage is that it is pharmacologically inert, its disadvantage that many people seem to suppose that it should be taken *in addition to* their ordinary diet.

Cephaloridine (Caporin): scientists have obtained antibiotics from all sorts of improbable sources. Oxytetracycline has the proprietary name of Terramycin because it was obtained from an earth mould, bacitracin came from a culture taken from a leg infection in a little girl named Margaret Tracey, and as everybody knows penicillin came from a piece of mould blown in from the dust of a rather grubby London street to enter the window of Alexander Fleming's laboratory and contaminate one of his culture plates. The origin of the latest of the important antibiotics, cephaloridine, was at least as strange; for it was picked up by Professor Brotzu of Sardinia in the sea just by the end of a sewage pipe. This is not so strange, however, as it seems because Brotzu was logically reasoning that sewage which contains a great deal of excrement might also be associated with something which could attack the organisms causing intestinal diseases and, in fact, his culture material when filtered did prove successful in treating typhoid fever and brucellosis. The discovery occurred in 1945 and three years later Sir Howard Florey asked for a specimen; the specimen proved to contain not one antibiotic but three, described as cephalosporin N, P, and the present one C. But it was not until 1964 that the immense amount of research needed to extract adequate amounts of this antibiotic, ascertain its properties and chemical structure, its toxicity, and so on, was completed. The substance proved to be like penicillin but (and this is important in view of the fact that various bacteria such as certain types of staphylococci have become penicillin-resistant) it was capable of destroying resistant strains. It is almost non-toxic, but the main defect was that its potency was rather low, so further work had to be done similar to that carried out in making the semi-synthetic penicillins (i.e. adding synthetic side-chains to the basic nucleus).

Cephaloridine has to be given by injection; as already mentioned is active against germs resistant to penicillin; it is one of the safest broad-spectrum antibiotics known (i.e. it kills with safety to the patient more different types of germs than almost any other comparable antibiotic) and, although at present its price is high, this may be partly offset by the lower dosage needed and the shorter period over which it has to be given.

Cerebrum, Cerebellum, Cerebro-spinal Fluid: (*see* Nervous System).

Cerebro-spinal fever, or Meningitis: (*see* Meningitis).

Cerumen: the wax-like secretion normally found in the human ear which, in excess, may cause blockage and temporary deafness (*see* Ear, Diseases of).

Cervical: concerned with the neck, as in cervical vertebrae or cervical nerves. Also connected with the cervix, the neck or entrance to the pear-shaped womb which lies at the top of the vagina.

Cervicitis: inflammation of the cervix of the womb (*see* Uterus).

Cetrimide: Cetavlon, Cetavlex, are proprietary names for cetrimide, the official title of a mixture of alkyl ammonium bromides either in liquid or powder form or incorporated in a cream. It is one of the best modern antiseptics and used in a 1% solution for cleaning wounds or treating burns. As it is also a detergent it is very useful in cleaning the skin in such conditions as acne and seborrhea which are characterised by excess grease formation and superimposed infection, or for cleaning and disinfecting lavatory wash-basins or baths.

Chafing: occurs in such areas as the armpits, the buttocks, or the groin both in infants and elderly or overweight people. It is brought about where two skin surfaces in a moist part are in contact with each other, or where clothing rubs in the presence of excess sweat, e.g. the feet and the groin following unwonted exercise or lack of hygiene. An element of infection is either present initially or develops later. The areas should be kept frequently washed and subsequently dusted with powder or, better still, a silicone preparation such as an aerosol can be used. In the case of the feet, washing can be followed by rubbing with spirit and subsequent dusting but spirit should not be used in the more sensitive parts.

Chalazion: a small round swelling of the eyelid due to the blocking of a duct with cyst formation (Meibomian cyst). It may settle down with hot bathing and antiseptic ointment but otherwise may have to be opened on the inner surface of the eyelid. No anaesthetic is necessary.

Chancre: the early ulcer or sore of syphilis or chancroid; the former feels hard, the latter soft (hence the name 'soft sore.') The chancre develops on that area where inoculation took place, usually the genitals, but occasionally around the mouth or elsewhere (*see* Syphilis, Chancroid). Both are venereal diseases.

Chancroid: a venereal but non-syphilitic infection caused by Ducrey's bacillus and taking the form of very small dirty ulcers on the sexual organs which develop 1–5 days after intercourse with an infected person. The glands in the groin may be enlarged. The condition should always be referred to a specialist to exclude other infections but clears up fairly rapidly after five days treatment with the sulpha drugs. No local treatment attention to general cleanliness is required.

Change of Life: (*see* Menopause).

Chapped Hands and Lips: (*see* Chilblains, Lips).

Charcot's Disease: the name given to swelling of the joints found in the later stages of Tabes Dorsalis, i.e. syphilis of the nervous system in one of its manifestations.

Chaulmoogra Oil: a volatile oil obtained from an Asiatic shrub by expressing the seeds (Taraktogenos Kurzii); it was used externally and internally in the treatment of leprosy but is now largely replaced by the derivative ethyl chaulmoograte which, given by intramuscular or intravenous injection, is much less iritant and more effective.

Cheiropompholyx: a skin condition of the hands and sometimes the feet in which tiny blisters appear typically along the sides of, and between, the fingers. There is intense itching. The rash may be a reaction to an irritant which is usually alkaline of either organic or inorganic origin and, if discovered, should be avoided; in some cases nervous sweating may be responsible. It may be cleared up with salicylate ointment or the use of a cortisone cream with antibiotic added.

Cheloid: is an overgrowth of scar tissue on the site of an old injury or burn. It occurs in some races more than others and is particularly common amongst some Negro peoples although by no means confined to them. The scar spreads, sending out claw-like offshoots which pucker up the surrounding tissues usually in areas where the skin is stretched, e.g. on the front of the chest. Sometimes the cheloid may disappear spontaneously, otherwise radiotherapy will be necessary.

Chemotherapy: the treatment of infectious diseases by chemical agents which deal with the specific organism, or as Paul Ehrlich described such drugs, 'magic bullets.' The first specific treatment was the use of quinine in malaria followed many years later by the discovery by Ehrlich in 1910 of salvarsan used in syphilis. Since that time there has been a constant flood of specific remedies beginning with the sulpha drugs and followed by the antibiotics.

Chenopodium Oil: an oil distilled from the American wormseed and used in the treatment of roundworms and hookworms.

Chest: or thorax is the upper part of the trunk with the breastbone or sternum in front together with the cartilaginous parts of the ribs at the point where they join the sternum. At the sides are the twelve ribs with two layers of intercostal muscles between them, and at the back the spinal column which is joined by the ribs in the centre. In addition there are the two pectoral muscles passing from the ribs to the upper arm in front and four thick layers of muscle together with the shoulder-blade or scapula and its muscles at the back. Underneath, it is separated from the abdomen by a large sheet of muscle known as the diaphragm or midriff, and at the top a relatively narrow gap permits the passage of the windpipe or trachea, the gullet or oesophagus, and the large blood-vessels. The intercostal vessels and nerves pass between the intercostal muscles. Inside the chest the main organs are the two lungs with the end of the trachea dividing into right and left bronchial tubes, the oesophagus, the heart, and the beginnings and ends of the great blood-vessels entering and leaving it; just as the abdominal organs are covered with a cellophane-like membrane of peritoneum so the heart is covered with two layers of pericardium and the lungs with two layers of pleura.

Chest, Diseases of: since the chief organs in the chest are the heart and lungs the main symptoms of chest diseases refer to these, and since all are so closely-packed it is obvious that disease of one part is likely to affect the others. *Pain* is found most often in relation to the pericardium and the pleura where infection causes roughening of the two surfaces which by rubbing together produce pain. Hence pleurisy causes pain on breathing and the pain present in pneumonia is caused by the overlying pleurisy rather than by the changes in the lungs. *Pericarditis* causes pain over the heart and a feeling of distress but, as in the case of pleurisy, fluid is exuded at a later stage between the layers and the pain then ceases; this is known as an effusion. The only two heart diseases of the muscle itself which cause pain are *angina pectoris* and *coronary thrombosis* both due to cramp of the muscle through interference with its blood-supply in the coronary vessels. With these exceptions, pain is not ordinarily a sign of heart disease and may be most frequently ascribed to dyspepsia or intercostal neuralgia. *Breathlessness* is a feature of nearly all lung and heart diseases of any degree of severity; in the former case it arises from interference with the air-flow to the lung tissues, in the latter to interference with the circulation which carries the oxygen round the body. A sign of poor aeration is *cyanosis* or blueness of the skin, and although much *sputum and cough* indicate something wrong with the lungs or bronchi, blood in the sputum is coughed up in both heart and lung diseases. Cough, too, may be due to pressure from outside the lungs as in an *aneurism* or even to wax in the ear which stimulates the coughing centre in the brain (*see* Lungs, diseases of, Heart diseases, Aneurism, Angina pectoris, Coronary thrombosis, Pleurisy, Pneumonia, Bronchitis, Tuberculosis, Actinomycosis). The only danger in fracture of the ribs is that a rough end may pierce the lungs, but a simple fracture without displacement soon heals up except in the very old. Wounds can only be surgically treated.

Cheynes-Stoke's Breathing: the type of breathing found in general in those who are about to die or are in deep coma which is not necessarily fatal. The breathing is shallow and gradually increases in volume till, reaching a peak, it proceeds to become shallow again, may stop altogether for a short period, and then starts the cycle over again.

Chickenpox: or varicella is a common infection of children at all seasons of the year caused by a virus which has been shown fairly conclusively to be related to that of herpes or shingles. Thus an adult with shingles can infect a child with chickenpox and vice versa. Chickenpox may also occur in infancy and in adults when its reaction is correspondingly severe. The incubation period is 10–15 days and the typical rash appears on the first day. This begins as tiny red spots in the area covered by the vest and spreads outwards to the limbs (unlike smallpox which starts on the limbs and moves inwards), the spots turn to blisters which finally become pustules and form scabs. Generally the rash is the first, and sometimes the only, symptom, but the child may be irritable, headachy, and have a slight temperature. No specific treatment exists (although if the child is irritable aspirin may be given and calamine lotion applied to the sores); there are no complications in the vast majority of cases. Quarantine period is three weeks from the beginning of the rash, but doctors are increasingly of the opinion that there is no reason why other members of the family should not be exposed to a harmless infection which confers immunity for life – other people's children are, of course, another matter.

Chilblain: or erythema pernio is an inflamed condition of the skin of the hands, feet, and sometimes the ears. It is related to poor circulation. The sores develop in three stages: (1) the skin of the little finger or toe becomes purple and itchy; (2) blisters may form on the area which can be very painful; (3) the blisters break leaving a sore which is open and often takes a long time to heal and other fingers are affected. The treatment is to improve the circulation with exercise and hot baths followed by a cold shower but drug treatment with or without Spartan measures is quite successful. There is little value in such older remedies as calcium and vitamin D, but cure may be effected by Pernivite tablets, nicotinic acid, or Vasculit all of which act by dilating the blood-vessels or decreasing their permeability.

Chills: (*see* Colds).

Chloral Hydrate: a powerful non-barbiturate hypnotic for producing sleep. Chloral syrup is one of the older drugs and is very safe but has the disadvantage of irritating the stomach; as it is a short-acting sedative it is sometimes combined with the bromides. More pleasant-tasting and less irritant proprietary preparations can also be obtained.

Chloramphenicol: or chloromycetin is a broad-spectrum antibiotic obtained from a specimen of soil collected in Venezuela by Burkholder in 1947; the fungus containing it is known as streptomyces venezuelae. This substance has remarkable properties the chief being its wide range of action, not only against bacteria, but also against viruses (which had previously failed to respond to any agent known to medicine); thus the Rickettsiae lying on the borderland between bacteria and viruses and causing Rocky Mountain spotted fever, typhus, and other serious diseases can be destroyed and so too can some of the larger viruses such as that of psittacosis (q.v.) and lymphogranuloma venereum which causes a venereal disease. The organisms of whooping-cough and typhoid fever respond particularly well. However chloromycetin is not without its risks and in 1952 a number of cases of agranulocytosis, a serious blood disease, were traced to its use in America. It is used with a certain amount of caution nowadays although there can be no doubt that the good it has resulted in vastly outdoes any harm. Employed with care there is very little risk, although even this is rarely justifiable.

Chloroform: was introduced into medicine as an anaesthetic by Sir J. Y. Simpson in 1847, being found in certain respects more convenient than ether which was in use rather earlier. Its main drawbacks are that it is irritant to the skin, sometimes produces collapse, and usually leads to post-operative nausea and vomiting. It is still used as an anaesthetic either alone or with ether. Internally, in minute doses chloroform remains a common component of cough and digestive medicines (*see* Anaesthetics for modern techniques in anaesthesia).

Chloromycetin: (*see* Chloramphenicol).

Chlorophyll: the green colouring-matter of plants which has the same structural formula as haemoglobin in the blood of animals except that the metal component is magnesium instead of iron. Taken internally, there is no reason to suppose that chlorophyll has any effect. It was given in the treatment of anaemia for a brief period on the continent but, lacking iron, it is quite useless for this condition as also for hardening of the vessels in old age for which purpose it was included in a well-known patent medicine. The belief that chlorophyll has some effect in reducing bad smells seems to be justified in respect of its local use by direct application, e.g. in the mouth or on foul wounds; there is no evidence for (and much against) the belief that it works when taken in tablet form to destroy body odour.

Chloroquine: a drug (4-aminoquinoline) introduced during the war for the treatment of malaria and since found useful in amoebic abscess of the liver and certain skin diseases.

Chlorpromazine: trade name 'Largactil,' is a drug used in mental disorders as a 'tranquillizer' and for various other purposes in medicine, e.g. to stop unnecessary vomiting, to potentiate the effect of pain-killing drugs. Although originally given for the minor neuroses, it has on the whole proved more successful in the serious mental illnesses and other tranquillizers are now available for the relief of mere nervousness. Chlorpromazine is chemically related to the anti-histamine drug promethazine and its use was suggested initially when it was noticed that the giving of allergy-suppressing drugs was often accompanied by a sedative effect and an improvement of mental symptoms.

Chlortetracyline: the official name for aureomycin (q.v.).

Choking: a state produced by blocking of the air passages usually by a piece of food which has 'gone down the wrong way,' i.e. the glottis at the entrance to the larynx or voice-box and breathing passages has failed to close as normally occurs when food or drink is being swallowed, probably because the individual was laughing or talking at the same time. The only remedies in mild cases or when no other help is available are the time-honoured ones of slapping the back to coincide with the patient's coughs, drinking water, or, in the case of children, turning upside-down. As death can occur when even quite small objects are caught in this way, immediate aid should be sought if they are not soon dislodged or if the patient is becoming blue in the face and collapsed-looking. If this is unobtainable, an attempt can be made to hook the body out with the fingers in the area behind the tongue. Choking is also brought about by neurological diseases which interfere with the nerves correlating the movements in the act of swallowing, by such conditions as angioneurotic oedema (q.v.) which cause swelling of the face and throat (this usually subsides at once with an injection of adrenaline), and in certain infections as in diphtheria.

Cholagogues: drugs which stimulate the flow of bile. There are few conditions where this is necessary and the whole rationale of drugs such as ipecacuanha, aloes, blue pill, calomel and rhubarb lies on the faulty basis of supposing that conditions to which the term 'liverish' might apply are frequent, or that they even exist at all. Most of these are rightly cast on the scrap-heap. However, in such conditions as cirrhosis of the liver it is conceivable, if unlikely, that cholagogues might help and the only true ones are bile and the bile salts, which because of their bitter taste are usually given in capsules or sugar-coated pills. Magnesium sulphate (Epsom salts) acts by drawing fluid into the bowel from the system hence it stimulates the flow of bile and may be helpful if laxatives are necessary. It has the great advantage of being safe and on occasion useful which the others have not.

Cholangitis: inflammation of the bile-ducts.

Cholecystitis, Cholelithiasis, Cholecystectomy, Cholecystography: (*see* Gall Bladder).

Cholera: or 'Asiatic' cholera had its original home in India, especially in the region of Bengal whence it began to spread in a series of epidemics throughout the 19th century. Thus an epidemic from India spread to Japan in 1817 and westwards to Astrakhan in Russia; another in 1826 reached Moscow and Berlin by 1831, and had invaded Paris and the British Isles by the following year. Thence it was spread by immigrants to Canada causing many more deaths. Other epidemics reached Europe in the years 1847–1855 and in 1865, when it was carried by pilgrims from India to Mecca, thence to Egypt and Europe; in 1884, travelling by the same route, it reached Europe and South America; but by 1895 it had almost disappeared in Europe although remaining in the other areas. Its mortality was terrifying, e.g. in 1892 there were nearly 17,000 cases, more than half of which died, in a single epidemic in Hamburg. The conquest of cholera began in 1883 when the German bacteriologist Robert Koch discovered its cause, the cholera vibrio, and showed that it was (*a*) spread very often by 'carriers', i.e. symptomless cases either of mild cholera or those who had just recovered and become immune whilst still carrying the germs, (*b*) spread by infected human faeces, primarily through the polluted water-supply, but also by flies which contaminate food. Crowding and disorganisation of communications with pollution of water predispose to its spread hence war and famine are often followed by cholera epidemics. Its removal from Europe and some other lands has progressed with the ensuring of a pure water-supply or the

111

boiling or chlorination of doubtful water more than by individual treatment. The incubation period of 2–5 days and the essential disease-process in cholera is a reduction of body fluids to a point at which the body can no longer carry on. The illness is described in three stages: (1) the first lasts from three to 12 hours and begins simply with mild diarrhoea and vomiting which however rapidly increases in frequency until the motions no longer contain any faecal matter and are described as 'rice-water' stools from their appearance. Soon severe pain arises which bears no direct relation to what is happening in the intestines being caused by cramps in the muscles of the limbs and abdomen owing to the depletion of salts. The temperature is raised but the skin is cold and bluish, the pulse weak, and there is a terrible thirst which, when satisfied by water, only makes matters worse by further diluting the body salts. (2) The second is the stage of collapse, and by this time the body becomes colder, the skin dry and shrunken, its colour dusky purple, the voice weak and husky, and the flow of urine ceases; these are nature's attempts to stop further loss of fluids. Death in cholera may happen during this stage, but it sometimes occurs in 24 hours and in epidemics people may practically drop dead in their tracks or die in 1–2 hours. (3) The third stage, in favourable cases, is the stage of recovery when all the changes appear to reverse themselves with the loss of fluid decreasing and the general condition improving. But even at this time relapses may occur or the patient may sink into a state resembling typhoid fever when he gradually deteriorates over a period of two or three weeks. The *preventive* measures in dealing with cholera have already been mentioned, and a protective vaccine (Haffkine's) is available but this is only effective for quite a brief period. In treatment of the individual case, nursing is of great importance the main efforts being directed to replacement of the fluids lost by means of saline solution (*not* of course water). Drugs are available to kill the germ, e.g. sulphaguanidine, chloromycetin and aureomycin, but as the progress of the infection can be rapid it is important to ensure that these are not given too late.

Cholesterol: (see Arteries, Coronary thrombosis, Gall-bladder).

Choline: one of the factors of the vitamin B complex which is found in egg-yolk, liver, and meat. As its absence in animals causes fatty liver ultimately leading to cirrhosis, it has been tried in this condition which usually appears either in gross malnutrition or in chronic alcoholism but without success. (Nevertheless chronic alcoholics should always be given vitamin B complex in view of the neuritis which is likely to develop.) Acetyl-choline, one of the derivatives of choline, plays a part in the conduction of nerve-impulses in the parasympathetic sections of the autonomic nervous system (*see* Nervous System).

Chondroma: a benign and harmless, although sometimes inconvenient tumour of cartilage.

Chordotomy: the operation of cutting the nerves which in the spinal cord carry impulses of pain usually done for the relief of severe and intractable pain, as in cancer.

Chorea: also called Sydenham's chorea (after the English physician who first described it) and St Vitus's Dance (after the saint at whose shrine those afflicted with the dancing mania occurring in epidemics during the Middle Ages in Germany were said to be cured, as they probably were, since this was a manifestation of hysteria totally unrelated to the present condition). The true cause of chorea is unknown, but most physicians believe it to be a form of rheumatism of the nervous system characterised by an inflammation of the brain and meninges and sometimes accompanied by the damage to the heart typical of rheumatic fever. Nevertheless it is peculiar that this heart involvement is neither very common nor very severe, e.g. the pulse-rate is often quite normal, that from being a very common illness of children at the school-going age it is now somewhat uncommon, that it was associated with insanitary and impoverished surroundings and occurred mainly in highly-intelligent and sensitive children, that it was unusual in adults except women after a first pregnancy. Cases are treated as for rheumatic fever with the addition of sedatives where necessary and a prolonged period of rest with good food and fresh air is advised. The symptoms are well-known and consist of jerky incoordinated movements which the child is unable to control; it is difficult to grasp glasses or other objects without knocking them over, and the child is often excitable and moody. The movements may be initially mistaken for wilful clumsiness and, by more intelligent observers for habit tics, but the latter can be excluded by the fact that the person with a tic can be of any age and always performs the same movements whereas the case of chorea makes widely different movements not located in any one part of the body. *Huntington's chorea* has no relationship to the ordinary type, being a progressive and hereditary form of mental defect appearing late in life and associated with choreiform movements.

Chorion: the outer of the two membranes enclosing the foetus (*see* Pregnancy).

Choroid: the middle of the three coats of the eye consisting mainly of blood-vessels (*see* Eye). Inflammation of the choroid is *choroiditis* (*see* Eye Diseases).

Christmas Disease: a hereditary blood disease similar to haemophilia in that coagulation is affected and bleeding readily occurs which is difficult to control. Named after the surname of the first case reported in this country, it is discovered in 1 in 10 cases diagnosed clinically as haemophilia from which it can be distinguished only by laboratory tests.

Chromium: a silvery, hard, metal which with its salts is much used in industry in making alloys, paints, ceramics, dyeing, tanning, and in the production of aviation petrol. Air contaminated with dust of chromates or bichromates is the chief source of exposure in industry and leads to a form of dermatitis with or without ulceration of the skin. There is often gross swelling of the face and severe itching. The ulcers are small (1 cm. or less in diameter) but penetrate deeply, sometimes right to the bone where the joints may become infected by germs free to enter in this way. Perforation of the septum inside the nose is common and usually causes no disability but helps in the diagnosis. *Prevention* depends mainly on adequate exhaust ventilation to remove dust and mist, in some cases the wearing of protective clothing, and the maintenance of cleanliness by frequent washing. The ulcers are treated readily with an ointment containing 10% edathamil calcium (calcium EDTA). Chronic acid, once applied where a caustic was needed, is now little used in medicine.

Chrysarobin: or Goa powder is obtained from concretions which form on the stems of the Araoba plant of Brazil. It is used in the treatment of certain chronic skin diseases, especially psoriasis (q.v.) and mainly in the form of an ointment. It is fairly effective, but has the disadvantage of staining skin and clothes a deep violet colour, which however can be removed with benzole or 'Milton.'

Chyle: the name given to the partly-digested food as it passes down the intestine, and to that part of it which is absorbed by the lymph-vessels through the lacteals in the intestinal wall to pass into the chief lymph-vessel, the thoracic duct, which discharges into the jugular vein in the neck (*see* Glands).

Chyme: the partly-digested food as it leaves the stomach.

Cicatrix: a scar.

Cinchona: several types of tree in South America in the bark of which quinine is found. It is known as Jesuit's bark, since it was the Spanish priests who first observed its use by the natives for malaria during the Spanish invasion of Central and South America. Cinchona itself is named after the wife of the viceroy of Peru, the Countess of Cinchon who brought it to Europe in 1640.

Cinchopen: also known by the proprietary names of 'Agotan' and 'Atophan,' is phenyl-quinoline-carboxylic acid, used in the treatment of gout. In this condition it seems to have an effect in relieving the pain and in prevention, but it should not be taken continuously as it can be dangerous and, apart from irritating the stomach and intestines, may cause serious damage to the liver. Properly used it is quite safe.

Circulatory System: the fact of the circulation of the blood was demonstrated in 1628 by the great English physician William Harvey who, however, did not understand how the blood flowed from the arteries to the veins and assumed that it must percolate through 'pores' in the flesh. But this gap was filled in thirty years later by Malpighi of Italy who was able to find the tiny capillaries under the microscope. The course of the circulation is as follows: blood from the rest of the body flows into the right upper of the four chambers of the heart (the right auricle) by way of the two great veins, the superior and inferior venae cavae. The auricle contracts, sending it through the tricuspid valve into the right ventricle (the lower chamber) which pumps it into the main pulmonary artery that soon divides into two branches, one to each lung; whilst the right ventricle is contracting the tricuspid valve closes to prevent the blood returning and the pulmonary valve simultaneously opened to let it pass, closing again once it has got through. In the lungs the blood, which has been dark in

115

colour from lack of the oxygen used up by the body, absorbs oxygen through the walls of the capillaries into which, like the small branches of a great tree, the artery has divided and lie within the walls of the sponge-like alveoli of the lung tissue filled with the breathed-in air. Carbon dioxide is given off at the same time for the processes of combustion in the body cells has given off this waste gas. The capillaries are continuous with the venules and these with the larger veins and soon the blood is being pushed back to the heart through the pulmonary veins to the left auricle of the heart (it will be noted that, although all over the rest of the body the arteries contain bright red arterial blood and the veins dull red venous blood, in the case of the pulmonary vessels this rule is reversed, the arteries containing venous blood and vice versa). From the left auricle the flow is through the bicuspid or mitral valve into the left ventricle whence it is sent through the aorta or great artery to every part of the body. Here again the valves regulate it, the mitral one closing as the ventricle contracts, and the aortic one opening then closing once more to prevent back-flow. The only complexity in this process is the small separate circulation known as the portal system of veins which carry blood from the intestines to the liver where it is purified and gives up some of its foodstuffs to be stored for future use (e.g. excess sugar is stored in the form of animal starch or glycogen). Having done this, the blood flows into the inferior vena cava which passes right up the back of the abdomen and part of the chest, next to the spine, joining the superior vena cava at the right auricle, just as the aorta passes downwards close to its companion vein (*see* Arteries, Blood, Heart, Glands).

Circumcision: the removal of the foreskin is (*a*) a religious rite of great antiquity and very widespread geographically being found, e.g. among the ancient Egyptians, the Coptic branch of the Christian religion which copied it from the Egyptians, the primitive Arabs, the Aztecs of Peru, all Muslims and Jews, the Kaffirs, and the Australian aborigines. Its religious function is not clear, but presumably it was both a form of sacrifice and a distinctive tribal mark. Female circumcision which involves the removal of the larger part of the external genitals is practiced by a few primitive peoples today; unlike male circumcision which is a trivial procedure medically, this is a cruel and barbaric rite. (*b*) As a medical operation, circumcision is performed usually in infancy on cases where the foreskin allegedly is so tight as to interfere with urination. That this is ever necessary is dubious and psychologists might query whether, even at this early stage age, it may not have harmful psychological effects.

Cirrhosis: a condition, mainly of the liver and the kidneys, in which the normal tissues are replaced by scar tissues (fibrous tissue) with consequent shrinking and inability of the organ to function adequately. Most commonly the word is applied to cirrhosis of the liver which will be discussed here. Cirrhosis of the kidney occurs in chronic diseases of the blood-vessels and sometimes with gout (*see* Nephritis). The causes of the condition in the liver are not fully understood but it is certain that malnutrition plays a part and toxic and infective elements may be relevant. It is, of course, well known that some chronic alcoholics suffer from cirrhosis which is the main direct cause of death in this state (*see* Alcoholism), but the general opinion today is that the effect of alcohol is only indirect and the real cause is the inadequate diet taken by the alcoholic and the inadequate absorption of what is eaten brought about by the gastritis which develops in those who drink strong spirits undiluted on an empty stomach. Infected hepatitis, a viris infection (q.v.) may lead to permanent liver damage. Cirrhosis is common in localities where malnutrition is endemic and frequently where alcohol is never touched, and in childhood it may be the result of congenital syphilis. Whereas in America a majority of cases of cirrhosis are alcoholic in origin many cases in Britain are not. The process may be accompanied by extreme enlargement of the liver or extreme contraction with the latter probably following on the former, there is rarely much jaundice although the bile pigment content of the blood is always raised on laboratory examination, and pain if present is limited to a dull, constant, ache over the liver area. The ankles swell owing to interference with the circulation and in the later stages there may be dropsy of the abdomen, enlarged veins in the region of the umbilicus and on the face around the cheeks and nose, loss of appetite, depression, nausea especially in the mornings and constipation. No specific treatment is available, but sometimes the operation of portocaval anastomosis or shunt is performed in which the portal vein is directed into the inferior vena cava so that the blood-supply to the liver is reduced. A diet rich in carbohydrate and protein should be taken, and vitamin B complex added; the physician may treat the symptoms as they arise with diuretics to reduce the fluid in the body, etc. Although cirrhosis is a serious disease, there are lesser conditions in which those who drink and eat too much suffer from similar symptoms to a mild degree which can be corrected if they stop drinking in time. No matter what its cause, alcohol and cirrhosis do not go together.

Claustrophobia: a phobia or irrational fear of enclosed spaces, e.g. lifts, being shut in a small room, travelling in a railway carriage or an underground train, etc. It is a symptom of neurosis which does not necessarily mean that anything need be done about it since plenty otherwise normal people suffer from the fear and avoid it by avoiding the circumstances which bring it about.

Clavicle: the collar-bone.

Claw-hand: a condition which brings about a state of affairs adequately described by the name. It is caused (a) by damage to the ulnar nerve or disease of the nerve leading to paralysis which is more obvious in the ring and little finger, (b) by the condition known as Dupuytren's contracture which is brought about by a contraction of the fibrous tissues in the palm of the hand, either as a result of rheumatic changes or constant pressure of an instrument upon the palm. Treatment depends upon the cause, but is usually surgical, although some believe that Dupuytren's contracture can be treated by the use of vitamin E or X-ray therapy. Vitamin E is used both in ointment and tablet form (proprietary name 'Fertilol,' etc.).

Climacteric: (*see* Menopause).

Climate and Disease: in recent years it is apparent that the enormous significance attached to climate in earlier times was somewhat overdone because people failed to see that many of the effects that seemed to be due to the climate in itself were really due to quite different factors only indirectly related to climate. It is true that one cannot get heat-stroke from the sun in Britain – but we can get it in an engine-room in Alaska; one is unlikely to get bilharzia and other tropical diseases here but that is not a direct result of climate; one *can* get bronchitis in the East end of London more easily than in the

Swiss Alps, but one is less likely to get it in North London too. Of course most people are better for 'a long sea-voyage' but how far this is due to the sea-breezes (which meant so much to the Victorians) and how much due to getting away from family, mothers-in-law, or responsibilties at work is not a question that would be found difficult to answer by modern physicians. Naturally we come back sun-burned and 'fit,' but the fitness lies partly in the sun-burn which makes most people look fit even if they have one foot in the grave and partly in the psychological effect. Only in a very small degree do direct physical effects of climate operate; otherwise, when we are all so wealthy (or so we are told), why has the long sea-voyage once recommended by doctors gone out of fashion? Much the same could be said of that other fixation of past days, hydrotherapy or balneotherapy, spas and baths and hydropathics – all gone for ever outside the few patronised by the very old in Britain and the many made use of in that in many respects curiously Victorian country, the Soviet Union. Generations of Englishmen struggled off to maintain the 'white man's burden' armed with spinal pads and solar topees and Heaven knows what equipment, but the last the British army of the last war saw of the solar topees with which a thoughtful government had supplied it was when they were all sadly floating in the sea around the troop transports in Suez harbour; the desert campaign in North Africa was won without them and even 'somewhere east of Suez' the Burma campaign was fought in the jungles with battered Australian-type hats or none at all. Probably it is a good idea to wear the polar bear-skin clothes dear to the heart of boys reading adventure-stories of exploration to the North or South poles but the American sailors who arrived by submarine at the North Pole played a game of baseball in clothes that were somewhat lighter than they were wearing at Lord's that season. On Everest these might be inappropriate, but we *do* know that underclothes made of string with a mesh of $\frac{1}{2}$–1 inch are warmer than woollen combinations. The great Swiss sanatoria, Davos, Montana, and Leysin, are gone too (or gone for the most part) to be turned into sporting resorts pure and simple: it is true that streptomycin and other drugs are well on the way to wiping out tuberculosis, but how many physicians really feel that their patients would benefit from sanatorium treatment in Switzerland? Very few one would guess. This is not to deny that climates have their own specific qualities or that nobody, if they could help it, would choose to live in Ghana, that dreadful Turkish bath supplied by nature, or in Death Valley or even Alaska, but what has this to do with health? The answer is: Nothing at all (*see* Hypothermia).

Clotting: (*see* Coagulation).

Club-foot: a deformity, primarily of the ankle-joint, brought about by conditions before birth (defective development, faulty position of the foetus) or after birth (diseases of the nerves or muscles producing spasm or paralysis as in poliomyelitis, scarring from severe burns or injuries) and resulting in an inability to place the sole of the foot flat on the ground when standing. The foot may be twisted in four directions or various combinations of these: heel pulled up so that the patient walks on his toes (talipes equinus); toes pulled up so that he walks on his heel (talipes calcaneus); sole turned inwards so that he walks on the outer edge of the foot (talipes varus); sole turned outwards so that he walks on the inner edge of the foot (talipes valgus). When these are combined we get, e.g. talipes calcaneo-valgus, i.e. the foot twisted so that the heel is on the ground and the sole turned outwards, or talipes equino-varus with the toes on the ground and the sole twisted inwards. The treatment is, of course, a matter for an orthopaedic specialist and may consist in the prescription of special appliances worn to correct the position, physiotherapy, or surgical operations.

Coagulation of Blood: blood-clotting is the means whereby haemorrhage from any area is normally stopped. The process takes place as follows: substances known as prothrombin (i.e. 'precursor of thrombin') and fibrinogen (i.e. 'capable of giving rise to fibrin') exist normally in the blood with calcium salts. Blood platelets (*see* Blood) and body cells contain an enzyme known as thromboplastin which is only released when the cell-wall is broken by an injury as happens when the skin is breached. Then in the presence of thromboplastin prothrombin is changed with the help of calcium to thrombin and this in its turn reacts with fibrinogen to form fibrin. Fibrin takes the form of needle-shaped crystals which form a network around the injured area where they are joined by blood platelets which become entangled in the net as soon do the blood cells themselves. This is the clot which gradually contracts to form a scab and, with the help of fibrous tissue, shortly becomes a scar.

Coal Gas: the constituents of coal-gas vary from place to place but its deadly constituent, carbon monoxide, is present normally in amounts which vary from 5-10% or more. The dangers of carbon monoxide alone (it may arise in any conditions where there is incomplete combustion, e.g. it is the cause of the blue flame often seen in slow-burning fires) is that it has no smell and its affinity for the haemoglobin of the blood is 300 times greater than that of oxygen. Normally oxygen is carried to the tissues in the unstable form of oxyhaemoglobin which readily gives up its oxygen component to the body cells, carboxyhaemoglobin on the other hand is stable and by retaining the carbon monoxide prevents the body cells from receiving any oxygen. In carbon monoxide poisoning, which includes coal-gas poisoning, the patient's colour is cherry-red and remains so even after death and the difficulty is that even with artificial respiration there may be very little unfixed haemoglobin left to transport the oxygen breathed in. Therefore it is essential to give oxygen with carbon dioxide to stimulate breathing through a mask which supplies it under pressure. Since nerve-cells cannot survive deprivation of oxygen for more than a short time and the higher and more complex the levels the shorter the time (e.g. the cells of the spinal cord can survive lack of oxygen for 60 minutes but those of the cortex less than 8 minutes without destruction); mental changes which may be permanent sometimes result in recovered cases of carbon monoxide poisoning.

Cobalt 60: a radioactive isotope used in the treatment of certain forms of malignant disease.

Cocaine: coco leaves come from two South American plants and contain the alkaloid drug cocaine which has the properties of paralysing nerve endings and therefore acting as a local anaesthetic, and stimulating the cells of the brain thereby inducing a feeling of euphoria and loss of fatigue. The South American Indians used to chew the dried leaves mixed with a little chalk in order to still the pangs of hunger and the remarkable postal system of the Incas of Peru which was maintained by runners who carried messages over long distances seems to have been due in part to the use of this drug which, however, taken in large amounts has harmful effects. Cocaine was introduced as a local anaesthetic towards the end of the last century by Karl Koller and Sigmund Freud, the founder of psychoanalysis, and it was even used to some extent for its general effect in various diseases. However, its tendency to cause serious addiction has virtually removed it from the field of medicine except sometimes in the form of eye-drops prior to operation. As a drug of addiction, cocaine is less used than opium and its derivatives but, with the exception of heroin, it is the most likely of all these drugs to lead to an addiction which is rarely cured. It is used in most cases in the form of snuff ('snow') although occasionally by injection and is usually found to be taken in combination with other drugs such as morphine. The addict is likely to be emaciated with no desire for food, unfitted for mental or physical work, sexually impotent, and sometimes there are hallucinations with very frequently a sense of creeping under the skin known as the 'cocaine bug.' When it is first given the addict is cheerful, witty, and inexhaustible, but the exhilaration is soon followed by depression. Death is usually due to the inability to resist minor infections, but suicide is also frequent.

Coccydynia: severe pain in the region of the coccyx, the lower end of the spinal column. This may be due to neuralgia of the spinal nerves, to injury by sitting down violently, being kicked, or to damage when giving birth. Coccydynia is one of those very troublesome and chronic afflictions which often comes to be associated with neurotic symptoms. Treatment depends on the cause, but sometimes an operation to remove the coccyx is necessary.

Codeine: an alkaloid (q.v.) obtained from opium which does not cause addiction and, apart from a tendency to produce constipation, is relatively harmless. It is used generally as tablets of codeine phosphate (which forms a constituent of tablets containing aspirin, phenacetin, and codeine), or as a syrup or linctus for the relief of cough. Official pronunciations have made it clear that codeine is not a very useful drug, although the general public will take some convincing to the contrary; it is probably useful in suppressing unproductive cough but its pain-killing properties are negligible either with or without aspirin.

Cod Liver Oil: is rich in vitamins A and D but much less so than halibut-liver oil. Although traditionally the thing which is 'good' for children, its nauseating taste (which, however, very young children do not seem to mind) makes it difficult to see why it need be used, save for reasons of economy, when so many other preparations of the vitamins are available, e.g. capsules of halibut-liver oil or the pure vitamins ('Adexolin') and 'Haliborange' tablets or liquid containing vitamins A, C, and D. Of course, as is pointed out elsewhere, there is no reason whatever why normal children should be given vitamins in ordinary circumstances.

Coeliac Disease: a disease of children beginning during the first two years of life of which the main feature is an inability to digest fats. The basic symptoms are: (1) infantilism, i.e. the child does not seem to grow up and is often mentally unhappy and querulous; (2) the bowel motions are unformed, of a porridge-like consistency, pale and offensive; (3) the child, although thin and underdeveloped, has a large and protuberant abdomen; (4) there is a chronic lack of appetite. The appearance of the motions is due to the failure to digest fats so that they are broken down into fatty acids and glycerol (*see* Digestion) but not absorbed and therefore the child, in spite of the food taken in, is really suffering from a severe state of malnutrition which explains the infantilism and wasting. The immediate cause of this is unknown, but it is necessary to obtain specialist advice and to let the child have a suitable diet which will include the foods it can absorb, extra vitamins, and iron for the anaemia which is always present. Over-ripe bananas in which the skin has turned black are very suitable for this purpose and are given usually two or three daily. There is a definite tendency for the child to outgrow the disease; bilesalts, which are concerned with the ability to absorb fats have been given with some success in treatment although the disease does not seem to be caused by any lack of bile. A type of coeliac disease known as 'idiopathic steatorrhea' occurs in adults.

Colchicum: is obtained from the bulb of meadow-saffron and used solely for gout. Used during the attack it markedly relieves the pain, but is useless as a prophylactic. It is a gastric irritant and may be given by intravenous injection in the form of colchicine, or by mouth as the extract or tincture. A derivative, demecolcine, has been used in the treatment of one type of leukaemia.

Colds: otherwise known as coryza, 'chills,' etc., are names given to a number of what are known to be quite separate conditions to which doctors have added the title 'coryza' which is the cold proper. 'Chills' means nothing at all except that people feel chilly when they are in the initial stages of any infection whatever and no more so in a cold than in anything else. Like 'catarrh' the word 'chill' would be better dropped and, as in that condition, the chronic cold sufferer frequently goes to his doctor in order to tell him what is the matter and how it should be treated rather than the reverse. It is necessary to start by clearing the air (if the term does not give the cold sufferer too much offence) by noting quite dogmatically that investigations have shown that: (1) the true cold is caused by a virus infection which, since it produces a very brief period of immunity, probably cannot be inoculated against; (2) the cold has nothing to do with cold or damp air, getting wet or wearing sodden clothes – nor, so far as scientists know, has any other disease; (3) there is no such thing as a 'cold-cure,' although there are numerous drugs which can relieve the symptoms of a cold until it gets well by itself; (4) colds have almost certainly as much connection with the sort of person who meets the germ as with the germ which meets the person and it seems likely that there is a large psychological and constitutional element involved in determining whether or not infection takes in a given individual. The proofs of these statements lie in such observations as that under scientific control people have been sent out in thin running clothes to walk for long distances in the rain, get soaking wet, and go to sleep in their wet clothes, yet not one developed as much as a sniff; that, when 'cold prevention' tablets were being tested out in industry, 'dummy' tablets containing nothing but chalk were given as controls and those who had the 'dummy' tablets shared as much as the others in the very considerable reduction in colds that resulted. The so-called 'summer colds' are not even colds or produced by infection but a form of allergy to dusts of various sorts arising in the same way that hay-fever does and relieved by antihistamine drugs in the majority of cases. Chronic colds are a contradiction in terms; for a cold is acute and in itself cannot become chronic and those who suffer from continual discharge and blocking of the nose are likely to be cases of chronic sinusitis. There are no vaccines or inoculations against colds, although there are vaccines which may or may not be effective against the secondary infection with bacteria which sometimes follows a cold; these are taken by injection and cannot be given by mouth so the claims made regarding a certain patent medicine cannot be substantiated since killed bacteria are as much 'food' to the stomach as any other form of protein and are digested just as readily. (The fact that people have gained advantage from these products is merely another proof of the suggestibility of human nature and the large psychological element in colds.) The experience of psychoanalysts, for example, shows that many people being psychologically treated for a neurosis stop having colds quite by the way since analysts are neither interested in, nor do they treat, colds. Are colds infectious? Presumably they are, although many people who have spent much of their lives associating with those who have colds have never been able to contract one. There is no specific treatment but aspirin will doubtless continue to be taken although it has no place in therapeutics except in the relieving of pain because reduction of temperature is rarely necessary or advisable. Frequent colds should be investigated since it is possible that sinus infection may be responsible, but otherwise colds are on the whole 'cured' by anything one believes in.

Colectomy: the operation for removal of the colon or large intestine. It is performed for the treatment of severe cases of ulcerative colitis or for the removal of various tumours. The operative recovery rate is over 90% (*see* Colitis, Digestive System).

Colic: pain in the abdomen caused by the attempt of one or other of the internal tubes, i.e. the intestines, the bile-ducts, or the ureter, to expel something which causes blockage or irritation. Typically, the pain of colic is spasmodic in that it comes to a peak, slowly lessens, stops, and then builds up again. What the tube is trying to expel may be the contents of a bowel which have become infected, irritant food, or tumours (which, of course, cannot be expelled, but the bowel acts as if they should) and other swellings; or the lining of the tube may have become inflamed and is therefore too responsive to stimuli which irritate its wall, as in colitis. In the case of the bile-duct what is being pushed down may be a stone (*see* Gall-bladder), and in the ureter between the kidneys and the bladder it may be a stone or even tiny crystals; but in both cases infection may have caused such irritation that any stimulus provokes colic. Occasionally, and particularly in children, colic may be largely nervous caused by fear of going to school or some other situation. Lead poisoning (q.v.) leads to colic, but is much less common today since lead is no longer used in paint manufacturing which was its main source, nor is lead much employed for containers. Colic, unless its cause is clear, should always be investigated; its pain is usually relieved by heat or giving antispasmodic drugs (e.g. atropine or belladonna). (*See* Intestines and Kidneys.)

Colitis: means inflammation of the major part of the large intestine or colon and is of two types: mucous colitis (mucomembranous colitis, spastic colon) and ulcerative colitis. Mucous colitis is a bowel neurosis characterised by the passage of mucus, diarrhoea alternating with constipation, and dull abdominal pain in the left lower abdomen. It is found mainly in middle-aged people (of both sexes) who are absorbed in their bowel-motions and caused by the excessive use of purgatives. Fortunately the condition is becoming rather rare as knowledge spreads and the danger of taking purgatives comes to be realised and perhaps another element in its disappearance is that the more drastic purges are now almost unobtainable. The treatment is to stop addiction and obtain advice about a sensible diet. Ulcerative colitis is a more serious illness of unknown origin which may arise either gradually or quite suddenly. It is more common in women and Dr. A. E. Clark-Kennedy, Dean of the Medical School at the London Hospital, writes that '. . . many cases seem to follow emotional stress and it is certainly true that all cases, whatever starts the disease, are aggravated by emotional stress of any kind.' In all probability the condition is a pyschosomatic disease (i.e. one in which emotional factors lead directly to organic illness) rather than a purely neurotic one (i.e. for our present purpose, one in which a neurotic outlook leads to the patient doing stupid things which in turn cause the disease as in the case of mucous colitis). Thus mucous colitis is caused by purgatives when the patient poisons herself, whereas it seems likely that ulcerative colitis is caused by mental stress which she cannot avoid. The symptoms of ulcerative colitis are frequent small stools which are liquid in consistency and contain mucus, blood, and pus. There is very little pain but some abdominal discomfort and the patient becomes anaemic and emaciated. A few cases are rapidly fatal, but most become chronic with relapses taking place over a period of many years. The sulpha drugs have been given since infection may occur with bouts of fever, but the basic condition is not an infectious disease. Specialist treatment is required and sometimes operations such as ileostomy or colectomy are performed to remove the ulcerated areas which are a feature of the local lesion.

Collagen Diseases: a group of diseases such as rheumatoid arthritis and rheumatic fever which are characterised by changes in the collagen or connective tissues of the body. The exact cause of these changes is not known, but they respond to treatment with cortisone and A.C.T.H.

Collapse Therapy: a means of treating diseases of the lungs such as chronic tuberculosis by collapse so that the infection is not disturbed by the constant movement of breathing and is given a chance to heal on the basis of the old adage that it is essential to 'rest the diseased part.' As the pressure inside the chest is lower than that outside, the introduction of air into the pleural cavity is followed by collapse of the lung (pneumothorax) and the same result may be achieved by the operation of thoracoplasty in which portions of the supporting ribs are removed.

Collar-bone: the clavicle which serves to give breadth to the shoulders and helps to support the arm is an f-shaped bone and the most frequently-fractured in the body. The usual type of injury is a fall on the shoulder or on the outstretched hand. The immediate treatment is to tie a bandage round the neck, bringing the wrist as close to the neck as possible.

Colles' Fracture: a common type of fracture which, like a fractured collar-bone, is often caused by a fall on the outstretched hand. The lower end of the radius or outer bone of the forearm is broken just above the base of the thumb. In view of the possibility of complications an X-ray should be taken and the bone may need to be 'set' under an anaesthetic with the subsequent application of plaster of Paris.

Collodion: or 'New Skin' is an old-fashioned remedy for small cuts which have stopped bleeding. It can also, and more appropriately, be used for chapping and cold sores or in shingles.

Colloids: a term applied in the mid-19th century by Thomas Graham to certain solutions which, unlike crystalloids or solutions of crystals, are unable to pass through a parchment membrane. In this sense glue and milk are colloidal solutions made up of tiny globules suspended in a liquid medium. However, it is now known that all substances can be obtained in the colloidal state; with metals, for example, when they are finely enough divided, the particles are electrically charged and remain suspended in the surrounding liquid being kept in that position by bombardment from its molecules. Hence colloidal sulphur, iodine, silver, etc., which are used in medicine.

Colour Blindness: a defect of the eyes which makes it impossible to distinguish certain colours or shades of colour. Colour blindness is always congenital and more common in men than women who transmit the defect to male children. Colour blind women are very rare but about 10% of the male population have some defect usually in distinguishing between red, green, and yellow those with this type being described as red-green blind types who can see the colours but have difficulty in distinguishing which is which. Less common is blue-yellow blindness in which blue, green, and yellow, are confused. The cause of colour-blindness is most cases is a defect of the functioning of the rods and cones in the retina (*see* Eye) and most boys with the condition grow up in complete ignorance of the fact that anything abnormal is present, most being discovered by the tests now carried out by many education authorities. Such tests are of importance especially in those jobs where the power to distinguish red and green is of particular significance as in the railways and Mercantile Marine. Tests for colour-blindness are the test-cards used by these bodies showing the colours of the spectrum which candidates are asked to pick out as they are named. Holmgren's test based on the matching of coloured wools, and the Ishihara test described under that heading which is the most efficient and now the most generally in use.

Colon: the main part of the large intestine excluding the rectum; from the caecum in the appendix region the ascending colon passes up, then across the upper abdomen (transverse colon), and downwards (the descending colon) on the left side where it joins the rectum in the pelvis.

Colostrum: the first fluid secreted by the breasts for two or three days after childbirth; it differs slightly from ordinary milk.

Coma: a state of deep unconsciousness in which even the reflexes are abolished, e.g. the eyeball can be touched without arousing the blinking reflex. The usual causes are poisoning from narcotic drugs, alcohol, an overdose of insulin, not enough insulin (diabetic coma), cerebral haemorrhage, chronic kidney disease (uraemic coma), also high fever, the after-effects of an epileptic fit, head injury, etc. It is important to be able to distinguish between the different types of coma so that, for instance, the smell of alcohol on the breath does not cause one to miss a case of cerebral haemorrhage or a diabetic down whose throat some well-meaning individual has tried to force brandy.

Compositor's Disease: (*see* Lead Poisoning). It is found in those who handle type.

Concussion and Skull Injuries: *concussion* is a general term referring to the state of affairs when a brief period of unconsciousness follows a head injury. In itself, it is not serious, requires no treatment, and recovers spontaneously. However, since even the slightest blow to the head may have complications, the patient should be kept under observation for some time for the danger signs which are mentioned below. *Fracture of the skull* is also not necessarily serious and provided the bones are not displaced (as would be shown if a dent can be felt) no further treatment is necessary. The real measure of danger is determined by the degree of underlying brain damage. Surgical aid is limited to dealing with open wounds, to the removal of pieces of bone which may press upon the brain, and to the stopping of haemorrhage should this have occurred within the skull. There are no specific means of dealing with brain injury, but fortunately most cases recover by themselves. The symptoms of haemorrhage should be watched for in even the mildest cases of concussion or head injury; ordinarily they make their appearance in a matter of hours after the injury and manifest themselves by increasing drowsiness and weakness of the limbs on one side of the body. A common and tragic incident is the case of the individual who whilst drunk falls and hits his head on the pavement; he may be arrested and put in a police cell where his increasing drowsiness is interpreted as a sign of his drunkenness although in fact it arises from haemorrhage from the middle meniningeal artery in the skull and by the morning he is dead. Haemorrhage inside the skull is a surgical emergency and necessitates immediate operation. Under local anaesthesia a small hole is drilled in front of, and above the ear so that bleeding can be arrested and blood-clot removed. This is a minor operation, but failure to carry it out when necessary leads to almost certain death. Occasionally, signs of haemorrhage may appear weeks or months after an injury with symptoms of headache, mental confusion, and drowsiness. Operation in this case is less urgent but none the less necessary. Since head injury is something most people fear, even slight injuries (in fact, more especially slight injuries) may lead to post-traumatic symptoms such as headache, inability to concentrate, irritability, and so on. These are almost entirely psychological in nature – that is to say, they are neuroses and are more likely to occur (a) when the person is already of a neurotic disposition, and (b) when the question of compensation is involved. Thus it is well known that those who are injured, however slightly, at their work or in some other position where compensation can be claimed often suffer from post-traumatic symptoms, whilst those who suffer the same or worse injuries on the football field or whilst hunting rarely do. The real disease in this case is conscious or unconscious resentment and the desire to get one's own back.

Congenital: a word meaning literally 'appearing with birth,' it has become almost synonymous with 'hereditary.' This is erroneous because, as we now know, every disease which is present at birth is not necessarily hereditary since it may arise after conception and prior to being born. Thus the child may be born with abnormalities owing to the mother having developed German measles whilst it was in the womb and numerous conditions, for which the word congenital is best used, come into this category. A hereditary disease, of course, is one which has been handed on in the germ-cells from parents to child. Thus, whilst every hereditary disease is, in some sense, congenital, all congenital diseases are not hereditary.

Conjunctiva: the thin transparent membrane covering the front of the eye.

Conjunctivitis: is inflammation of this membrane (*see* Eye).

Conovid-E: one of the British oral contraceptives which is norethynodrel with ethinoyloestradiol-3-methyl ether. These drugs are taken under medical advice (or should be), and the usual method of administration is to take one tablet a day for 21 days followed by 7 days without them, repeating this each month. Extensive trials have shown (*a*) that in the correct dosage the drugs are successful in preventing pregnancy in almost all cases, and (*b*) that later fertility is not affected. The main side-effects have been nausea (which was by far the commonest and disappeared spontaneously after the first three menstrual cycles); less frequently reported were vomiting, headache, and weight increase. More recently, the medical journals have reported a few cases of thrombo-phlebitis (i.e. clotting of blood in a vein of more or less seriousness) in those taking these tablets, but it is not at all clear that this was due to the drug since, obviously, when thousands of women are being tested some are bound to become ill during the time involved and there need be no necessary connection between the illness and the pills.

Constipation: like 'catarrh' constipation is a difficult subject, not because we do not know enough about it, but because (apart from the constipation which arises from intestinal obstruction and a few other diseases) it is a disease largely invented by the individual himself. Whereas duodenal ulcers are found in people who are guilty of indiscretion, self-sacrifice, and mental stress, constipation in general in complained of by those who take far too much care of themselves. It will be noted that the phrase 'is complained of' was used rather than 'is suffered by' and this was quite deliberate because, although anyone may certainly 'suffer from,' or have constipation, not everyone *complains* of it. Those who do are mostly chronic neurotics who have not the slightest intention of taking advice, who pester their doctors with a complaint which they themselves propose to describe and prescribe for, who are concerned with all the more morbid aspects of their condition (not excluding the infrequency, consistency, colour, smell, and shape of their motions), and who have so thoroughly 'studied themselves' that all life, all relationships, all beauty, revolves around the lower end of their intestinal canal. In a word, they are selfish hypochondriacs to whom anything said by their own or any other doctor is as peas shot at an aircraft carrier. Most end up finally poisoned by their own purges taken in spite of, or with the despairing collusion of, the unfortunate physician. It is, therefore, to those who want to know about constipation, rather than to those who already know all about it, that the following is addressed. There are diseases of which constipation is a symptom, but very few of these exist and, with a single exception, they are all conditions in which constipation makes its appearance in previously normal people (e.g. intestinal obstruction). In itself, constipation produces no diseases and no symptoms except those brought about (a) by thinking of its 'evil' effects, and (b) by the discomfort the physical distension may cause in the abdomen. There is no such thing as 'auto-intoxication' from the intestines. As evidence we may produce the observations of Professor Samson Wright whose 'Applied Physiology' is almost the Bible of students of medicine. 'The symptoms of constipation,' he says, 'are largely due to distension and mechanical irritation of the rectum' and he goes on to show that an enema which clears out the bowel stops these symptoms *immediately* which would not be the case if they were due to poisoning from the bowel contents. Indeed, stuffing the rectum with cotton-wool produces the same symptoms. How long can a person remain constipated? Well, to judge by the views of the purgative addicts, the answer should be 'about two days,' but Professor Wright mentions that in one of his cases the condition lasted for *just over a year* without any bowel movement whatever and all that the patient felt was slight discomfort and a distended abdomen. There are quite a number of people who have movements about five or six times a year yet their general health remains good and certainly much better than that of the sad cases with mucous colitis caused by purgatives. Normally, motions depend upon habit; they may occur once a day, twice a day, or twice a week without being in any sense out of the way. But, since most people have been reared on notions of 'inner cleanliness,' 'regularity,' and the vague notion that there is something dirty or evil inside which must get out it is not surprising that those who think in this way feel ill when 'regularity' fails. Genuine constipation means that something is defective about one's habits, diet, or outlook on life, and should be treated by meals which contain more bulk (e.g. breakfast cereals or porridge), more fluids, and, if artificial aids are really necessary, a dose of salts before breakfast or 'Senokot' tablets or granules at night, in gradually decreasing doses. There is no reason at all why one should not take almost any purgative on the odd occasion, but there is very little reason why one should unless it is feared that the desire may come on at an awkward time or when recommended just prior to an operation. The regular use of purgatives is condemned by all medical men although, as has been mentioned, most family doctors are under constant demands to give their addicts drugs of which they do not personally approve. It is not in the patient's personal interest that he should get them. One cannot die of constipation but one can become very ill with pills designed to treat it.

Contact Lenses: are lenses shaped to fit the surface of the eyeball and virtually invisible on ordinary examination. Their advantages are: (a) they look better on those who do not like themselves in ordinary glasses and, for obvious reasons, are much in demand by actors and actresses who, apart from their cosmetic value, may have to play parts which do not go well with glasses although their vision is defective; (b) for some purposes they are more efficient than glasses, e.g. they do not steam up in warm moist atmospheres, they can be worn to play quite violent games, and in certain disturbances of vision they give better results than ordinary lenses. On the other hand, they are not suitable for all visual disturbances since powerful lenses suitable for reading blur distant vision and vice versa; also many people find the process of inserting and removing, or even wearing them for more than a short time, unpleasant. The decision should be made with the advice of an experienced ophthalmologist.

Contraception: is the artificial prevention of pregnancy by one or several of four main methods (or five, if one counts the 'safe period' method which is the only one permitted by the Roman Catholic Church because it is claimed *not* to be artificial): these are (1) the use of chemicals either in the form of foaming tablets, capsules and pessaries or jelly squeezed from a tube through a special applicator into the uppermost part of the vagina; (2) the use of mechanical means such as the sheath of rubber or other material used by the man or the Dutch cap used by the woman which covers the entrance to the womb; (3) the use of douches etc. after intercourse has taken place; (4) the use of the new contraceptive tablets which are sex hormones taken by mouth to suppress the menstrual cycle, and particularly ovulation; (5) the use of other means concerned with the technique of intercourse such as withdrawal or coitus interruptus and the 'safe period' which, by means of tables, enables one to calculate the days of the month on which conception is unlikely to happen, i.e. a varying number of days on either side of the midperiod when ovulation occurs. It is important to emphasise that information about contraception and the best method to apply it in the individual case should invariably be obtained either from a gynaecologist or a birth-control clinic since, if the principle of contraception is accepted, it is obviously essential that it should be efficient. However, the following general points may be made: chemical contraceptives are, in general, the least reliable method and unless recommended by an expert should never be used alone. Mechanical means if used properly and usually in combination with a chemical contraceptive are the safest of all; their disadvantages are that not all people find it easy to use them, and that there are aesthetic grounds for objection by some. The use of douches, although time-honoured, is extremely unsafe and never to be recommended, nor, except for religious reasons, is the safe period which may be wrongly calculated, varies because not all women have regular periods, and there is some evidence that strong emotions (as in those who have been parted for some time) may in themselves bring about ovulation. Coitus interruptus is undesirable, unreliable, and bad for psychological health. The new oral hormone pills seem to be very effective, but queries have been raised about their safety (although there seems to be little justification for these), and some women dislike the idea of their menstrual cycle being interfered with. Several brands are available in Britain (*see* Conovid).

Convulsions: or fits are accompanied by unconsciousness (in most cases), falling to the ground if standing, a preliminary period of jerking movements in which the muscles alternately contract and relax whilst the face becomes blue, a period of relaxation with heavy breathing when the colour returns to the face and it may be noticed that the tongue has been bitten and urine or faeces passed. In minor fits (petit mal) there may be no loss of consciousness but merely peculiar twitchings or single involuntary movements during which the eyes may be staring and the patient, although not unconscious, is just 'not there.' Fits are very dramatic and often frightening to the onlooker but their occurrence, especially in young children, should not necessarily be a cause for concern. Death rarely occurs during a fit and its seriousness is to be measured by the seriousness of the condition that brought it on. The following are the main causes: (1) In children or infants fits are extremely common during a fever and especially in the common infectious diseases when they need be of no special significance; a child may be fevered, delirious, and have a fit yet look quite well the following day when the temperature has gone down. (2) Fits occur in brain disease such as meningitis, abscess, tumours, or cysts in the brain, after a birth-injury or later head-injury, etc. (3) Certain poisons circulating in the blood because of disease or the lack of normal substances may produce fits, e.g. uraemia complicating serious kidney disease, cholaemia complicating liver disease, an overdose of insulin where there is lack of glucose, in tetany where there is lack of calcium. (4) Certain types of heart disease or heart failure may cause fits, although not very frequently. (5) Idiopathic epilepsy (which simply means fits whose causes, in general, are unknown). The following figures by Peterman give some indication of the most frequent causes in children: fever and acute infections, 34%; idiopathic epilepsy, 23·6%; birth injury. 15·5%; tetany (q.v.) 8·9%. Except in those cases with a history of fits, it is always wisest to call the doctor when a fit occurs (*see* Epilepsy).

Cornea: (*see* Eye).

Corneal Graft: the operative technique of treating certain cases of disease of the cornea (the clear membrane in front

135

of the eye through which light passes) by cutting out the part where vision has been obstructed and replacing it by a piece of cornea from a dead body or from an eye which has been removed at operation but has a healthy cornea. An Act of Parliament of 1952 allows the removal of the eyes from a dead body for this purpose unless the deceased prior to his death or a surviving relative expresses objection. The eye or cornea, if removed within ten hours of death, can be kept for up to twenty days in a corneal bank similar in conception to the blood banks used to store blood for transfusion which have saved so many lives. The procedure involves the removal of the scarred or diseased opaque area from the patient's eye and replacing it by the transplant under a local anaesthetic, and this gives successful results in about 60% of all cases. Of course, only those people in whom blindness or partial blindness is due to corneal disease and whose eyes are otherwise healthy can benefit, i.e. about one in every twenty-five cases of blindness.

Corns and Bunions: a corn is a localised thickening of the skin, pyramidal is shape, with the top of the pyramid pointing inwards; thickening over a larger area is a callosity which is not necessarily a defect and is frequently protective in function; a bunion is a callosity over the base of the big toe in which there is not only thickening of the skin but also a pressing outwards of the head of the metatarsal bone of the toe (i.e. the long bone which joins the smaller ones at the toe's base.) All these are produced by the pressure of ill-fitting shoes however much this may be denied, with the exception of callosities which may occur in any part exposed to pressure even when no shoes are worn at all, e.g. the natural thickening which occurs on the soles in those accustomed to go about barefoot. 'Hammer-toe' which results in the joints of the second toe being bent in hammer form is produced by the pressure of boots or shoes which are too short or pointed. Most of these conditions are best treated by a chiropodist or, where necessary, by an orthopaedic surgeon. They should not be dealt with at home except in the most minor cases, nor is there much point in doing so whilst the same footwear continues to be worn. Verrucas of the sole of the foot are painful and infectious and it is important that they should not be mistaken for corns.

Coronary Thrombosis: is caused by clotting of the blood in the small coronary arteries which supply the muscles of the heart and a coronary attack is very similar to that found in angina pectoris, i.e. there is pain of varying degree over the heart region radiating to the shoulder and often down the left arm. The patient is distressed and suffers from some measure of shock with pallor and cold sweat in the cases which survive although about half of all cases result in sudden death. Coronary thrombosis is, in fact, the most common single cause of instantaneous death, but provided this does not happen the outlook (as in the case of President Eisenhower) is not at all bad, especially when active treatment is undertaken. It is worth noting that, although there appear to be far more cases of the disease than formerly and it is undoubtedly the case that this increase is real, it is also true that mild cases occur which would not have been diagnosed previously. Thus, whilst coronary thrombosis may cause immediate death, it is also true that it frequently comes in the guise of what would at one time have been diagnosed as an attack of indigestion which does not respond to the ordinary treatment. In such a case it is likely that only a small branch of the arteries has been affected, the so-called branch-block. Coronary thrombosis occurs chiefly in men in their forties and fifties and is uncommon before or after these years; it is commoner in the industrialised countries and seems to be basically a disease of civilisation; and the man who develops it tends to be the driving, ambitious, aggressive, stoutish, worrying, and sometimes over-eating and drinking type. Thus it is in most countries commoner in the well-to-do than the poorer classes. Two theories have been advanced to account for these observations: (1) that coronary disease is a stress condition caused by tension and prolonged anxiety in a driving, aggressive, type of character; (2) that it is a disease of the over-indulgent, who drink too much and eat too much food, particularly food containing large amounts of cholesterol. Such foods are animal fats (not vegetable or fish fat or oils), eggs, liver, and most of those things which our parents probably told us were healthy and good for the body. In part these observations are obtained from the medical evidence that such cases have an excess of cholesterol in their bloodstream and that cholesterol is what forms the 'furring' material lining narrowed arteries in arteriosclerosis, in part it comes from that most fallible of sources, statistics. Of course, what statistics show are *correlations* not *relations* and certainly not causative relations; thus, although it could probably be shown that the incidence of coronary disease correlates closely with the number of cars in one's garage, we do not necessarily deduce that the number of cars *caused* the thrombosis because having two or more cars is correlated with many other factors: perhaps with more money, more food, and too many material goods, but also with more worries, more ambition, more drive, less exercise. Which is the usual factor? The worry, the food and lack of exercise, or both together? It may be the case (and there is some evidence for this) that whilst excess cholesterol in the blood, and coronary thrombosis or the liability to it, is due to an excess of cholesterol-containing food, stress may be the factor which causes it to be deposited in the arteries as it is certainly the frequent cause of an immediate attack. But we know that during the war when fats were rationed coronary attacks dramatically diminished in Norway, that the condition is also uncommon in countries where the diet is mainly vegetable or where vegetable oils rather than animal fats are used in cooking, e.g. Southern Italy. The treatment of the disease once it has started is a matter for the doctor whose advice will depend upon individual factors; the main thing to begin with being to get the patient over his first attack. After that, depending on the results of blood tests and electrocardiograms, etc., he will set about ensuring than no more attacks occur. Prevention depends upon remaining at the optimum weight for one's age, taking regular daily exercise in the form of walking or such excuses for walking as golf, and reduction in the intake of animal fats; anticoagulant drugs may be used under supervision.

Corpus Luteum: the mass of cells which fills the follicle in in the ovary when the ovum itself has been expelled. In pregnancy it persists and produces the hormone progesterone (*see* Endocrine Glands).

Corticotrophin: (*see* A.C.T.H.).

Cortisone: was isolated from the cortex of the adrenal glands in 1936 at the Mayo Clinic but was not commercially available until about 1949 when it was shown to have a dramatic but brief effect on cases of rheumatoid arthritis. Broadly speaking, cortisone or its activator A.C.T.H. (q.v.) has an effect in preventing the proliferation of the connective tissues which are those mainly affected in rheumatism, and in suppressing the similar changes which take place in inflammation and allergy. Therefore it is mainly used in the treatment of the rheumatic diseases, allergic manifestations, e.g. of the skin, and in unnecessary inflammation. It is also, of course, given where the suprarenal glands are diseased or have been removed by operation. In ulcers, although soothing, it has the bad effect of slowing-down the healing process.

Coryza: (*see* Colds).

Counter-irritants: (*see* Blisters).

Cow-pox: the disease of cows' udders with which one is infected in vaccination as a protection against smallpox. It is probably a modified version of the human disease.

Coxalgia, Coxa Vara: the former means pain in the hip-joint, the latter is a bending outwards of the thighs causing lameness.

Coxsackie Viruses: a group of viruses originally isolated from the throats of two patients with symptoms resembling poliomyelitis in the village of that name in New York State. Sixteen or more types have now been isolated which are divided into two groups: group A which appear to be concerned with throat infections and group B from patients with Bornholm disease (q.v.).

Cramp: a painful spasmodic contraction of the muscles either in the limbs or in certain internal organs (when it is usually described as 'colic'). Ordinary cramp may occur in anyone, usually in the calves of the legs and often at night; its cause is a temporary interruption in the blood-supply to the muscles and the odd attack can be ignored as it is universal. If cramps occur frequently, the doctor's advice should be sought as it is possible that some disease of the arteries is present and treatment may be necessary. The treatment in ordinary cases is to give vasodilator drugs, the classical one of which is quinine, but many more efficient ones have been discovered since and these, taken at night, usually stop the cramps instantly. The cramp of swimmers arises from the same cause, aggravated in this case by anything that temporarily removes blood from the muscles, i.e. the cold water, exhaustion, and especially the taking of too much food before swimming which draws blood to the digestive organs and therefore away from the limbs. (Colic in the internal organs is dealt with under that heading). The *occupational cramps* are quite a different matter and occur in those who do work where repetitive and fairly delicate movements of the fingers are necessary: they affect classically writers (as in 'writer's cramp') but also telegraphists, cotton twisters, tailors, drapers, seamstresses, sailmakers, knitters, hairdressers, ironers, metal workers, turners, diamond cutters, pianists, typists, violinists and every kind of musician and, indeed, every kind of work in which too much repetition may lead to boredom. It is typical of these cramps (*a*) that they prevent the individual doing his work, (*b*) that no organic or bodily disease has ever been found, and (*c*) that they rarely prevent the sufferer from doing anything else, e.g. the man with writer's cramp is quite able to eat his meals and use his fork and knife (which makes use of the same muscles) unless he has taken as much distaste to his food as he has to his job. In other words, these cramps are purely psychological and can be dealt with either by a holiday from work (against which the unconscious mind is so busily rebelling), or by self-realisation with or without psychotherapy. The only physical disorders which are associated with cramps are those in which the arteries of the limbs or their nervous control is affected (*see* Arteries, Diseases of) and those in which there has been excessive loss of salts from the body (Heat-stroke, Cholera, etc.).

Crisis: apart from its ordinary use implying a state of emergency, the word may be used to mean (*a*) a sudden paroxysm of pain in certain diseases, e.g. 'tabetic crisis' in tabes dorsalis, (*b*) the condition in lobar pneumonia and some other diseases which, if allowed to run their course, resolve suddenly by a rapid fall of temperature to normal, in this case about the eighth day. Naturally, since the introduction of the sulpha drugs and the antibiotics, the crisis is rarely seen.

Croup: a popular word not generally used in medicine which applies to any condition in which there is difficulty in taking in breath, usually in infants and children. The cause is any disease affecting the larynx and narrowing its entry, whether inflammatory (as in acute laryngitis, diptheria in the area) or due to spasm (laryngismus stridulosa). The latter condition is not very common in these days since it is a manifestation of rickets. Occasionally in congenital laryngeal stridor the difficulty of inspiration may be present from birth and is probably caused by nervous incoordination. All of these states require early medical attention.

Crural: connected with the leg.

Crush Syndrome: a type of injury first discovered in 1941 during the air-raids in Britain when it was noted that injuries caused by, e.g. falling masonry, in which crushing of muscular tissues played a large part, were often followed by chemical damage to the kidneys from absorption of toxic products of cellular break-down. In the syndrome blood-pressure falls with a decrease in the blood volume, the blood urea and potassium rise, and death (if it occurs) happens from renal failure.

Crymotherapy: treatment by refrigeration used either in the form of *hypothermia* (q.v.) where the need of the tissues for oxygen, particularly in the heart and brain, is reduced by freezing during surgical operations to make prolonged surgery possible, or *refrigeration anaesthesia* where a gangrenous limb is kept at a temperature of 5 degrees Centigrade for 1–5 hours in order to lessen the risk of infection and shock. In cases due to gangrene in diabetics or arterial disease this is done by packing the limb with ice-bags.

Cupping: a technique once, but no longer popular, in which diseases characterised by congestion of underlying tissues, e.g. the kidneys in acute nephritis, or heart disease, pneumonia and bronchitis, were treated by the application of a special cup which drew blood to the surface. This was done by putting a piece of cotton-wool soaked in methylated spirits and lighted over the area, when a vacuum was created which brought blood to just beneath the skin and away from the affected tissues. In 'wet cupping' the skin was first scratched with a scalpel to increase the withdrawal of blood and lymph.

Curare: a drug obtained from the juice of certain trees and used by the South American Indians for poisoning their arrow-tips. The active principle is d-tubocurarine which deadens the nerve-endings in muscle causing universal paralysis with complete retention of consciousness. Since the general effect is to produce great relaxation of the body muscles and this is very important to the surgeon during an operation it is used for this purpose also enabling smaller amounts of anaesthetic to be given; it is used too in the treatment of certain diseases characterised by muscle spasm (spastic paralysis), and in psychiatry prior to convulsant therapy (E.C.T., q.v.). This reduces the risk of fractures which sometimes occurred during the fit which is deliberately induced in the treatment of certain mental illnesses.

Curette: a spoon-shaped instrument used in surgery for scooping out the contents of a cavity when this is necessary, as in curettage of the womb.

Cushing's Syndrome: one type of reaction to disease of the anterior lobe of the pituitary gland at the base of the brain. It occurs usually in the younger age-groups and is characterised by excessive tallness in men and shortness in females, high blood-pressure with sugar in the urine and sexual defects (impotence or amenorrhea), there is excess of fat on the face and trunk but not the limbs, excessive hairiness of the body, and red lines or striae on the lower abdomen and thighs. The cause is an adenoma (q.v.) of the anterior lobe which, as in most pituitary swellings, may be associated with defects of vision. Cushing was an American surgeon who described the condition.

Cyanides: are salts of hydrocyanic acid (prussic acid) the active principle of oil of bitter almonds, although not commercially obtained from this source. They were formerly employed in medicine as antiseptics or in high dilution as sedatives but are little used now; being one of the most deadly and rapidly-acting poisons known, prussic acid or cyanide was used in the capsules issued during the war to those who might find suicide preferable to capture, e.g. those likely to be tortured or accused of war-crimes.

Cyanocobalamin: the approved name for vitamin B12, isolated from liver in 1948, and used in the treatment of pernicious anaemia. It is now mainly obtained as a by-product of the production of streptomycin. Although available in liquid and tablet form for use in vitamin deficiencies and (wrongly) as a 'tonic' for children, it is not in these forms suitable for treating pernicious anaemia when it must be given by injection. (Proprietary names 'Cytacon,' 'Cytamen,' etc.).

Cyanosis: blueness of the skin appearing when the blood is not properly oxygenated in the lungs as may occur when the lungs are diseased or when there is a local or general defect in the circulation of the blood.

Cyclopropane: a modern anaesthetic gas (*see* Anaesthetics).

Cystitis: inflammation of the urinary bladder (*see* Bladder, Urinary).

Cystoscope: (*see* Bladder, Urinary).

Cysts: are hollow swellings containing fluid. They may be (*a*) retention cysts, as when a space normally containing fluid with a duct to the exterior (e.g. the glands in the breast) develops a blocked duct and the fluid being retained causes a hard lump; (*b*) developmental cysts, usually in the ovary or kidney, are due to some unknown cause which shuts off particular groups of cells in the course of development with the result that at a later stage they may proliferate and sometimes produce fluid; (*c*) hydatid cysts are produced, mainly in the liver or brain, by the larval stage of a tapeworm (*see* Worms); (*d*) cysts may appear in hard tumours of any sort when the breakdown of tissue inside leads to fluid formation. Some cysts are best removed surgically, others can be dealt with by aspiration (i.e. drawing-off the fluid). The diagnosis, of course, is a medical matter.

Dacryocystitis: inflammation of the tear-sac at the inner and upper angle of the eye nearest the nose where it causes a swelling. The duct of the tear-sac communicates with the inside of the nose whence excess tears are normally drained (hence in crying we usually sniff), and any infection spreading up from the nose or down from the eye may block the duct causing inflammation. The condition may appear only once or become repetitive and treatment depends on the circumstances; in simple cases hot bathing and antiseptic eye-lotions usually suffice otherwise a physician should be seen.

D.A.H.: means 'disordered action of the heart' as it was described during the First World War or 'effort syndrome' as it was described during the Second. The condition is described under Effort Syndrome.

Dandruff: (*see* Seborrhea, Baldness).

Dapsone: a modern drug effectively used in the treatment of leprosy.

D.D.T.: with a complex chemical formula is officially known as dicophane. Its use is now so universal in destroying insect pests that few people realise that it was first synthesised in 1874 although it was not until 1940 that its value as an insecticide was discovered by the Swiss. It became an extremely important feature in the war and post-war years when there can be no doubt that it played a major part in preventing outbreaks of typhus spread by the louse which it readily destroys. It is also effective against a wide range of other insects such as the mosquitoes which carry malaria, the house-fly, fleas, moths, bed-bugs, and agricultural pests. Unfortunately, its efficiency is part of its danger because (1) it kills harmless and even useful insects like bees, and (2) in killing both good and bad ones on such a vast scale it is prone to upset the balance of nature. For practical purposes D.D.T. is not poisonous to human beings and large amounts have been swallowed experimentally without harmful results; however it is said to be more poisonous to domestic animals on which it is used to kill parasites especially if used in the form of an oily suspension which the animal may lick off its skin. It is generally used as a 5% dust or spray.

Deafness: is usually, but not always, associated with localised disease in the ear which is divided into three parts: the outer middle ear, and inner ear. The former extends from the outside to the ear-drum and is about $1\frac{1}{2}$ inches in length; since the only connection it has with hearing is to remain open so that sounds may pass to the ear-drum, the one type of deafness associated with the outer ear is that caused by blockage which may be from a boil (in which case there will probably be severe pain), a polypus or other kind of lump, sometimes skin irritation of the lining due to infection or allergy which causes closure by swelling, in children the insertion of beads or peas, and most commonly a plug of wax. The middle ear lies between the inner ear and the ear-drum, but its most important connections so far as disease is concerned are with the mastoid antrum, the spongy bone behind the ear, and, through the Eustacian tube, with the throat. The function of the tube is to keep the air-pressure within the ear equal to that in the surrounding atmosphere, hence gunners are advised to keep the mouth open when a heavy gun is being fired to prevent the ear-drum being ruptured by a sudden increase of pressure through the outer ear, and the temporary deafness noticed when descending quickly in an aeroplane which is dispelled by 'blowing' whilst holding the nostrils closed thus forcing air up the Eustacian tube. The tube is liable to become infected from disease of the throat or nose and this may spread to the middle ear and then to the mastoid antrum. Slight temporary deafness is common during colds in the head and mild fevers, and in chronic or acute tonsillitis infection may spread to the middle ear causing otitis media so that the space becomes filled with pus, causing great pain from tension and sometimes rupture of the ear-drum with discharge coming from the outer ear. Disease of the antrum can be spread from the middle ear, or the infection may be in the reverse dirction, but in any case such suppurative conditions can cause permanent damage in the middle ear by damaging the three tiny bones which transmit the impulse from the ear-drum to the inner ear. Perforation of the ear-drum, however, which may be caused by sudden loud explosions or a blow on the outer ear does not in itself lead to any hearing defect and when pus is accumulating in the middle ear the usual procedure is to slit the eardrum to let it out before it does permanent damage to the bones transmitting the impulse or spreads to the mastoid antrum. Middle ear deafness and chronic ear-discharge usually go with a history of sore throats and adenoids or tonsillitis. It is typical of this type of deafness that hearing is often better when there is a background of loud noise, e.g. traffic noises, the noise of a train, etc. Infection of the middle ear should be treated by a doctor and in the acute stage its symptoms are those of a fever with more or less severe earache. Pain and swelling behind the ear associated with fever are signs of infection of the mastoid antrum. Those who are aware of having a perforated ear-drum should be very careful of having their ears syringed for wax, but it is safe enough to use oils such as the proprietary 'Cerumol' or hydrogen peroxide drops to loosen the wax which may then come out without the need for syringing. Olive oil, although often used, and quite in order when warmed as a treatment for earache, is too thick for removing wax and thinner oils are preferable. The inner ear is the part where hearing impulses collected by the outer ear and transmitted through the middle ear are received by the nerve to be passed on to the brain; it also contains the balancing equipment for orientating the body in space. Disease and deafness in this part is caused by such fevers as typhus and typhoid, meningitis and mumps, by injuries such as fractures of the base of the skull, occasionally tumours of the brain which interrupt the hearing pathways, and Menière's disease of the balancing apparatus. In some trades persistent and especially high-pitched sounds may cause deafness within the range of the noise (boilermaker's deafness), and drugs such as quinine or salicylates can cause temporary nerve deafness. Sometimes deafness is hereditary (otosclerosis). Advice about hearing-aids can be obtained from the National Institute for the Deaf, 105 Gower Street, London, W.C.1, who also advise on other matters relating to the problem. Help in this respect is particularly important as each person has different requirements. Operative treatment helps types of deafness (*see* Fenestration, Mastoiditis).

Debility: or weakness is a symptom of many diseases or none at all. From the strictly medical point of view the two diseases in which debility is a striking factor are certain types of pulmonary tuberculosis and cases of Addison's disease (q.v.) or pernicious anaemia (q.v.). These are comparatively rare compared with the number of people who complain of debility or the number of patent medicines which mention the word on their wrappings. Scientifically speaking, it is clear that anyone who feels weak is either (*a*) suffering from some specific illness which must be diagnosed and treated appropriately or (*b*) simply 'feels' weak without any specific organic disease being present. In the latter, which forms probably the large bulk of cases in this country, the real cause is the withdrawal of interest from one's surroundings or one's person typical of many neurotic conditions. It is notable that those who may be extremely ill with a serious physical disease do not, on the whole, frequently complain of weakness as a main symptom. However, when one is feeling ill in a non-specific way (which is what debility usually means) it is important to have a proper medical check-up before resorting to 'tonics' which are for the most part valueless (*see* Tonics) and there is not the slightest use in treating 'anaemia' which has not been proved to exist or 'feeding' nerves which do not need to be fed since psychological troubles are unrelated to undernutrition of the physical nerves of the body.

Decapsulation: an operation performed upon the kidney which is stripped of its capsule in order that it may expand and its blood-supply be improved in certain types of nephritis (*see* Nephritis).

Decholin: or dehydrocholic acid is obtained from bile salts and used as a cholagogue (q.v.); at one time it was thought to be of value in *expelling* (not *dissolving*) gall-stones, and it may do this when they are very small.

Delhi Boil: also known as Dermal Leishmaniasis, Oriental sore, Baghdad sore, or Aleppo sore. It is caused by Leishmania tropica, a protozoon which is carried by sand-flies and takes the form of ulcers on the skin and mucous membranes; it is also found in S. America. Treatment is with a short course of injections with antimony tartrate as in kala-azar (q.v.).

Delta Waves: the name given to certain abnormal waves found in electroencephalography (q.v.). They may indicate a mass in the brain or some forms of epilepsy.

Delusions: are false beliefs or judgments usually thought to be associated with serious mental illness. However, a little thought will make it evident that we should be very cautious in ascribing them to this cause even if it is true that they do so occur, e.g. a person may exaggerate the significance of a true belief (such as that his body-odour is objectionable) by supposing that everyone notices it (which may not be true at all) without being legally or medically insane because we all tend to exaggerate certain of our feelings when mildly depressed. Similarly, a delusion must be taken in its social and cultural context, e.g. a native of East Africa who thinks that he is being poisoned by a witch-doctor may have a belief which, although untrue, is quite usual in the circumstances, whereas a European with a good education who thought the same would probably be deluded in the sense of being mentally ill. Yet there are people who believe the earth to be flat; the fact that they have formed a society to propagate this belief is, on the whole, a sign of relative normality since insane people do not ordinarily form societies. Delusions should not be confused with hallucinations which are not false *beliefs* but false *sense-impressions*, i.e. seeing, hearing, feeling, or more rarely smelling, what is not there. But even here other factors must be taken into account such as the individual's beliefs and cultural background (*see* Hallucinations, Mental Illness).

Dementia: is a symptom in mental illness the typical feature of

147

which is regression, i.e. a return to more primitive forms of behaviour. It occurs in serious physical diseases of the brain where a large number of nerve-cells are destroyed by inadequate blood supply, toxins, or primary degeneration (e.g. chronic alcoholism and drug addictions, syphilis and other infections of the brain, arteriosclerosis); in old age to varying degrees; in the delirium of fevers; and in the functional psychoses such as schizophrenia. Its main features are poor memory, rambling talk, indifference to the feelings of others or unawareness of their disapproval of certain behaviour, sometimes incontinence of urine and faeces – 'second childishness and mere oblivion' as Shakespeare described it. The outlook depends upon the cause, since the functional psychoses sometimes recover with treatment and temporary states of delirium recover with their accompanying disease, whereas in old age and long-drawn-out physical disorders of the brain where structural changes to the arteries or nerve-cells have occurred the outlook is poor (*see* Mental Illness).

Dengue: also known as breakbone fever, dandy fever, and three-day fever is an unpleasant but not serious disease caused by a virus spread by the mosquito Culex Aegypti and found in the Mediterranean countries especially in the Middle East, in Africa, South America and the West Indies, and in New South Wales and some of the Pacific Islands. It closely resembles influenza with fever and aching in the back and limbs but in other respects it is like measles with a rash on the third day accompanied by redness of the eyes as in that disease. There is no specific treatment and no complications save occasional swelling of the joints; aspirin is the main standby.

Depression: (*see* Mental Illness).

Dermabrasion: a method of scraping off the superficial layers of the skin to remove surface deformities as, e.g. tattoo marks or the scars of chronic acne.

Dermatitis: like the word 'eczema' dermatitis, in spite of the dread significance often attached to it in industry and elsewhere, is not the name of any specific disease but merely means 'inflammation of the skin' and strictly speaking any skin disease could properly (if not very meaningfully) be given the title. Yet many doctors must have had the experience of writing a name such as 'flexural eczema' (which, if it is not a disease entity either, at least describes the location of the rash) on a certificate only to be practically accused of trying to do the patient out of the compensation which he proposes to claim for 'industrial dermatitis.' It must be repeated that the word is a general one, like 'fever', and that 'industrial dermatitis' is in practice a rash allegedly arising at work although no more *necessarily* caused by the work than a cold caught in the army would be a 'military cold.'

Dermographia: a symptom found in hysteria and certain allergic states where 'writing' on the skin with one's fingernail leaves the written word or mark imprinted on the skin in the form of raised weals caused by an over-active secretion of histamine from the capillaries. It is probably connected with various 'miracles' in which the stigmata of the cross or the raised circle on the forehead of the Buddha are simulated in those who have long meditated on them or the fact that these can be produced under hypnosis.

Diabetes: a word referring to two separate conditions: (1) diabetes insipidus, and (2) diabetes mellitus, the latter being what is usually understood by the term. *Diabetes insipidus* is a rather rare disease in which a constant sense of thirst is accompanied by the passing of large amounts of urine, which, apart from being dilute, is otherwise normal. It is caused by diseases which interfere with the production of an antidiuretic hormone normally produced by the posterior part of the pituitary gland at the base of the brain. In some cases this is hereditary but in others such conditions as tumours, inflammation, or syphilis at the base of the brain can bring it about and in these the treatment obviously depends upon the underlying cause. In the simple types pituitary extract is either injected or given in the form of snuff. *Diabetes Mellitus* or ordinary diabetes is caused by a disorder of the pancreas which fails to secrete insulin, the hormone which makes it possible for the body to utilise sugar and therefore the unused sugar accumulates in the blood until the excess overflows into the urine to be excreted. Various symptoms may draw attention to the disorder, and because all of these can be found in other diseases their presence or absence can only suggest the possibility of diabetes which is diagnosed with certainty by blood and urine tests alone; amongst them are, general weakness, loss of weight and wasting, irritation of

149

the area around the genital organs with which the urine may come into contact, pains in the legs, numbers of boils or carbuncles, constipation, gangrene of a toe, relatively sudden failure of eyesight, and impotence. But *no single one of these can be taken as a definite sign of diabetes* and, even if all were present, it would still be far from proving the nature of the case. However, the continuing presence of any one should be regarded as an indication for having the urine tested. Diabetes is a more serious disease in younger people whilst in the aged it is less dramatic. The complications in untreated or inadequately treated diabetes are: coma, frequent sepsis, gangrene, cataract and other eye diseases, and neuritis, but coma may be caused by too much as well as too little insulin. The treatment of diabetes is a matter for skilled advice (e.g. even the presence of sugar in the urine does not always indicate the presence of the disease) and testing which may be followed by treatment with diet alone, treatment by diet and various types of insulin administered at the times found most appropriate, or in a few cases especially of the older or mild types, treatment with tolbutamide ('Rastinon,' etc.) which is taken by mouth. The nature of the defect in the pancreas which causes diabetes is unknown for the Islets of Langerhans which secrete insulin are not always noticeably damaged.

Diaphoretics: remedies which promote perspiration such as hot baths, the taking of spirits, and the use of aspirin as taken ordinarily in the treatment of a cold. Many other methods and drugs produce this effect: hot packs, tepid bathing, phenacetin, quinine, Dover's powders, ipecacuanha, etc., but, although there is no harm in taking these measures, nobody today finds any special virtue in producing perspiration which is generally a *sign* of a temperature coming down rather than its *cause*, even if there were also a case for reducing temperature which, apart from heat-stroke or delirium, there is not.

Diarrhoea: diarrhoea means looseness of the bowels, i.e. both of the consistency of the motions and their frequency. It can be either an extremely serious symptom or a relatively trivial one which may exist in the total absence of any disease in nervous individuals. But although diarrhoea may be nervous in origin it is advisable to regard most cases as infections and if some are due to indiscretions of eating (as in the frequently-mentioned 'collywobbles' after eating green apples) there are very few people nowadays who seriously believe that the weather or heat has much significance in this respect in temperate climates. Weather, of course, can often have an indirect effect, in that hot weather allows germs to multiply in food, but in itself is irrelevant. In infants gastro-enteritis (diarrhoea accompanied by vomiting and fever) is common when hygiene is neglected and should always receive immediate medical attention as it may be serious and children who lose fluids very quickly become dehydrated and really ill. The causes of 'summer diarrhoea' are in general those associated with contamination of food, and various germs may be found such as the Sonné bacillus and others. Treatment depends on the doctor but may be symptomatic such as the use of kaolin and morphine or chalk and opium to stop the diarrhoea and relieve the colic, or sulpha drugs or antibiotics may be used in the more serious cases. In adult diarrhoea, the same drugs either separately or together may be given but in this country there is less cause to worry about those beyond the stage of infancy during the 'summer diarrhoea,' although a less frequent cause of death than it was, is still more frequent than it should be. Tropical diseases cannot be discussed here and typhoid is relatively uncommon, but in those who have been abroad and occasionally those who have not, dysentery, cholera, and other causes of diarrhoea have to be considered. Nervous diarrhoea is, as mentioned already, not particularly uncommon and nervous colic without diarrhoea is quite frequent; in these cases no pathological organisms are found in the motions, there may be no vomiting, the emotional cause is usually fairly obvious, and there is unlikely to be fever. Chronic or periodic diarrhoea occurs in colitis (q.v.) and the frequent use of strong purgatives produces the same result since many lead to the after-effect of constipation which is then 'treated' with a further dose. Indeed, castor oil used to be employed for this reason since its purging effect in diarrhoea was followed by constipation for which the patient was by this time grateful. Bulky, offensive, motions are passed frequently in coeliac disease (q.v.). The various forms of diarrhoea suffered by Britons on arriving in Mediterrainean countries or the East are frequently attributed to the 'rich food' that is supposedly typical of these lands but most cases are due to food contamination to which the local populace has become inured (*see* Dysentery, etc., Food-poisoning).

Diastase: an enzyme found in malt which is capable of converting starches into sugars. 'Taka-diastase' is a proprietary preparation of this designed 'for the treatment of amylaceous dyspepsia, flatulence, and hyperacidity' and its value depends upon whether we believe that a condition exists in which starches in particular are poorly digested and that flatulence has some connection with this. Since most authorities today believe that flatulence of the stomach is a neurosis produced by swallowing air and 'amylaceous dyspepsia' is not a term in general use, it is unlikely that diastase is particularly helpful in dealing with them.

Diathermy: is a method of physiotherapy employing electricity which (1) is used in order to create heat in the deeper layers of the body tissues, and (2) in another form destroys warts, tumours of the various sorts, and diseased areas bloodlessly.

Dick Test: a test for discovering the individual's susceptibility to scarlet fever (e.g. in the case of contacts) by injecting a small amount of scarlet fever streptococcal toxin into the skin and comparing the result with a similar amount of a control heated toxin. The test is positive in about 90% of cases in the first three days of the illness and becomes negative in about ten days.

Dicoumarol: (*see* Anticoagulants).

Diet: food is one of those things we either accept as being simply a part of living which may be arranged pleasantly or unpleasantly or, on the other hand, as a matter of the utmost importance (which it is) containing the key to all disease and health (which it does not). It may be said at once that a normal individual taking the kind of food in the kind of quantities usual in western Europe has no need to think about his food except for the reason that, as he gets older, he may have to reduce its amount, and the view is also expressed here that dietetics except of the most ordinary and common-sense kind plays little part in the treatment of disease. It would be difficult to think of more than half-a-dozen or so important diseases which need dietetic advice of any specialised sort and it would take a psychoanalyst to analyse why so many people think otherwise and evidently believe that an endless number of diseases and the maintenance of health itself depend upon diet or why they accept totally unverified statements from a series of dieticians ranging from Dr Hay to Mr Gaylord Hauser and the gentleman who tells us that most ailments can be cured by the administration of cider (or is it cider vinegar?) and honey – i.e. by a mixture of acetic acid and sugar. Like some people's attitude to constipation, these attitudes are not based on objective study but on primitive emotional reactions dating from early childhood. We symbolically take in love with our mother's milk, so, as is now fairly generally recognised, emotionally starved people are the ones who overeat; we feel as babies that something 'bad' (really our own bad feelings) is shut up inside us and this is later equated with constipation which also is thought of as something 'bad' inside. We repress our aggressiveness and become superficially gentle so some of us must become vegetarians to prove that we are not blood-thirsty. These are some of the conflicts which rage around the background of people's minds when they talk about food although it is a matter perfectly susceptible to scientific study. The non-scientific attitude is well illustrated by the remarks made to a medical committee by a presiding layman who announced that his cure for a cold was to starve himself for three days and eat nothing but grape-fruit three times a day. When it was pointed out to him that he could have obtained 10–100 times the amount of vitamin C in the more concentrated form of tablets, he was quite annoyed yet it is obvious that he was making a number of absurd claims: (1) that he alone had discovered the cure for a cold, a cure which, incidentally, happens to have no rationale; (2) that grape-fruit, and not oranges or lemons which also contain vitamin C, was a necessity for the cure thereby implying either that vitamin C was not the curing agent, that it took a different form in the other fruits and in the pills, or that a mysterious 'something else' undiscovered by chemists and capable of curing colds lurked in the grape-fruit; (3) that feeling better is a criterion of cure in a disease when it has been known from the earliest times that entirely inert substances (such as the 'tonics' given with such good effect by doctors) can make people feel better and even cure them if they have sufficient

153

confidence; (4) that colds, apart from complications, last longer than three days when they do not. Most of the fad diets that people go in for have no firmer basis than this: they simply state that a certain food is better without saying why or without saying so in a way that science can accept and they assume that feeling better is the same as being better. We need have no doubt that many business men and professional men would be the better of a couple of weeks on nothing but orange juice – but why orange juice rather than water? If the answer is that oranges contain sugar, then by all means give him sugar and water; if it is that they contain vitamin C then one has to ask, why bother about vitamin C and not vitamins A, B, and D? It is not that a diet of this sort may not do good, it is that the good is done in an unscientific way and because one would not attract so many wealthy business men if you said that the diet was tea without sugar or milk or tea and a little sugar. Similarly with Hauser's 'black-strap' molasses, the old country doctor's cider, vinegar and honey, the Queen-bee jelly or Royal jelly (or is that something for rubbing on one's head?). If they are not sheer humbug, then it is up to the deviser to show why in a way which does not simply involve saying that people felt better since there is not a manufacturer of patent medicine who could not say as much. For present purposes we shall say as briefly as possible what is known about diet, the facts which can be proved or disproved.

In order to be adequate any diet must first of all supply enough energy and energy is measured in calories (q.v.). Thus a ten-stone man leading a moderately active life will require about 3,000 calories daily in order to avoid living on his stored-up food. The number of calories needed varies with age, size, and the amount of work done, from 1,500 calories for the light-weight sedentary worker to three or more times that amount for the heavy manual worker. Now, in theory, this could be supplied by sugar, starch, or fats alone since calories are merely a measure of energy which could be supplied by any food. But, in practice, an individual who tried to do so would not live long because he needs for body maintenance certain kinds of food in correct proportions. Just as one cannot run a car on petrol alone whilst ignoring lubricating oil and engine maintenance or water for the cooling system, so the body cannot be run simply by taking in calories. There must be adequate quantities of the three basic food-stuffs: carbohydrates which are sugars and starches (the fuel), fats and oils (for insulation and other purposes), and proteins (for body-building purposes). Proteins are necessary to replace the parts of the body when they become run-down, and whereas fats and sugars can be transformed into each other as the obesity produced by eating too many sweets shows, protein, which contains the elements of nitrogen absent in the others, can not. We could live on a diet of protein but not on a purely fat or carbohydrate one, and in this country the average man or woman eats a diet which consists of one part of fat, one of protein, and three of carbohydrate; this is partly conditioned by economic factors, since fat and protein are relatively dear whilst carbohydrates are relatively cheap, a rule which, by and large, is true all over the world. The following foods are classified according to the predominating basic foodstuff they contain:

(1) **Carbohydrates:** bread, sugar, and all starchy or sweet things such as confectionery, pastries (which are also rich in fat), puddings either of the sponge or custard variety, cakes, and certain fruits such as bananas or root vegetables such as potatoes, swedes, parsnips, and carrots.

(2) **Fats:** animal fats such as fat meat, lard, dripping, anything fried, and butter or anything containing it; vegetable or fish oils such as margarine, olive oil, peanut butter, nuts and olives, certain fish which contain more fat than others, e.g. herring in its various forms.

(3) **Proteins:** lean meat, cheese, steamed, boiled or grilled fish, eggs, oatmeal, and to some extent milk and wholemeal or crispbreads. Most fruits do not contain any significant amount of protein but they do contain upwards of 90% of water with vitamins and a little sugar; they are therefore not usually excessively fattening.

In addition to these basic foods the body requires vitamins in proper amounts (unless an actual deficiency exists which is comparatively rarely vitamins taken over and above the normal amounts in the food have no effect), and certain minerals such as iron, manganese, calcium, copper, sodium, and potassium. Water, of course, is also necessary, but it is rubbish to suppose that large amounts have any special virtue in 'cleaning out the inside' since no such process exists although it is true that constipation can be caused by taking too little water. On the other hand, too much water retained in the tissues can cause people to be overweight and look fatter than they are. So far as one knows these are the essentials of a balanced diet and in what form the substances are taken does not seem to matter, even if there is some evidence that vegetable and fish oils may be safer than animal fats, since on the other hand vegetarians who are strictly vegetarian are likely to have difficulty in obtaining adequate supplies of protein, which is why cows have to spend all day eating. The conditions for which special diets are *known* to be needed are obesity, gastric or duodenal ulcer, diabetes, coeliac disease and sprue, nephritis, colitis, some of the allergies, and gall-bladder disease; apart from these (and many would doubt whether in all of these it is necessary) diet is not a major factor in medicine although, of course, one could invent a 'fever diet,' a diet for gout, and goodness knows what else if one wanted to when all that is really necessary is to tell the patient to eat or not to eat or drink certain foods (*see* disease diets under the various conditions mentioned here). Finally, many people have emphasised the timing and the technique of eating, at one period to a quite absurd degree since the real reason why we eat at certain times is purely a matter of convenience. There is no medical reason why anyone should eat 'three square meals a day' rather than eat in between mealtimes. On the contrary, if we were really concerned about our digestion (which Heaven forbid!) there is evidence that eating small amounts frequently is precisely what we should do just as the sufferer from a gastric or duodenal ulcer is recommended to see that his stomach is 'never empty, never full.' But like the baby's feeds and hours of sleep, whether they are well or ill-advised, meals are arranged primarily at times to suit convention rather than the individual. Again, it is doubtful whether anyone today is told to take eighteen chews to each bite but the easily observed fact is that some people have dyspepsia and others do not and that the latter can swallow down food in large gobbets without chewing them at all whereas the former will get indigestion, chewing or no chewing, whatever they do. In these matters those who have been granted a reasonably healthy body and a cheerful temperament will follow the advice of the Book of

Ecclesiastes: 'Go thy way, eat thy bread with joy, and drink thy wine with a merry heart;' for this rather than selfish faddism is the way of life for those who are well and wish to remain so.

Digestive System: the digestive system begins at the mouth and ends at the anus where the waste products are excreted. Food taken in at the mouth is moistened by saliva secreted from the salivary glands of which the largest are the parotid glands in front of the ear (the ones affected in mumps) and the smaller the submaxillary (under the angle of the jaw) and the sublingual (under the tongue). Saliva contains an enzyme called ptyalin which, whilst the teeth are cutting and grinding the food into a pulp which can be easily swallowed, mixes with the mass and begins the process of digestion by turning some of the starch into sugars. This process is not of major importance and the main function of saliva is to lubricate the food on its way down. Since the stimulus to the secretion of saliva is basically psychological through the senses of sight, smell, and taste, or even through expectation, the importance of food looking and smelling appetising will be appreciated for without saliva, i.e. when the mouth is completely dry, food cannot be chewed or swallowed. This happens when such emotions as fear, anxiety, or disgust inhibit the flow or when the individual is preoccupied with something else, e.g. reading the papers. The food then passes to the oesophagus whilst a reflex action normally closes the glottis to prevent it finding its way into the windpipe or the lungs; when someone is suffering from certain diseases of the nervous system, is laughing and eating at the same time, or unconscious, the failure of this reflex causes food or drink to 'go down the wrong way' and this is one of the reasons for not giving drink to an unconscious person. The oesophagus is about two feet long and passes the food on to the stomach by a series of rhythmic movements which make it quite possible for someone to drink whilst standing on his head. The gastric juice of the stomach is acid because of the presence of hydrochloric acid which helps the action of the enzymes carrying out the actual process of digestion and, although it is usual to blame an excess of this acid for the various types of dyspepsia and in cases of peptic ulcer the acid content is usually raised, it must be remembered that (a) some people suffer from severe dyspepsia in the total

157

absence of hydrochloric acid, and (*b*) that it is by no means proved that it is the raised acid content which causes pain in ordinary indigestion. Alkalies work as much by relaxing muscular spasm as by neutralising acid and there are drugs such as belladonna which relieve indigestion without affecting the acid content of the stomach. The main enzymes (q.v.) in the gastric juice are pepsin which digests proteins into their constituent parts, and rennin which curdles milk. As the stomach finishes its work, the semi-liquid food is passed through the valve at the end of the stomach known as the pylorus into the duodenum, the beginning of the small intestine, where it comes under the influence of the alkaline intestinal juices with their enzymes and other factors which are: (1) the bile collected from the liver and gall-bladder into the common bile-duct that, together with the duct from the pancreas, enters the duodenum shortly after its beginning where the bile aids in the breakdown of fats; (2) the pancreatic juice which contains the enzymes lipase to break down fats, amylase which completes the digestion of starch, a milk-curdling substance, and trypsin which completes the breakdown of proteins begun in the stomach; (3) the juices secreted from the walls of the intestine itself which help in the breakdown of protein into amino-acids, act upon complex sugars (disaccharides) such as sucrose and maltose to convert them into the monosaccharide glucose, and split fats into fatty acids and glycerin; (4) the bacteria of the small intestine have an action similar to that of the enzymes and break down sugars to some extent into acids, those of the large intestine decompose the residual matter into such products as indole, skatole, cresol, and phenol which gives faeces their characteristic odour. In both small and large intestine they play a major part in synthesising components of the vitamin B complex. Only one substance is absorbed directly from the stomach, i.e. alcohol, but by the time the food has got to the end of the small intestine everything eaten, no matter how complex, has been broken down into a few simple chemicals. The proteins into amino-acids, the fats into fatty acids and glycerin, and the starches and sugars into glucose. It is probably the fact that glucose is the end-product of carbohydrate digestion and therefore easily and rapidly absorbed that has provided its quite unjustified reputation as an energy-provider with some sort of scientific basis. Of course, glucose (q.v.) is absorbed quickly and does supply energy but the fallacy attaching to its use in normal people is that they are not ordinarily suffering from lack of energy but rather from the psychological inability to put their energy to work. The duodenum is about a foot long and continues into the jejunum and ileum which together are about twenty-three feet long. At the end of the ileum the small intestine joins the large intestine or colon whose beginning is situated under the right lower part of the abdomen where lie also the caecum and the appendix. Finally, the five-foot long colon reaching the pelvis joins the rectum which is only six inches long and leads to the anus where waste products are discharged; the main material absorbed in the large intestine is water, hence stasis during this part of the process may lead to dry motions and constipation. In the small intestine, the fatty acids and glycerin enter the lymph channels (*see* Glands) passing from the intestinal walls and thence to the blood-stream where they may move to the fat-deposits in the body, but the amino-acids and glucose pass through the portal system of veins (*see* Circulatory System) to the liver to be stored for later use, the glucose in the form of glycogen or animal starch (*see* the various parts of the system under their individual names and the individual disorders similarly listed).

Digitalis: is the leaf of the wild foxglove (Digitalis purpurea) gathered at a particular time, dried and powdered, to be used in various forms in the treatment of heart disease. The preparations used today are either standardised tinctures (i.e. alcoholic solutions) or the pure substance known as digoxin (proprietary names, Digitaline Granules, Crystodigin, Lanoxin) since in the case of the natural leaf one could not be sure of the dose being given. From the strictly scientific point of view digitalis (and the similarly-acting drugs strophanthus, squill, and ouabain) has an action which is almost specific in certain types of heart disease, but is not something to give automatically in all cases. Digitalis and the other rather rarely used drugs are useful only if given in the correct conditions and in the correct way; the correct conditions being disorders of the heart's beat, e.g. auricular fibrillation or auricular flutter, and less significantly congestive heart failure. The correct way is to give enough, under observation, to produce the desired effect but the mere automatic prescribing of a minute

159

dose in all cases of heart disease is not enough. Digitalis acts by influencing the nerves to the heart or in the heart in such a way as to block abnormal impulses and it is a complete waste of time to give it in conditions other than those mentioned.

Dill: is only mentioned because it is doubtless still being given for various complaints of infancy which, so far as one hears, include those of the whole digestive tract. Dill is pleasant with pickled cucumbers for adults and, unless children have a taste for pickled cucumbers, it is not known to have any other useful applications.

Diphtheria: this disease represents one of the many triumphs of bacteriology because, although once one of the great killers of childhood, its cause has been found and immunisation against it has produced dramatic effects (in spite of the efforts of antivivisectionists and G. B. Shaw). The infection used to be extremely common in childhood mainly between the second and the fifth year and is spread by coughing, sneezing, kissing, or objects which have been handled by an infected person; the incubation period is 2–8 days, and carriers who carry the germs (the Klebs-Loeffler bacillus) without suffering from the disease may play a large part in its dissemination. Immunity conferred by an attack is short-lived and subsequent attacks are by no means uncommon. The quarantine period is ten days. The symptoms of diphtheria arise primarily from the absorption of toxins produced in one particular area affected which may be the throat, the nose, the larynx, and in rare cases the eye, the genitals, or wounds as in the case of 'desert sores.' Since absorption of poisons is the main method of attack, the mere destruction of bacteria, unless done at a very early stage, is not the major concern and penicillin which kills the germs can do nothing to the toxins to which the devastating symptoms are due. These are: sore throat, typically a blood-stained nasal discharge, swollen glands under the neck, and later extreme difficulty in breathing with enlargement of the neck. The most usual sign is a greyish-white membrane in the throat which bleeds when touched, but the later complications include neuritis, heart disease with a pulse more rapid than the usually low temperature seems to justify, and various secondary infections of the lungs, ears, and glands. Treatment involves the use of diphtheria antitoxin in appropriate amounts as soon as possible; preventive measures are the giving of toxoid antitoxin (T.A.M. and T.A.F.) or purified toxoid alum phosphate precipitated (P.T.A.P.) of which two injections at four weeks interval are given after the third month of age and maintenance doses at the fifth and tenth years. In view of the danger to the heart complete rest is of great importance in diphtheria.

Diplopia: or double vision is caused by some incoordination of the muscles moving the eyeball which results in the eyes being placed so that the light coming from the observed object does not fall upon corresponding parts of the two retinae. This is brought about by certain organic nervous diseases, bacterial toxins as in diphtheria, fatigue when the eyes are too tired to focus, and the temporary effects of alcohol and other drugs. It is a symptom and therefore treatment must be directed against the cause, but transient diplopia is neither unusual nor is it ordinarily necessary to do anything about it.

Dipsomania: (*see* Alcoholism).

Disinfection: (*see* Antiseptics).

Disinfestation: (*see* D.D.T., Antiseptics).

Disorientation: a symptom in mental disease (whether with or without an organic basis) in which the patient has difficulty in locating himself in space or time.

Disseminated Sclerosis: a disease of the nervous system of unknown cause in which small areas of scarring (sclerosis) where the covering of the nerves has been removed are scattered (disseminated) throughout the brain and spinal cord. The onset is gradual and the young adult who is usually affected may first notice one of a number of apparently unconnected symptoms the diffuse nature of which are obviously related to the nature of the disease: these include, weakness in a leg, numbness or tingling, difficulty in starting to pass urine, sudden loss of vision in a single eye, paralysis of half of the body, i.e. the left or the right side, double vision, or fits. Although the symptoms may lead the family doctor to think of this disease, the certain diagnosis depends upon neurological examination. Rather characteristic is an unduly cheerful attitude of mind which is in contrast with the unpleasantness of the symptoms and it is not uncommon for the condition to be mistaken for a psychological one in which widely diverse symptoms are often present too. Treatment is a matter for the specialist, but the illness may be long drawn-out with apparent

161

remissions in which it seems to disappear. This is one of the reasons for very carefully evaluating what seems to be a cure.

Disulfiram: (*see* Antabuse).

Diuretics: are drugs which increase the flow of urine. This may be necessary when the heart or the kidneys are working inefficiently so that fluid accumulates in the body; in certain liver diseases which produce a similar effect; or in infections of the bladder where a 'washing-out' effect is needed as, e.g. in cystitis. Many drugs produce this effect, but notably (*a*) drugs which increase the blood-flow to, or stimulate, the kidneys such as caffeine, theophylline, aminophyllin, theobromine (Diuretin), and oil of juniper with most of the other essential oils; (*b*) many salts such as potassium citrate and ammonium chloride produce diuresis because, by changing the salt concentration of the blood, they have to be expelled and this can only be done by passing them in a sufficient amount of urine; (*c*) drugs which act by diminishing the process of reabsorption which takes place in the kidneys (q.v.) such as the organic mercurial substances (e.g. Mersalyl); (*d*) the modern diuretics which are considerably more effective than the foregoing and include the various forms of chlorothiazide (Saluric) and hydrochlorothiazide (Hydrosaluric, etc.). In certain types of fluid retention special drugs may be required as in cirrhosis of the liver which does not always respond to the others. Diuretics are also used in reducing weight, since much of the total weight of the body is due to water, and in the treatment of premenstrual tension which in part is due to temporary fluid retention.

Dolichocephalic: long-headed (*see* Brachycephalic).

Douche: theoretically the treatment of any part of the body by a continuous flow of (usually medicated) water. It has been used in the treatment of wounds and burns, in washing-out the bladder or irrigation, and for cleansing the vagina. It is in the latter sense that the word is now almost invariably used. Douching is regarded by most women on the continent as an ordinary and necessary part of female hygiene, but in this country many seem to think of it as unnecessary or even potentially dangerous. In fact, no danger whatever attaches to the procedure and normal women should douche once or twice a week with plain warm water. Disinfectant is unnecessary as the main effect of a douche is a mechanical one removing discharge and dead tissue, but if thought necessary added disinfectant should be of the everyday modern type such as 'Dettol' employed according to the instructions on the label. Special medicated douches for specific conditions may be prescribed by the doctor, but their application is rather limited since most forms of abnormal discharge come from the womb and are obviously not affected by douching and local infections in the vagina are more usually treated by pessaries which keep the medicated material in contact with the infected area for longer periods.

Dover's Powder: a powder composed of potassium sulphate with 10% each of powdered opium and ipecacuanha and once one of the most popular remedies in medicine. It was devised by the pirate Captain Thomas Dover whose main other claim to fame rests upon his rescue of Alexander Selkirk, the original Robinson Crusoe, from his desert island of Juan Fernandez. Used for colds and fevers generally, Dover's powder is quite suitable for pirates; ordinary people may prefer aspirin.

Dramamine: a proprietary drug known officially as dimenhydrinate used for travel sickness and the vomiting of pregnancy.

Drop-Foot: a condition in which there is difficulty in raising the foot which hangs limp from the ankle-joint; it is caused by those circumstances which cause neuritis or by poliomyelitis (in the former case there are disturbances of feeling such as 'pins and needles' or loss of sensation, in the latter there are not). The common causes of neuritis (q.v.) are: injury, diphtheria or typhoid fevers, alcohol, lead poisoning, etc., and vitamin deficiencies. Treatment is a matter for a specialist, although the types due to neuritis tend to pass as the condition causing them is relieved.

Dropsy: technically known as oedema, is an abnormal accumulation of fluid in the body which may be localised (as in some cases of allergy or interference with the local circulation) or general (as in heart, kidney, or liver disease). Oedema occurs most frequently in heart or kidney disease, occasionally in allergy or interference with the local circulation, as in phlebitis, and somewhat rarely here in malnutrition and the anaemias. The treatment is that of the cause, and in general it is true to say that kidney disease causes oedema which is worse in the mornings and is noticed at first beneath the eyes and in

163

the face, whereas in heart disease the swelling tends to be worse in the evenings and begins in the lower parts of the body such as the ankles. In liver disease which is often the result of chronic alcoholism, the swelling is in the legs and abdomen. It should be noted that (*a*) localised oedema with pain is likely to be due to interference with the circulation whilst with itching allergy is likely to be the cause; (*b*) that most normal people as they grow older have some swelling of the ankles during the evenings which is of no significance whatsoever, and in hot weather everybody's ankles are swollen (*see* Angioneurotic oedema, Heart, Diseases of, Nephritis, Cirrhosis, Allergy, Varicose Veins).

Drop-Wrist: (*see* Drop-Foot).

Drug Addiction: for practical purposes addiction means a state in which physical symptoms are produced by stopping the drug. Thus it is possible to stop smoking or drinking tea or coffee, not without wishing that the drugs were there, but without such symptoms as the trembling of the alcoholic, the diarrhoea of the morphine addict, the weakness and depression of the cocaine-taker. Someone who has stopped taking cigarettes or tea may be irritable and nervous, but he can carry on as the alcohol, morphine, or cocaine addict cannot do, because these drugs create a real physical need. What is accepted as a drug of addiction is defined by this physical demand which is something different from the psychological hunger for anything we have got used to (*see* Alcoholism, Cocaine, Morphine, Cannabis Indica). It is possible to become addicted to the strangest drugs, e.g. to chloroform and ether, the benzedrene in inhalers, and opium in the form of chlorodyne in cough medicines. But it is not correct to refer to drugs of addiction when all that one means is that the person is in the habit of taking them and feels uncomfortable without which would imply that a cup of malted milk at night is a form of addiction.

Drugs, their Dangers, and Commercialism: in Britain dangerous drugs, legally defined, are those which are scheduled under the Dangerous Drugs Act. The only three classes relevant so far as medicine is concerned are (1) the drugs of addiction such as opium, heroin, morphine, cocaine, etc., of which a record must be kept by the doctor and his prescription must state the total amount supplied; (2) common poisons such as arsenic not necessarily used for medical purposes saleable to anyone known to the seller provided that the buyer enters his name and address in a book kept for the purpose; (3) drugs such as the barbiturates, sulphonal or tridione, dangerous when misused, for which a prescription is required and, unless specifically stated that they can be repeated a given number of times, must not be supplied on the same prescription more than once. Here, however, we are basically concerned with the problems aroused by modern drugs, their safety or other-wise, but most of all with the vast increase in the production and consumption of what are (perhaps quaintly) known as ethical preparations, i.e. those proprietary drugs prescribed solely by physicians in contrast with the 'patent medicines' which anyone can buy. The ethics of the drug firms have been under suspicion for some time, and amongst the arguments brought against them are the following: (1) they make in-ordinate profits (e.g. in America there were such dollar net increases as 677% in one firm and a phenomenal 2,208% in another over a period of five years, whilst in Britain a well-known company had a trading profit of just over £3 million in 1950 rising to £8.5 million in 1960, and another over the same period had advanced from just over £3 million to nearly £11 million); (2) in Britain the cost of these (and other) drugs caused the drug bill *on practically the same number of NHS prescriptions* to rise from £20 millions in 1950 to £70 millions in 1960 – how many patients realise that the proprietary pills they so casually consume may cost from 2/6 to 5/- or more *each*?; (3) many drug firms advertise their products to doctors in ways which are almost unbelievably importunate, vulgar, and imbecilic (the average doctor gets 'information' at the rate of about a hundredweight yearly which ranges from the reasonably truthful to plain lying) – in the U.S. he gets free golf lessons, duck shooting, and barbecues thrown in; (4) proprietary drugs range from the genuinely useful, the useless but harmless, the useful but dangerous, to the useless, un-necessary, and positively harmful; (5) there is a quite unneces-sary reduplication of drugs under various proprietary names whereby, for example, a preparation of an antibiotic and cortisone or one of its derivatives may appear under more than a dozen different names according to the firm producing it; (6) finally, it is alleged, many firms are so keen to get a

165

drug on the market before their competitors that it is often inadequately tested before being released. Some of these observations have been substantiated beyond doubt. Thus Dr Louis Lasagna, Associate Professor of Medicine and Pharmacology at the great American medical centre, the Johns Hopkins University School of Medicine, says: 'Every year 300 to 400 "new" formulations hit the market, each with an average life span of well under five years. Many of these are merely combinations of old remedies – there are 300 antibiotic preparations on the market, but only a dozen or so useful single antibiotics.' Most advertisements reaching the physician contain references to publications which, it is claimed, show the usefulness of the drug following actual clinical experiment; many of these are genuine references to standard medical journals known to every doctor, but others refer to articles in foreign medical journals often published in countries in which the standard of scientific medicine is, to say the least of it, dubious. Some come from 'personal communications' (i.e. articles not published at all), and in America, some from doctors who do not even exist at all. No secret is made of the fact that drugs are advertised on the same basis as any other commodity. Indeed, a British firm, proudly announces in one of its advertisements in which an imaginary dialogue takes place between a 'man in the street' and a drug manufacturer with the former asking whether the public interest is 'the lodestar of pharmaceutical firms': 'No more than it is for lawyers, say. Apart from such public spirit as we have, and the many controls that affect us, *what we do for the public good is a by-product of what we do for our own private good.*'

Of course, something is to be said for the manufacturers: (1) their apparently excessive gains are said to be necessary in order to carry on further research; (2) many of them have pioneered the way in the great revolution in medical treatment which has arisen with the discovery of the newer antibiotics, cortisone, the tranquillisers and other psychiatric drugs thus changing the whole face of medicine; (3) most drugs put out by reputable firms are very carefully tested, but the ultimate test of safety depends upon their results on human beings which only the doctors themselves can evaluate; (4) good firms do not rely on the vulgar advertising methods described above. Turning now to a consideration of the useful new drugs which have mostly been discovered since the last war and include both the valuable proprietary ones and those, such as chlor-promazine, which have already found their way into the official Pharmacopoeia, it is necessary to make certain points quite clear to the lay reader. Firstly, these are extremely potent preparations which have saved millions of lives (so many, in fact, that their use has played no small part, together with the specific drugs for tropical diseases most of which were discovered rather earlier, in bringing about the population explosion (q.v.), one of the serious problems facing mankind today). Secondly, their potency is often – although, of course, not invariably – accompanied by side-effects which may be dangerous. This does not mean that they should not be used, but it *does* mean that they should not be used lightly. One does not refuse a serious surgical operation if one is almost certain to die without it. Lastly, we should not be misled by early glowing reports of a new drug until it has been subjected to exhaustive clinical trials (in this connection, see the remarks in the Introduction). The thalidomide tragedy of 1962 when thousands of children in Britain and Germany were born without arms or legs was not, in the writer's view, one in which much of the blame can fairly be attributed to the very reliable firms manufacturing the preparation; for here was a drug which, apart from a few cases of neuritis, was used by literally millions of people without any ill-effects as a sedative so safe that would-be suicides who swallowed as many as fifty or more tablets together survived unharmed. Furthermore, the only real damage, terrible as it was, happened to the children of mothers who had taken the drug in the first fifty days of pregnancy and damage to the unborn foetus was something that few had ever foreseen. But it should be a warning. For the injury done to the child seems to have been the result of interference by thalidomide with the absorption or utilisation of the B vitamins, and we already know that certain antibiotics in common use can produce just this effect. They, too, may be dangerous to mothers in early pregnancy. Of course, there is nothing which, in certain amounts, or in certain people, may not be dangerous: water drunk in large quantities can produce intoxication as readily as smaller amounts of alcohol. Aspirin, one of the safest drugs we have, produces minute bowel haemorrhages detectable only on biochemical

167

investigation of the motions in quite a high proportion of people and may be dangerous to those suffering from bowel complaints or peptic ulcer. Tranquillisers, obtainable without a doctor's prescription in some countries, can lead to fits, depression, fainting attacks, and in a minority of cases to serious blood and liver diseases. Penicillin, non-toxic in the largest amounts, can lead to sensitisation by creating an allergy, or even worse in those who have used it too often to the development of resistance so that it is no longer effective, and, lastly, by killing off harmless or 'good' germs, it may allow others which have previously been kept under control to multiply and bring about a new disease.

The solution to this problem is that the patient should always choose a doctor he can implicitly trust and never (unless he has serious grounds for doubt) interfere with his treatment; that he should never try to obtain medicines – even if he regards himself as an important business executive to whom 'time is money' – which are more potent than the complaint for which they are intended justifies (e.g. the useless taking of antibiotics for colds); that he may *ask* his doctor about any drug but should never press to get it against the doctor's better judgement; that, by and large, he should never buy patent medicines at all; and that, if he wants to save his money, he can avoid wasting it on vitamins, glucose preparations, and nerve tonics, which are rarely necessary.

Ductless Glands: (*see* Endocrine Glands).

Dumbness: the primary cause of dumbness is the total inability to hear because a person who is deaf is unable to learn to speak even when his voice mechanism is normal. However, a few cases are due to either defects in voice production or mental defect generally (i.e. the inability to learn from experience). All such cases should be referred to Child Guidance Clinics to discover whether the condition is due to deafness, problems of speaking, or dullness of intellect. The treatment will depend upon the cause.

Duodenal Ulcer: (*see* Stomach Diseases).

Duodenum: (*see* Digestive system).

Dupuytren's Contracture: (*see* Claw-hand), a condition in which the fibrous tissue of the palm contracts with subsequent bending of the fingers beginning with the small and ring fingers. It may arise from pressure of a tool in the palm of the hand but generally develops from no obvious reason at all, the hand becoming increasingly claw-shaped. Treatment is either by operation, or in the view of some by drugs (vitamin E) and X-ray, both of which may lead to complete cure.

Dwarfism: (*see* Achondroplasia).

Dysentery: a form of diarrhoea associated with bleeding from the bowels which is caused either by an infection with bacteria (bacillary dysentery) or an infection by amoebae (amoebic dysentery). Both types are discussed here. Bacillary dysentery is primarily a tropical disease caused by different organisms (Shiga, Flexner, Sonne) which may in some cases be found in Europe; in England the Flexner and Sonne strains are most common and, except in infants, are fairly harmless. In infancy all diarrhoeas are potentially dangerous. The symptoms may vary from those of a mild attack of diarrhoea to those of severe colic, fever, blood and mucus passed in the motions which in those who are very young, very weak, or very old, may lead to death. Bacillary dysentery is cured by the drugs sulphaguanidine and sulphasuccidine, but the really important thing is to deal with the causes: bad sanitation, flies, poor methods of garbage disposal, and to realise that dysentery is very infectious. The original mortality of about 50% has been completely altered by the use of sulpha drugs, and in most cases bacillary dysentery is now a rather minor disease. Amoebic dysentery is, for all practical purposes, confined to tropical countries and is caused by the Entamoeba histolytica introduced by uncooked vegetables or unpurified water. It differs from bacillary dysentery in almost every respect except that it leads to very much the same symptoms: the incubation period is three weeks to three months rather than the one week or a few days of bacillary dysentery, there are potential complications such as the common abscess of the liver and the less frequent abscesses of the lungs and brain, and it does not respond to the sulpha drugs. Treatment is with emetine, a derivative of ipecacuanha, which is given as emetine-bismuth-iodide; this is usually presented in the form of capsules at night, but when infection of the liver is feared, by injection. Chloroquine is also sometimes used in the treatment of amoebic hepatitis, and antibiotics are given when there is infection by secondary organisms.

Dysmenorrhea: painful menstrual periods (*see* Menstruation).

Dyspareunia: painful sexual intercourse, due either to physical or psychological causes.

Dyspepsia: means quite simply discomfort in the process of digestion and may apply (*a*) to simple difficulty in the process (functional dyspepsia); (*b*) to actual physical changes in the stomach or duodenum such as ulceration; (*c*) to intestinal disease; (*d*) to nervous complaints; (*e*) to temporary complaints. It is necessary therefore to distinguish between the individual who has over-indulged in food or drink the night before or may have a slight infection whilst not being prone to digestive disturbances and the one who has frequently had such troubles. The former case is quite satisfied with a dose of baking-soda or some other alkali whereas the latter may need a more complex investigation. Then it is necessary to be sure of the site of the trouble since a very great deal of indigestion is caused by intestinal disease such as that brought about by excessive use of purgatives or chronic appendicitis or colitis; these will obviously not be helped by medicines containing alkalies since their cause has nothing to do with hyper-acidity. Typical of gastric diseases or diseases of the duodenum are a regular pain coming on after a specific period and in the same place, usually 1½–2 hours after eating, and in the upper part of the abdomen on the right-hand side. The pain is relieved by taking more food or by the taking of alkalies. Nervous dyspepsia is accompanied by such neurotic complaints as flatulence or 'bringing up wind,' which are pure neuroses and have no relationship to real disease (by and large it is found that the more dramatic the complaint the less the danger of trouble). So the significance of abdominal pain is to be judged by whether it has been present before, how regular it is, how far it can be removed by ordinary remedies, how far it is accompanied by bizarre symptoms such as 'wind' or 'queer feelings' – the more specific the symptoms, the more real the disease, e.g. if someone has a pain just above the right eye which comes on at five in the evening one would in general believe him, but the man who has a 'terrible' pain 'all over the head' which lasts 'all the time' is generally exaggerating. People with organic disease are very calm in describing symptoms which occur in a particular place at a particular time, they are specific symptoms not just 'funny feelings,' and they have no connection with conditions which one knows to be neurotic such as flatulence. Duodenal ulcers tend to occur in the period of the thirties or forties and most commonly in men; they occur in ordinarily healthy people and those who have a particular type of character. The sufferer is the man who is 'lean and hungry, lives strenuously, driving mind and body hard,' as one physician describes him. On the other hand the sufferer from gastric ulcer tends to be weak, older, with a poor appetite, bronchitic, and with too little rather than too much acid in the stomach. The fact is that some people can eat anything, chewing or no chewing, teeth or no teeth, others can eat almost nothing (*see* Stomach Diseases, Digestive System, Colitis).

Dysphagia: difficulty in swallowing which is either hysterical or due to a blockage in the oesophagus (*see* Throat).

Dyspnoea: difficulty in breathing (*see* Breathlessness).

Dysuria: difficulty in passing urine or pain on urination (*see* Bladder, Kidneys, Prostate Gland).

Ear: the ear consists not only of the outer part visible to the observer but also the middle and inner ear which lie within the bones of the skull. Its functions are hearing and the maintenance of equilibrium which is located in the semi-circular canals of the inner ear. The outer ear, apart from the visible part or pinna whose function is to collect sounds, consists of a short canal leading from the external auditory meatus for a distance of about an inch and a half to a blind end at the eardrum. It is lined with skin and in this there are implanted hairs (to exclude dust) and glands which secrete wax in amounts which vary with the individual. The middle ear is about one third of an inch wide and one sixth of an inch deep; its only important contents are the three tiny bones, the malleus (hammer), the incus (anvil), and the stapes (stirrup), known collectively as 'ossicles.' These are arranged in a chain and their function is to transform the vibrations caused by soundwaves on the ear-drum into mechanical movements which are transmitted to the fluid of the inner ear by the 'foot-piece' of the 'stirrup' which fits into one of the two holes connecting the middle and inner ear (the fenestra ovalis). Two other connections of the middle ear are of great significance: the Eustachian tube, which runs between the upper part of the throat and the middle ear and has the function of keeping the external air-pressures equal, and the opening connecting the middle ear with the mastoid antrum, the mass of spongy bone which lies behind the ear. It will be seen from this that infections from the throat are very liable to spread to the middle ear whence they may pass to the mastoid; furthermore, when the Eustachian tube is blocked by infection in the throat, it is possible to have deafness without the ear itself being affected. The internal ear consists of a system of spaces in the temporal bone filled with a fluid known as perilymph and containing a membraneous duplicate filled with the so-called endolymph. The part nearest to the middle ear is a small bag or saccule at the end of a coil shaped like a snail's shell known as the cochlea and associated with the sense of hearing, whilst further back lie the semicircular canals attached to a larger sac or utricle, each of the canals being in a different plane of space. Disease of the semicircular canals leads to difficulty in maintaining balance with consequent sensations of giddiness. The most central part of the inside of the cochlea contains the organ of Corti, a system of rods and cells carrying fine hairs of varying length and this is where sounds are received. It has been thought that this acts like a piano in which the rods represent the keys which are set into action by vibrations of varying frequency representing the sounds entering the ear but more recently it has been suggested that sounds set the whole organ into vibration and that the process of analysis into separate sounds takes place in the brain. The main symptoms of ear disease are deafness (q.v.), earache, discharge, and attacks of giddiness. *Earache* is usually caused by acute inflammation of the middle ear which frequently spreads up the Eustachian tube from the throat and hence is a common complication of such fevers as measles and scarlet fever; in this condition, known as otitis media, pus may accumulate and finally burst through the ear-drum into the outer ear. Since it is necessary for the pus to escape and it is better that this should happen through a proper opening rather than that the result should be a ragged hole, it is sometimes necessary to make a small incision in the ear-drum, but this is much less frequently done since the discovery of antibiotics and sulpha drugs. The procedure does not subsequently affect hearing.

The symptoms of otitis media are severe earache accompanied by fever, but when the discharge escapes through the ear-drum there is a sudden relief of pain and the discharge appears on the outside. Earache may also be caused by chronic otitis media when there is interruption to the flow of discharge, by a boil in the outer ear, by skin conditions of the outer ear, by hard wax, and by conditions which have nothing to do with the ear such as neuralgia in this region or decaying molar or premolar teeth. Treatment obviously depends on the cause which must be diagnosed by a doctor but the pain is relieved by aspirin and the application of heat externally as with a hot-water bottle or internally as with warmed olive oil poured into the ear. More effective are phenol drops or the proprie-tary drugs containing a local anaesthetic such as Auralgicin, Otalgan, or Sedonan. *Discharge* is in the great majority of cases due to chronic otitis media and therefore must always receive attention, otherwise there is a grave danger of a spread of infection to the mastoid antrum or progressive deafness. In a few cases it may be due to disease causing irritation in the outer ear, e.g. a hard plug of wax, a foreign body, or a skin condition or boil. Treatment is a specialist matter and may consist in daily mopping-out and cleaning with the instillation of antiseptic drops or powder, the administration of anti-biotics or sulpha drugs, or an operation to clear out the whole middle ear removing the ossicles and leaving an empty cavity which is unlikely to become infected. The degree of deafness resulting from this process is negligible and much less than that produced by the chronic infection itself. *Noises or ringing in the head* are a common accompaniment of ear disease and are generally known as 'tinnitus.' They are found in chronic middle-ear disease and in Menière's disease (q.v.) when they are accompanied or followed by attacks of giddiness. General conditions such as anaemia or high blood-pressure can cause tinnitus (although recent investigations suggest that high blood-pressure is likely to have no symptoms accompanying it at all until the patient becomes aware of his state), and cer-tain drugs such as large doses of quinine or salicylates also cause noises in the ears. There is no doubt that a great many cases of noises in the head are wholly neurotic in origin and may be compared to the spots sometimes seen before the eyes without any organic disease being present, i.e. the noises, like the spots (which are the red-blood cells in the vessels of the eye) are really *there* – what is abnormal is that the individual notices them when the normal person does not unless he concentrates on doing so. An important function of the human brain is cutting out irrelevant stimuli, since our consciousness would be deluged with impulses all the time if we did not automatically ignore most of them; but the neurotic being both anxious and introverted often fails to do this and misinterprets the irrelevant stimuli as disease thus leading to a vicious circle of more anxiety and further concentration on the stimuli. The only treatment for this is sedatives or tranquillisers together with an acceptance of the fact that the stimuli indicate no disease and a determination to concentrate on other people and things in the environment rather than on the self. *Giddiness* together with other symptoms of ear disorders is a sign of Menière's disease. Wax in the ear is treated by syringing carried out by the doctor, although in a few cases the use of a thin oil such as 'Cerumol' may suffice. Olive oil is best not used as it is too thick. Foreign bodies are often pushed into the ears or nose by children and these, too, should be removed by syringing; on no account should any attempt be made to remove them by poking in the ear with an instrument. Boils and eczema of the outer ear may be the cause of slight discharge and both are best referred to the doctor. Chronic discharge may lead to the formation of polypi which sometimes have to be removed surgically, although they usually disappear spontaneously when the discharge is dealt with (*see* Menière's Disease, Mastoiditis, Deafness).

Eclampsia: convulsions associated with the later stages of pregnancy or just following childbirth. They are a serious complication occurring in about 1 in 500 pregnancies and appear to be caused by absorption of substances from the placenta which damage the kidneys leading to the retention of waste-products and further poisoning of the system. In milder cases there are relatively few fits with full consciousness in between but in the more serious cases one fit follows another without return to consciousness. Treatment is a matter for the obstetrician and will include the giving of anti-convulsant drugs and sometimes the induction of premature labour although this is less frequently done than formerly. The maternal mortality is about 10% but the risk to the life of the child is very much greater. Early warning signs (pre-eclamptic) are oedema, high blood-pressure and albumen in the urine.

Ectopic Gestation (or Pregnancy): the ovum is normally fertilised on its descent down the Fallopian tube which connects the ovary with the womb, but sometimes it fails to get down and implants itself in the tube. In this case, as the fertilised egg grows, it is obvious that after about six to eight weeks of pregnancy either the tube will rupture or discharge the embryo into the abdominal cavity. This is a serious surgical emergency requiring immediate treatment to prevent death from haemorrhage and shock. Provided that this is done in time, the operation (which involves removing the affected tube and sucking out the accumulated blood from the abdominal cavity) is almost always successful, recovery prompt, and the patient home within a week or ten days.

Ectopic gestation is a common complication of pregnancy occurring in about one of every 300–400 pregnancies. Among the causes are previous inflammation of the tube (Salpingitis q.v.), deformity of the tube from birth, endometrosis (*see* Ovaries), and adhesions from previous operations or peritonitis. Warning symptoms before the tube has burst are the usual symptoms of pregnancy accompanied by slight bleeding on and off for a few weeks, and occasional pain in the lower abdomen – these, of course, may equally mean nothing abnormal at all. But when the tube bursts the symptoms are those of acute abdominal emergency: i.e. sudden and intense abdominal pain, shock and collapse with increasing pallor, sighing respiration, weak fast pulse, and restlessness. Often there is some vaginal bleeding, and pain over the shoulder-blades. As already indicated, this condition is serious, but death in a modern community where proper hospital accommodation exists is very rare indeed. Later health and fertility are unaffected.

Eczema: or dermatitis simply means inflammation of the skin and is not a specific disease as so many people seem to suppose since it can be extended to include the vast majority of all skin diseases. In practice it is used for all non-specific skin conditions and in this sense eczema is usually caused by allergy or irritants applied to the skin. Treatment depends on the cause (*see* Dermatitis, Skin).

Effort Syndrome: the name given to a group of symptoms

175

wrongly attributed by the patient to disease of the heart, e.g. palpitation, breathlessness, pain over the heart, etc. During the First World War the condition was known as D.A.H. (disordered action of the heart) and it is also known as Da Costa's syndrome. It is mainly associated with military life in which heart disease would, of course, be a serious drawback to further service and naturally the symptoms, which are emotionally caused, are not unrelated to this fact; however, it is quite common in civilian life to find people with similar symptoms although in this case the patient is more willing to be reassured that nothing is organically wrong. Treatment, after eliminating genuine heart disease, is to give plenty of exercise which should be as violent as possible and to ensure that the patient understands the nature of his condition.

Elbow: is the joint formed by the humerus of the upper arm and the radius and ulna of the forearm. It is protected by strong lateral ligaments and powerful muscles cover it at the back and front, hence dislocation is a rare event. The ulnar nerve which passes down the inner side of the arm when the palms are turned forwards is in an exposed position as it passes over the humerus and therefore a blow in this area (the 'funny-bone') is liable to cause considerable pain, even a slight blow leading to a tingling pins and needles effect right down the arm. Miner's elbow, beat elbow, or bursitis of the elbow, in which there is pain and swelling over the point of the elbow developing in those whose work entails resting on the joint (this includes school-children and clerical workers as well as miners) is a condition similar to housemaid's knee and treated by heat and rest. Tennis elbow is a term applied to pain over the lower end of the humerus caused by the strains and joltings when playing tennis or similar games.

Electrical Injuries: may be brought about by electrical currents or by lightning and the amount of upset produced varies greatly with a number of factors which are only partly dependent on the voltage of the current. Thus the amperage is more important than the voltage and alternating current more dangerous than direct current. A current received through dry clothing is less dangerous than one received through wet clothing or on the bare skin, and obviously all currents are more dangerous when the body is earthed than when insulation is provided by rubber-soled shoes. The most dangerous room in the house from the point of view of risk from electrical apparatus is the bathroom; for if a shock is received from a faulty switch or electric fire when the body is naked, wet, and earthed through the bath-tub, conditions are perfect for the passage of a current and such shocks are nearly always fatal. The effects of electric shock are both local and general. The spasm of the muscles may lead to fractured bones and the flesh at the point of entry may be damaged to a degree which ranges from a mild burn to severe destruction of muscles and internal organs; these injuries take a long time to heal because the mass of dead tissue has to have time to separate itself from the living tissues. Sometimes the muscular spasm makes it impossible for the individual to leave go of the object producing the shock and it passes for a longer period producing damage to the brain or paralysis of the heart or respiration. Since a state of suspended animation may last for some time it is important that artificial respiration should be carried on even for hours.

Electricity in Treatment: from the time of its discovery to about twenty or thirty years ago electricity was much used in medicine especially in conditions which did not respond to other forms of treatment. But, like the use of water and ultra-violet rays, its range has been greatly reduced in the last two or three decades since we no longer believe that electricity has some magical effect upon neurasthenia or insomnia, nor is it usually accepted that electric shocks applied to a paralysed nerve speed its recovery – although it may prevent the muscles supplied by the nerve from wasting whilst healing is taking place spontaneously. Nobody now uses electrical belts and really the only field where electricity has much scope is in the use of diathermy for muscular pains or in shock treatment in psychiatry (*see* Diathermy).

Electrocardiogram: the record of the changes in electrical potential which occur in the heart when it contracts and relaxes. In practice this is taken whilst the patient is at rest with the arms and legs or various points on the chest connected up to an electrocardiograph which is an instrument in which a silvered wire vibrates in a strong magnetic field in response to the currents from the heart. The movement is photographed on a moving film and gives indications of any heart abnormality.

Electro-Convulsant Therapy: a form of treatment in psychiatry

177

devised by the Italian Cerletti to replace the use of drugs in convulsant therapy introduced in 1934 by von Meduna of Budapest. The history of the method is rather strange; for its original rationale was the belief (no longer held) of von Meduna that schizophrenia and epilepsy were antagonistic conditions such that one could not exist in the presence of the other. It was argued that the induction of artificial fits by the injection of the drug cardiazol would have a beneficial effect in schizophrenia, and initially, as is so often the case, very good results were obtained. Later it was found that many of these cases relapsed and, although E.C.T. is still used discreetly in some types of schizophrenia, alone or combined with insulin treatment, the main field of use for convulsant therapy is in depressive conditions for which it is almost specific, clearing up severe depressive states in 10–14 days. The main risk of E.C.T. was that fractures were sometimes produced by the muscular spasms, but since the introduction of curare and general anaesthesia during the treatment this risk has been removed.

Electro-Encephalography: a method of diagnosis in brain diseases where the changes of electrical potential over the surface of the brain are recorded by a method analogous to that of the electrocardiograph. The normal alpha or Berger waves (q.v.) occur with a frequency of 10 per second when the eyes are closed, the delta waves with a frequency of 7 or less per second occur in the presence of epilepsy or brain tumours.

Elephantiasis: meaning gross swelling of the leg leading to an elephantine appearance is a symptom of the disease known as filariasis caused by a minute worm which lives in infected human beings throughout Asia, N. Africa, and Central and South America and tends to block their lymphatic channels leading to gross oedema. Its larvae come out into the bloodstream at night when they are withdrawn by mosquitoes (which bite mainly at night) and carried to other human beings in the embryo form, the asexual phase taking place within the mosquito. Filariasis is now successfully treated with diethylcarbamazide (Hetrazan).

Embolism: the blocking of a small blood-vessel by material which has been carried through the blood-stream from another part of the body. The material may be a fragment of blood-clot, a portion of a diseased valve in the heart, a piece of tumour, a mass of bacteria, globules of fat, or bubbles of air. The immediate result is a loss of the blood-supply to the affected part with subsequent softening and death of the tissues; if the material contains bacteria an abscess will arise in the new site and if it be cancerous tissue a secondary tumour will be started. Fat embolism sometimes occurs in severe fractures of bone; air embolism occurs occasionally in operations on the neck and may be fatal.

Emetics: are drugs which cause vomiting and are now rarely used except in cases of suspected poisoning. They belong to two categories: (1) those which act by directly irritating the stomach such as salt in warm water, mustard in cold water, copper and zinc sulphate in water, (2) those which act on the vomiting centre in the brain such as apomorphine, ipecacuanha, and tartar emetic. Since nausea is accompanied by increased flow of secretion from mucous membranes, those substances which are used as emetics are also capable of being used in sub-emetic doses as stimulants in cough medicines in order to liquefy the secretions in the bronchial tubes and thus aid their expulsion. It is not entirely certain, however, whether in the doses given they have much effect in this respect. By far the safest and best emetic is common salt in warm water; large amounts of water should be taken and, if necessary, this may be accompanied by tickling the back of the throat with the finger.

Emetine: one of the active principles in ipecacuanha used in the treatment of amoebic dysentery, (q.v.).

Emphysema: the abnormal presence of air in any part of the body. This may be caused by a knife injury to the chest or a fractured rib, but in practice the word is generally used of a condition of the lungs secondary to some other disease in which the air cells are distended and the partitions between them broken down with consequent breathlessness, wheezing respiration, and the development of a barrel-shaped chest. The most common form attacks the air-vesicles themselves which become distended with air owing to material blocking the bronchioles, e.g. in chronic bronchitis where the secretion produces a valve-like effect in that the air is prevented from leaving the vesiscles but is constantly forced in by the stronger force of inspiration. Finally the breaking-down of the partitions between the vesicles leaves a decreasing amount of

179

lung-tissue available for aerating the blood so that the patient is breathless even whilst at rest. Much less common is acute interstitial emphysema in which the air initially infiltrates into the tissues below the pleura and between the vesicles producing the same final result. Emphysema is caused (1) where some local disease such as an embolism or tumour has destroyed part of the lung causing the surrounding tissues to swell in order to replace the vacuum, (2) in chronic bronchitis and bronchial asthma where the vesicles are broken down by the valve-like action mentioned above taking place in the bronchioles, (3) in diseases such as whooping cough where there are violent and frequent attacks of coughing or in processes involving great muscular strain or blowing wind-instruments which some, probably wrongly, believe can lead to emphysema. The condition ultimately leads to dilation of the right side of the heart which has to overwork to push the blood through considerably diminished channels and this in its turn is likely to lead to heart-failure with oedema or dropsy of the legs and elsewhere. Treatment is that of the primary condition in order to prevent further damage being done although obviously damage already done cannot be repaired. Asthma or bronchitis must therefore be dealt with, and any other treatment is merely alleviative.

Empyema: an internal abscess. In practice a collection of pus within one of the pleural cavities caused by the extension of an infection from elsewhere, e.g. following pneumonia, in chronic pulmonary tuberculosis, or from septic wounds of the chest, tumours in the chest, or abscesses due to the inhalation of foreign bodies. Empyema is diagnosed by the recurrence of temperature after a case of pneumonia has apparently subsided, profuse sweating, laboured breathing, and an area on the chest wall which is dull on percussion (*see* Auscultation). The treatment is usually surgical, although if the pus is not too thick it can sometimes be withdrawn through a needle attached to a syringe; antibiotics or sulpha drugs are also given. The outlook in most cases is excellent.

Encephalitis Lethargica: sleepy sickness (*not* sleeping sickness, (q.v.) or epidemic encephalitis is a virus disease of the brain occurring in epidemics usually in spring-time and attacking both the brain and the brain-stem. It begins as a fever accompanied by drowsiness and lethargy which may progress to complete unconsciousness although this may be preceded by a stage of restlessness or even of maniacal excitement. As the drowsiness progresses various types of paralysis appear in the region of the face and neck, e.g. quint, drooping of the eyelids, facial palsy of one or both sides, difficulty in swallowing due to paralysis of the throat muscles. Less frequently, the spinal cord is affected with pain in the limbs and partial paralysis. There may be haemorrhages under the skin, in the muscles, or from the stomach. In those cases which recover improvement is slow and may take many months or the clinical picture known as 'Parkinsonism' may make its appearance with the development of an expressionless face, rigidity of the muscles, festinant gait (i.e. the patient walks with the body bent forwards and the legs moving as if trying to catch up with it), coarse tremor, and 'pill-rolling' movements (i.e. the thumb and the first and second fingers are constantly rubbed against each other). The patient's intellectual ability may become greatly deteriorated, and encephalitis in children sometimes leads to delinquent behaviour. There is no specific treatment, but Parkinsonism is alleviated by such drugs as stramonium, atropine, hyoscine, amphetamine sulphate, and Artane. Sometimes surgical treatment has been used with excellent results. Other forms of encephalitis occur rarely as complications of measles, mumps, or following vaccination.

Endocrine Glands: or ductless glands are a number of organs scattered throughout the body which secrete substances direct into the blood-stream instead of through a duct and play a fundamental part in the control of growth, sexual development, metabolic processes, and intellectual and emotional development. The main ones are the pituitary at the base of the brain which plays a leading part in development and is, indeed, 'the conductor of the endocrine orchestra,' the thyroid in the front of the neck which influences the speed of metabolism and intellectual development in childhood, the suprarenal glands above each kidney which prepare the organism for emergency and in the form of cortisone and its derivatives produce substances essential to life, the pancreas which secretes insulin thus controlling the sugar content of the blood, the ovaries and testicles which control sexual development. Other glands are the parathyroids situated in the region of the thyroid which control calcium metabolism and the thymus, also in the neck, which has no known function (although its persistence into adult life is believed to be the cause of sudden death under an anaesthetic in the condition known as 'status lymphaticus'). The pineal gland in the brain is an evolutionary relic of the third eye which is not known to have any function but was at one time thought by the philosopher Descartes and others to be the seat of the soul. (For more detailed information about the glands see under the heading of each separate organ).

Endometritis: inflammation of the lining of the womb.

Endometrosis: (*see* Ovaries).

Enema: the injection of fluid into the bowel through the anus for various purposes, e.g. as a purgative, as a sedative, to supply nourishment when feeding by ordinary means is impossible or inadvisable, to heal local diseases of the bowel, or in the treatment of worms. It is probably true to say that, apart from cranks addicted to colonic lavage for the treatment of intestinal neuroses, enemata are no longer as popular as they once were because what they are capable of doing can be more easily done and with greater efficiency in other ways. They are still sometimes used after abdominal operations where it is undesirable to stimulate the whole bowel by the use of purgatives taken by mouth but nobody would willingly have an enema for constipation which is purely temporary and the habitual use of enemata is just as harmful as the regular use of purgatives since it leads to distension of the rectum and an increased tendency to constipation. Nutrient enemata are unsatisfactory because one is left in doubt as to how much has actually been absorbed and glucose is now usually given intravenously, and, if sedatives are given by rectum, it is usually in the form of suppositories which are also used for purging. Purgative enemata depend for their activity on the bulk of fluid injected rather than upon what is injected and therefore consist of 1–2 pints of water at body temperature with about 1 oz. of soft green or yellow soap to the pint; to expel flatus two tablespoons of turpentine may be added to each pint of water. Therapeutic enemata for ulceration of the bowel usually contain starch or silver nitrate; enemata for thread-worms often contain quassia but are now rarely necessary. During administration of an enema the patient lies on the left side with the knees drawn up and a thick pillow under the hips to keep them raised, but the use of the enema is dying out.

Enteric Fever: (*see* Typhoid Fever).

Enteritis: inflammation of the intestine usually, but not always, caused by infection (*see* Diarrhoea).

Enterostomy: an operation in which an articial opening is created in the intestines. This may be to the surface, as in colostomy, or between the stomach and the small intestine in peptic ulcer when the operation is known as gastro-enterostomy or gastro-jejunostomy. In the former the faeces are discharged on the surface of the abdomen and the major part of the large intestine is by-passed or removed, in the latter the alkaline intestinal juices enter the stomach and help to reduce its acidity.

Entropion: a condition in which disease causes the eyelid to be turned inwards towards the eyeball (*see* Eye, Diseases of).

Enzyme: meaning 'in yeast' where the first enzyme 'zymase' was found which changes sugar into alcohol. Enzymes are biological catalysts (i.e. they have the effect in very small amounts and without change to themselves of bringing about chemical reactions between other substances) and in this way resemble such inorganic catalysts as platinum black used in gas-lighters where it causes the gas to unite with the oxygen of the air thus igniting it without itself being affected. Best-known are the digestive enzymes such as ptyalin in saliva, pepsin in the gastric juice, and trypsin and diastase in pancreatic juice (*see* Digestive System), but in fact all the processes of living matter take place through the intervention of enzymes, e.g. the thrombin of the blood which causes coagulation is an enzyme.

Ephedrine: an alkaloid (q.v.) from the Chinese plant Ma Huang which is similar to adrenaline (q.v.) in its action although this is more prolonged and less dramatic than that of the biological substance. Its main function is in asthma and bronchitis where in tablet or linctus form it is used to dilate the bronchi and thus facilitate breathing.

Epiglottis: a leaf-shaped piece of cartilage covered with mucous membrane which lies between the back of the tongue and the voice-box or larynx at its entrance or glottis. Its function is to close the glottis whilst foods or liquids are being swallowed; if this does not happen food may 'go down the wrong way' and gain entry into the respiratory system when it may be coughed up again or go further down and sometimes cause damage to the lungs.

Epilepsy: idiopathic epilepsy is only one of many causes of fits and its existence is largely diagnosed (apart from the findings of an electroencephalogram) by the absence of other diseases which might cause them. Thus fits frequently occur in young children during a fever without necessarily being of any serious significance, and, more ominously, in apoplexy, in coma caused by diabetes and liver or kidney disorders, in brain tumours and other forms of brain disease, and they sometimes follow accidents in which the brain has been damaged or there is pressure upon it from a blood-clot or scar. Epileptiform fits also occur in hysteria (q.v.). Idiopathic or true epilepsy is caused by none of these and no organic cause has ever been found although it seems clear that something is wrong with the functioning of the brain so that, instead of a steady and controlled release of energy, spasmodic and uncontrolled releases occur which take the form of fits. A typical fit is preceded in 50% of cases by an 'aura' or sensation which is peculiar to the individual (eg. pain in a particular part of the body, strange sensations, tremor, a mysterious smell or vision unrelated to anything in the surrounding environment, a feeling of panic). He then falls down unconscious, with or without this warning, and all the muscles of the body go into spasm, the breathing stops so that he is at first pale and then turns blue in the face. After about half a minute this 'tonic' phase is followed by a so-called 'clonic' phase in which the limbs rythmically contract and relax, the bladder or bowels may be emptied, or the tongue may be bitten until the contractions gradually cease and the patient lies breathing heavily and unconscious for a varying period of time. Sometimes he gets up almost at once and resumes what he was doing before, but in other cases a state of confusion may last for several hours. Obviously the danger from such fits lies in the possibility that the patient may injure himself (e.g. by falling in the street or burning himself in the fireplace) and clearly epileptics should not drive a car or accept employment in any job where they would be in any danger should an attack come on suddenly. Death rarely occurs in a fit except in the comparatively rare status epilepticus where one fit follows another with no return to consciousness in between. What has been described so far is what is known as 'grand mal' or the great sickness, but there are two other types of epilepsy: petit mal (the little sickness) and Jacksonian epilepsy. In petit mal there is alteration of consciousness but no spasms and the individual may not even be noticed as he perhaps breaks off in the middle of a conversation and suddenly seems to be 'not there,' returning to full consciousness after a brief period with or without some mental confusion. Sometimes he may stagger whilst walking, turn to one side or the other, grimace, and pay no attention to what is said to him. In Jacksonian epilepsy there is usually no loss of consciousness but spasms occur in particular groups of muscles, e.g. beginning in the fingers and slowly passing up the arm which writhes and becomes contorted as if it had a separate existence. The fits in epilepsy may occur at any time of the day or night and be of any degree of frequency but the pattern tends to be characteristic of the individual; they may occur only at night in which case their existence may be unknown for many years, and daily, weekly, or only once or twice in a lifetime. Sometimes they begin in early childhood (although they are not to be confused with the fits which may accompany high fever in almost any young child) and sometimes quite late in life. No physical disease seems to accompany epilepsy and, apart from the fits, the individual remains in perfect health, but in some cases there may appear to be some deterioration over the years, the patient becoming dull, irritable and impulsive, forgetful, and self-centred. It is probable that this deterioration is basically due to the social situation the epileptic has to face. Thus it is often difficult for the epileptic to get a job – even one that is not a danger to himself – since many employers do not like the distress occasioned to other employees by the individual who may have fits during working hours. People tend to be afraid of him and he not unnaturally feels that he is shunned by society whilst being in all other respects a normal person. This, in part, may be a cause of the so-called epileptic personality just as many of the symptoms of senility are caused by the social isolation of the old. One form of epilepsy which is of medico-legal importance is the attack which takes the form of extreme violence whilst in an altered state of consciousness; this is known as an 'epileptic equivalent' or automatism and may take the place of a fit or follow one so that the individual may carry out murderous attacks which are quite pointless without knowing what he is doing. Fortunately, however, these are not very common. Numerous great men have been epileptics and in many respects the novelist Dostoevsky who was a sufferer is typical of the epileptic character with its violence, its love of mysticism, its persecutory beliefs and impulsiveness. In the treatment of epilepsy anti-convulsant drugs are given and formerly these were substances such as the bromides or phenobarbitone which acted by virtue of their general sedative effect causing the patient to be sleepy at the same time but today increasing knowledge has led to the use of substances which are anti-convulsant whilst having very little sedative effect, e.g. phentoin sodium (Epanutin), Mesontoin, and primidone (Mysoline) which may be taken alone or in combination with phenobarbitone. There is no condition which needs greater individual attention to medication than epilepsy: for individuals respond very variously to the same drug and it is necessary to find out which drug is best for the individual patient as well as how the doses should be distributed throughout the twenty-four hours, e.g. in a case where the attacks are most frequent at night the largest dose should obviously be taken before retiring. Troxidone (Tridione) is very useful for petit mal attacks. The problems of the epileptic are dealt with by the British Epilepsy Association, 27 Nassau Street, London, W.1.

Erysipelas: a serious streptococcal infection of the skin usually supervening on a small wound or abrasion and characterised by a red area with a raised advancing margin. Formerly known as the Rose or St Anthony's Fire, it was one of the common epidemics of the Middle Ages and, until the discovery of germs and antiseptics, was one of the scourges of surgical wards and maternity hospitals where it would spread like wildfire and, especially in the latter, often lead to death. None of this happens in technically-advanced countries nowadays, where the condition is rather uncommon and usually affects middle-aged people. The raised edge of the advancing red area may resemble the outline of a map and occurs most often on the head and face, although any part of the body may be attacked, and as the edge advances the parts first infected tend to become less inflamed. There is a fever which may be as high as 104–105 degrees F. or more and complications in earlier times were delirium, infection of the deeper tissues especially in surgical wounds leading to gangrene, peritonitis, pericarditis, and so on. But the use of the sulpha drugs and antibiotics have revolutionised the situation and erysipelas is rarely serious. It should always be remembered, however, that the disease is extremely contagious.

Essential Hypertension: is high blood-pressure which is not secondary to some other disease, e.g. to the toxaemia of pregnancy or kidney diseases. It is therefore synonymous with primary hypertension (*see* Hypertension).

Ethisterone: a drug which can be taken by mouth and has the same effect as the ovarian hormone progesterone which, generally speaking, has a sedative and relaxing effect on the genital tract. It is therefore given in uncomplicated cases of excessive menstrual bleeding and to prevent a threatened miscarriage.

Ethyl Chloride: a volatile liquid which is used both as a local anaesthetic (in which case it acts by 'freezing' the part by virtue of its rapid evaporation) and as a general anaesthetic (usually only in the initial stages when anaesthesia is being induced) (*see* Anaesthetics).

Eucalyptus: an oil obtained by distillation from the leaves of the eucalyptus tree, originally from Australia, but now found in many parts of the world. It is a favourite remedy for coughs and colds applied either externally as a rub or inhaled as a vapour, but there is little evidence that it has any very marked medical effects although it may give symptomatic relief.

Eugenics: the study of conditions that may improve the hereditary qualities of a species which largely originated with the work of Sir Francis Galton (1822–1911), a cousin of Charles Darwin. Today eugenics is viewed more critically, firstly because we no longer believe that heredity is all-powerful or our knowledge about it capable of giving accurate prediction, and secondly because of our unpleasant experience of the uses to which eugenics can be put in totalitarian countries. The same criticism applies to eugenics as to the concept of euthanasia (i.e. that once we accept the principle that we have the right to control inheritance or put some suffering individual to death there is no logical stopping-point and we may well end up making value judgments as to who we think should breed or die). Certainly there are circumstances in which it is highly inadvisable that people should have children and some diseases such as haemophilia which are directly inherited but in many theoretically transmissible diseases the chance of the individual having offspring is anyhow small, e.g. schizophrenia and certain forms of idiocy. In other cases ailments which are largely hereditary may be accompanied by great intellectual brilliance and even genius as in manic depressive insanity. It is easy to see that, if the eugeneticists had had their way, many people who have contributed much to human progress and understanding would never have been born; for the incidence of insanity, neurosis, epilepsy, and physical defects among geniuses has been quite high. It is generally accepted today that, certain disease being transmissible, it is reasonable that in individual cases those who carry these diseases should be advised against having children or even (with their own consent) sterilised. The real danger comes when scientists leave the field of physical disabilities and enter the psychological field to make judgements as to what sort of people are desirable, or when they want to apply positive eugenics in the form of selective breeding to human beings, a procedure which most people rightly view with disgust and which, in any case is scientifically unjustifiable since the human person is primarily a product of society and upbringing, not of heredity alone, and it is quite possible to get a physically perfect specimen who, like Hitler's supermen, would be nothing but a smashing bore or a moral imbecile. In fact, there is reason to believe that, at least in part, genius is a response to the individual person's awareness of physical incompleteness.

Eumydrin: atropine methyl nitrate is a long-action derivative of atropine which has been used successfully in the treatment of pyloric stenosis in infants (q.v.) and in a certain number of cases avoids the necessity for operation.

Euthanasia: the recommendation that it should become legal to put to death those who are suffering from incurable, painful, or distressing disease by some painless method as an overdose of morphia or similar substances. As noted in the case of eugenics, the most obvious danger of any such recommendation is that, once the principle is allowed, there is no knowing where it will end and there are very good medical reasons for treating human life as, for practical purposes, sacred. The main argument put forward by believers in euthanasia is that it is intolerable that people should be allowed to suffer needlessly when they are in any case doomed, but it is noteworthy that those who recommend it are not for the most part medical men who have seen much of death but laymen who are over-dramatising the real state of affairs. In fact death is rarely accompanied by pains so severe that they cannot be controlled by drugs and to put to death, even with his own permission, someone who is still in a clear state of mind is simply murder and should be regarded as such. It is sad when a parent kills an imbecile child on the grounds of suffering but it is even worse than that – it is stupid sentimentality because the imbecile child is, in all probability, a good deal happier than either its father or mother and there is no justification whatever for taking its life at no matter how lowly a level it may be lived. That it is on the whole unusual for death to be accompanied by severe pains is confirmed by a book entitled *The Day's End* written by Pamela Bright, a nurse with long experience of incurable cancer, whose views are those of the vast majority of medical men. Other reasons against euthanasia are that it would be intolerable should the general public come to associate the doctor with the role of public executioner instead of healer; that one has no right to perform euthanasia without the permission of the patient and no right either to perform it with the permission of one who, by reason of suffering, is not in an unbiased state of mind and might well ask for something which in his normal state he would abhor; and, above all, that there are many diseases in which the general application of euthanasia would mean the complete cessation of any attempts to find a cure. Who, after all, is entitled to say that a disease is 'incurable' in view of the fact that it is not unknown for a patient to be found to be suffering from 'incurable cancer' which proves to be inoperable and yet recovers spontaneously without any treatment? Are we to put to death those who are suffering from leukaemia because it is regarded as incurable when there is every reason to believe that, like pernicious anaemia and diabetes which were once incurable and are now easily treated, so will leukaemia be conquered also? When there are so many ways of relieving severe pain including, when necessary, the severing of the pain-bearing

189

nerves there seems to be little justification for euthanasia and many who are not Catholic will agree with the position taken by the Church that it is wrong to kill but, when a state is reached in which pain can only be relieved at the risk of the patient's life, that risk should be taken. Or, as a secular poet has it: 'Thou shalt not kill, but needst not strive officiously to keep alive.' The headquarters of the Euthanasia Society is at 13 Prince of Wales Terrace, London, W.8.

Exercise: to the primitive man or even to the manual worker on the land or in mines or factories it must seem strange that exercise should present itself as a problem at all. Nevertheless, there exists in modern society a large number of workers whose work is sedentary and who therefore feel a need for exercise or even a sense of duty in relation to it. But it is necessary to preserve a proper perspective since this is one of those subjects to which some people attach a quite disproportionate significance and others, perhaps, not enough. The idea that, in general, exercise is not only a duty for the sedentary individual but that it has a remarkable effect on the health of the body is a reversal of the truth which is that those who are healthy already will wish to take exercise from an overflow of physical energy, and many paralysed or otherwise immobilised individuals who are quite unable to walk have been noted for their longevity. For the normal person the best reason for taking exercise is to obtain pleasure and compulsive exercising is a miserable and futile form of puritanism. There are two possible exceptions to this general rule: (1) it has been suggested in recent years that lack of exercise is associated with the risk of coronary thrombosis but few doctors accept this view without reservations (e.g. some groups of miners who obviously have very heavy manual work have also a high rate of coronary thrombosis), (2) specific types of exercise are necessary in certain ailments (e.g. breathing exercises are very important in certain types of chest disease, and clearly wasted limbs need exercise to prevent further deterioration in the condition of the muscles). It will be noted that these cases have no bearing whatever on the general problem of exercise since the purpose of breathing exercises is basically to overcome bad habits of breathing, the purpose of exercising the limbs to prevent wasting, not some vague idea that the process exerts some magical tonic

effect on the body as a whole. So far as the possible connection, dubious as it is, between lack of exercise and
coronary thrombosis is concerned, it is quite sufficient that
the individual walk for five or ten minutes on his way to and
from work. Lastly, it should be pointed out that the effect of
exercise on reducing weight is often grossly exaggerated since
it would be necessary to climb up and down Ben Nevis twice
in order to lose even a couple of pounds of weight apart from
fluid loss. None of this, of course, has any bearing on the
problem of exercise in training for a specific purpose as in
sports and athletics.

Exophthalmic Goitre: (see Goitre).

Expectorants: substances used in cough medicines which have
an opposite action to sedative drugs which suppress cough,
i.e. their action is to liquefy the sputum and so enable the
patient to cough with more effect. In general, they are substances which in larger doses would have an emetic effect (*see*
Emetics) such as ipecacuanha, tartar emetic, ammonium
chloride, and common salt and one of the most effective expectorants used by Brompton Chest Hospital is simply a
solution of salt in water. To a certain extent inhalations of
steam with or without Friar's balsam, menthol, eucalyptus,
turpentine, or Balsam of tolu, together with hot drinks have
an expectorant action. Patients with chronic bronchitis or
bronchiectasis are often advised to carry out 'postural coughing' especially on getting up in the morning. This is done by
lying across the bed with the head down towards the floor
and deliberately coughing whilst the chest is in a position for
the sputum to run towards the throat.

Extra-uterine Gestation: (*see* Ectopic Gestation).

Eye: the eyelids are composed of skin stretched by a thin
layer of dense fibrous tissue at the margins; they are closed
by the action of the orbicularis oculi muscles surrounding
the eye and the upper lid is raised by the action of the levator
palpebrae. At the margins of the eyelids the Meibomian
glands secrete sebum or grease and sometimes become
blocked to form a small Meibomian cyst which may need
to be opened on the inner surface of the eyelid. Near the
outer canthus or angle of the orbit both above and below lie
the lachrymal or tear glands whose function is to secrete the
liquid which keeps the surface of the eye clean and moist;

normally the tears pass across the surface of the eye, being constantly distributed by the action of blinking, and leave it by the lachrymal canals which can be seen as two tiny openings above and below at the inner canthus of the eye. The ducts open into the lachrymal sac at the upper and inner angle of the orbit and from this a duct passes down into the nose. Strong emotions or irritant vapours and foreign bodies cause an excess flow of tears which is more than can be carried away by the duct and it overflows on to the cheek, but a similar result occurs when for some reason the duct is blocked, e.g. by a cold which causes the lining of the nose to swell thus blocking its exit – hence the watery eyes of coryza or hayfever. When the duct is blocked for any length of time the lachrymal sac swells and the condition known as dacryocystitis results in which the swelling at the inner and upper angle of the orbit can be clearly seen. The eyeball itself consists of three coats: (1) the external sclerotic and cornea of strong fibrous tissue which is opaque over most of the eye (the sclerotic) and transparent in front (the cornea); (2) the middle muscular and pigmented layer with many blood-vessels which forms the choroid and, in front, the iris: (3) the internal nervous and epithelial layer known as the retina. The retina contains the expanded termination of the optic nerve which may be seen radiating from a point slightly to the nasal side of the centre, whilst right in the centre is the yellow spot, a slight circular depression. No less than eight layers have been described in the very complex structure of the retina, but here it is enough to mention from without inwards the layer of nerve fibres, the layer of nerve cells, a layer of rods and cones, and a pigmented layer. Except in the yellow spot the rods greatly exceed the cones in number and there are differences of opinion as to their presumably separate functions; it is generally agreed, however, that each rod or cone sends a single impulse so that the picture on the retina is broken up into 'dots' in much the same way as a picture in a newspaper so that the image as seen is the combined impression of many individual stimuli. The chamber of the eye is divided into two by the crystalline lens which lies behind the iris or pupil in an elastic capsule and suspended by ligaments which can exert varying tensions thus making it more convex (by relaxation of the ligaments) or (by their contraction) less convex. Thus in accommodation for near objects the ciliary muscles relax making the lens more convex, the pupil contracts, and the eyes are made to converge by the six external eye muscles including four recti and two oblique. In accommodation for distant objects the opposite actions occur. Between the surface of the eye and the lens lies the aqueous humour which is virtually a saline solution of the same specific gravity as the blood whilst behind the lens in the larger chamber of the eye is the vitreous humour which has the consistency of jelly. Both, together with the lens, act as a very delicate and sensitive water-camera. In infancy the lens is almost sperical, but in old age it becomes less convex and therefore we tend to become long-sighted as age advances. The impressions on the retina pass along the optic nerves which in the substance of the brain become the optic tracts and finally pass it to the visual centre in the occipital lobe at the back of the brain. It follows that blindness whether partial or complete may be due to damage to the retina or optic nerve as in optic neuritis; to damage to the optic chiasma where both optic nerves meet just above the pituitary gland to become the optic tracts, as in a pituitary tumour; to damage to the tracts from a tumour or abcess of the brain; or, finally, to damage to the visual centre in the occipital lobes from a tumour or wound. In addition to the three coats mentioned the surface of the eye and the inner surface of the eyelids is covered by the thin transparent outer membrane known as the conjunctiva; this is the part most frequently subject to infection from without which is known as conjunctivitis.

Eye Diseases: the pupil reacts by contracting to both light and accommodation to near objects and absence of the light reflex indicates some disease of the central nervous system; the *Argyll Robertson pupil*, named after the Edinburgh physician who first described it, reacts to accommodation but not to light and is generally taken to be a sign of syphilis of the nervous system although it is now realised that it may occur in the absence of any disease at all. Double vision or *diplopia* may be due to an error of refraction in one eye in which case it will remain when the other eye is closed, but true diplopia is caused by weakness of the ocular muscles which should bring the eyes to converge accurately on an object and this type disappears when one eye is closed. True diplopia may be transient, e.g. it frequently appears in extreme fatigue, after too much alcohol, or with certain drugs and sometimes after an attack of migraine; but when it lasts for some time it is of urgent importance and a doctor should be consulted since diplopia may be a sign of disseminated sclerosis, myasthenia gravis, or various serious diseases within the skull causing interference with the 3rd, 4th and 6th cranial nerves which regulate these muscles. *Nystagmus* means that the eyeball flutters from side to side or up and down generally when the patient is asked to look at a finger held to the side of the head. It is a sign of many nervous diseases (e.g. disseminated sclerosis) or none at all (e.g. it is found in those who have had poor eyesight from childhood and was once notorious in the form of Miner's nystagmus now generally recognised to have been a neurosis). *Spasm of the eyelids or flickering* occurs, of course, when there is a foreign body in the eye, but flickering is most commonly a sign of nervous tension or fatigue. It is usually transient, but sedatives may be necessary. Epiphora or watering of the eyes so that tears run down the cheeks may similarly be due to an irritation of the conjunctiva which is merely temporary but can result from a scar on the cheek or weakness of the lower eyelid in old age when the duct which should carry the tears away is turned outwards. It may also happen when there is an over-secretion of tears or when the ducts or tear-sac at the side of the nose are blocked by inflammation; in the latter case (dacryocystitis) there is a swelling at the inner and upper corner of the eye. Dacryocystitis may be treated by hot bathing or if necessary by passing a probe through the nose along the duct in order to open it and wash it out with antiseptics, and in bad cases the tear-sac may have to be surgically removed. *Conjunctivitis* or 'red eye' is one of the commonest eye diseases and in nearly all cases is caused by bacterial infection. Although usually trivial and easily treated it should not be neglected as this may lead to the formation of a corneal ulcer which is much more serious. Some types are extremely infectious and epidemics occur in schools where the germs are passed on by towels used in common. In all cases there is redness of the eyes and a sensation of irritation as if particles of grit had gained entry; in more severe conjuctivitis the watery secretion may be replaced by pus and it is difficult to open the eyes on waking in the morning. Conjunctivitis is treated by hot bathing the eyes and the use of an appropriate eye-wash which will vary with the germs causing the infection. Two serious forms of conjunctivitis, fortunately not very common in this country, are conjunctivitis of the newborn or *ophthalmia neonatorum* and *trachoma*. Ophthalmia was at one time responsible for nearly 50% of blindness in children and is caused by infection of the eyes by gonorrhoea in the mother, but better diagnosis and the compulsory bathing of the eyes after birth with silver nitrate solution has caused it to disappear almost completely from this country. Trachoma is a chronic severe form of conjunctivitis found in Egypt and various Eastern and Mediterranean countries. Since it is so difficult to cure and leads to partial blindness people suffering from trachoma are forbidden entry into many countries such as the U.S. and the British Dominions. In this condition nodules which have been compared with sago grains appear on the conjunctiva lining the eyelids and later a film of blood-vessels spreads over the cornea obscuring vision and causing shrinking of the conjunctiva thus drawing the eyelids inwards (entropion) and bringing about further irritation of the surface of the eye from the eyelashes. Treatment is, of course, a specialist matter. *Xerophthalmia* is an inflammation of the cornia and eyelids leading to blindness and caused by lack of vitamin A in the diet. It is, of course, rare in civilised communities today. *Injuries and foreign bodies in the eye* should always be treated with the greatest caution. Ordinary dust or grit should be treated in the following way: on no account rub the eye, but blow the nose hard in order to dislodge the particle and then try to remove it with the corner of a clean handkerchief. If this fails put a drop of bland oil such as castor oil in the eye, then lift the upper lid outwards and downwards at the same time pushing the lower lid upwards under it; release the upper lid and the particle may be carried away on the eyelashes of the lower lid. If these attempts are unsuccessful, a pad should be placed over the eye and the patient taken to see a doctor. When the foreign body is metallic or hard and sharp it is likely to become embedded in the cornea and a doctor should always be seen as it may have to be dug out with a special instrument or an electromagnet. A *black eye* is simply a bruise in the eye region and cold compresses applied immediately after a blow may prevent the bruise from forming, but after it has appeared it is best treated with hot compresses. A black eye from a direct blow should on no account be confused with the black eye resulting from a blow elsewhere on the skull which has the much more serious significance of haemorrhage within the skull itself. Wounds of the eye, unless very trivial, should always be referred to the doctor. Treatment for shock may be necessary in severe cases (*see* Blepharitis, Blindness, Keratitis, Retinitis).

Facial Nerve: the seventh cranial nerve which supplies the muscle of expression of the face after passing from the hind part of the brain in close relationship to the middle and inner ear and leaving its bony covering just below the external ear where it is liable to injury from cold or a cut or blow leading to facial paralysis (*see* Bell's Palsy).

Faeces: the waste-products from the bowels.

Fainting: or syncope is a transient loss of consciousness caused by temporary lack of blood-supply to the brain. It is therefore brought about by conditions which produce this state such as very hot baths, long standing in one position as on military parades, getting up for the first time after a long period of being confined to bed, certain drugs such as an overdose of tobacco or alcohol, blows on the head or in the solar plexus region of the abdomen (when fainting really begins to shade into shock), and, possibly most frequently, from strong emotions in nervous people. Rarely, fainting occurs in heart disease (e.g. in heart-block and auricular flutter), and it may also occur in severe anaemia, low blood-pressure and vaso-vagal attacks, but by far the commonest causes are emotional and postural when it happens in otherwise normal adults. The fainting of a postural type which occurs in soldiers on parade results from more or less prolonged standing with inactivity of the leg muscles which ordinarily aid blood to return to the heart by the massaging effect of movement; the blood collects in the veins of the leg and the lower parts of the body and is therefore not available to supply the brain adequately. Such fainting may be prevented by contracting and relaxing the muscles of the calves whilst standing for

196

any length of time but, when the premonitory signs of pallor, rapid and weak pulse, a 'sinking feeling,' and cold sweat or dimming of vision and hearing occur, the individual should lie down or sit with the head bent forward between the knees which, even on parade, is better than falling down unconscious. Strong stimuli such as pungent smelling salts are also used and sometimes slapping of the cheeks but, once a faint has occurred, much the best thing to do is to let the patient lie flat on his or her back with any tight clothing loosened. The other precedures are more for the benefit of the onlookers than that of the individual who will recover without their help. When fainting attacks are at all frequent the doctor should be consulted to find whether some physical or emotional cause requires treatment. As in other types of unconsciousness, no attempt must be made to force an unconscious or partly unconscious person to drink; the brandy is best saved for the period of recovery or for the spectators who by this time probably need it more than the patient.

Fallopian Tubes: the two tubes, between four to five inches long, which pass from a position close to the ovaries on each side of the pelvis to the upper corners of the womb. Their function is to carry the released ovum at or about the mid-period to the womb so the end near the ovaries is wide and furnished with cilia or moving hairs which draw the ovum into the funnel but the other end is very narrow and only just sufficient for the ovum to pass. Inflammation of the tubes is known as salpingitis from the Greek word for 'trumpet' because of their shape (*see* Salpingitis).

Farcy: another name for glanders (q.v.).

Fastings: the length of time it is possible to exist without food varies with the circumstances. Thus without water most people would die within a week or ten days, but resting and kept warm it is possible to exist for about two and a half months if water be given. Terence McSwiney, the Mayor of Cork, died on hunger strike in prison in 1920 after a fast of 74 days and others have survived after fasting for fifty days or more. Professional fasters rarely subsist on water alone and their fluids usually contain fruit juice or glucose which naturally prolongs the period for which they can go 'without food' considerably. Fasting as a health measure is recommended by many people and it is probably quite a good idea for stomachs which are usually over-full to rest for a week or two on orange juice in a brief period of low living and high thinking. However, it must be remembered that it is always inadvisable for older people to change their way of life suddenly as when the over-fed and sedentary indulge in violent exercise or a fast with the quite mistaken notion that the change will inevitably be good for their health when it may merely result in a coronary thrombosis or a stomach ulcer from the unemployed acid.

Fatigue: fatigue is of two types (1) physical fatigue due to heavy muscular exercise in which recognisable waste-products appear in the blood such as lactic acid resulting from the breakdown of muscular tissues; (2) psychological fatigue in which no such waste-products appear since nerve tissue does not become exhausted in the ordinary sense and the results are really the result of boredom, e.g. in doing monotonous work against which the mind revolts or in doing work unwillingly with a feeling of resentment. The first type of fatigue is not at all common in our basically sedentary society and psychological fatigue plays a large part in all tiredness; it is, for example, at the root of most of what used to be called 'industrial fatigue.' Therefore someone who feels fatigue for psychological reasons when doing a particular form of work is usually quite capable of doing something he or she likes immediately the work is changed; the man who is tired on sentry duty and cannot see in the dark is quite able to meet his girl friend on the darkest night. Thus interest has a potent influence on the subjective feeling of tiredness and we are always tired when doing something unwillingly. There is no treatment for tiredness along the lines usually advertised in the press since nerves never need to be 'fed' nor are they soothed by nerve tonics or milk drinks although there are many stimulants which cover up the feeling of fatigue such as amphetamine and even alcohol. The advertisements recommending glucose are another piece of humbug because although it is quite true that glucose supplies energy in the completely academic sense that it is the main fuel of the body, it is not true (*a*) that glucose is in any way superior to a cup of sweet tea with ordinary cane sugar, (*b*) that anybody lacks glucose, or (*c*) that the person suffering from fatigue is usually suffering from the sort of tiredness that glucose could relieve

– they are not lacking energy but inclination. Most fatigue is a form of boredom mixed with resentment and results from doing something when all one's natural impulses are revolting against it. This sort of fatigue due to warring impulses is common in neurosis (q.v.).

Fat Necrosis: is caused by disease or injury to the pancreas in which the fat-splitting enzyme lipase escapes into the abdomen and destroys fatty cells.

Fatty Degeneration: occurs as a result of anaemia of certain types, interference with the blood or nervous supply (as in diseases causing an increase of fibrous tissue such as cirrhosis of the liver where the blood-vessels are crushed), or from some poisons such as chloroform and carbon tetrachloride or phosphorus. The organs most frequently affected are the heart, liver, and kidneys in which the cells degenerate with the appearance of fat globules which cause them to lose their normal function.

Fauces: the narrow opening between the mouth and throat bounded above by the soft palate, below by the tongue, and on either side by the tonsils. The two ridges of mucous membrane behind the tonsils are called the pillars of the fauces.

Favus: the name given to one type of ringworm (q.v.).

Febrifuges: an older name for antipyretic drugs or remedies.

Feeble-mindedness: (*see* Mental Deficiency).

Feeding: the details of the *kind* of foods necessary to health are described under the heading of Diet and here we are only concerned with the other factors such as timing and quality. There is no evidence that regular meals are of any importance except in cases of peptic ulcer where the rule has been a stomach 'never full, never empty'; otherwise the hours of adult feeding are simply a matter of social convenience as are the rules of infant feeding which are, like their bed-times, arranged for the convenience of grown-ups. Time has dealt harshly too with the belief that one should take 'eighteen chews to each bite,' for, although it is advisable to chew food thoroughly before swallowing it, the fact is that some people are prone to peptic ulcer no matter how carefully they eat whilst others could swallow all their food in large lumps without suffering in the least. Indeed many people who are wholly without teeth have never had indigestion in their lives although there is no doubt that in their presence digestion would take place much more rapidly. Because of the infantile association between food and love many people in adult life unconsciously associate the two with the result that they may, when anxious or unhappy, overeat (anxiety is an important cause of obesity), or they may attach undue importance to food and accept peculiar ideas about its potency to cure all ills (i.e. become food cranks). Thus, apart from vegetarianism, we have in recent years had two diets or forms of treatment one based on the belief, for which there is no medical evidence whatever, that proteins and carbohydrates should not be eaten together in the same meal, and the other on the equally absurd belief that meals are improved by the addition of something which is quaintly described as 'black-strap molasses' (presumably treacle). Yet another individual described as an old-fashioned American country doctor advocates the use of sour cider and honey as a cure for nearly every disease under the sun, although why sugar and vinegar should have this remarkable effect is not known – in any case it enabled him to become a best-seller among unscientific readers. It can be said categorically (*a*) that *how* one takes one's food does not matter from the medical point of view so long as enough of the essential food materials are available from either animal or vegetable sources; (*b*) that *when* one takes one's food does not matter in normal people; (*c*) that most people eat too much and their food tends to be too rich, too soft, not bulky enough, and not fresh enough. There would be healthier teeth and no need to worry about constipation if people would eat hard foods which require biting and chewing and with enough roughage to give bulk to the motions and stimulate the bowels. Most of us would be much the better for a period of fasting and yet one finds that anyone who has the temerity to miss a meal or even, when not feeling inclined, chooses to fast for a few days is immediately put under strong social pressure (which ranges from that of the lunatic fringe which apparently believes that anyone who fasts even for a single day is in danger of imminent death to that of the disgruntled housewife who feels that any refusal of a meal is an affront to herself) to eat whether he wants to or not. An improved appetite is a *sign* of better health in the invalid, not the *cause* of it, and nobody should eat (except in certain nervous illnesses) if he does not feel inclined. Vegetarianism (q.v.) is an example of a belief which can be perfectly well justified on the grounds of humanitarianism, personal taste, or even health, but is all too often held in the form of an absurd obsession amounting almost to a religion. There is no reason at all why people should not be vegetarians but neither is there any reason why they should read magazines about it, preach it, and try to convert others whilst shutting themselves off from intimate social intercourse with the rest of the world in the process. A man who was obsessed with a desire for inch-thick steaks or caviare would rightly be judged a sensualist but so is the vegetarian who allows himself to think that his practice is more than a matter of preference and in effect centres his life around food which, in ordinary civilised life, does not justify more attention than that due to any other cultural commodity. What disconcerts the ordinary man about vegetarians is not what they believe but the way in which they believe it for he not unjustly senses that here is someone who is prepared to give up the ordinary pleasures of company in order to save his own soul or body. It is worth while pointing out that at a time when vegetarians and other food faddists are ever more vehemently insisting on the importance of diet in curing disease, orthodox medicine tends to pay rather less attention to it than in the past; there are very few detailed diets in medical treatment today and even in the treatment of peptic ulcer it is sufficient in most cases to require the patient to leave out fried foods, spicy or rich foods, and to eat little and often. Obesity, diabetes, gastric and some intestinal diseases, and kidney diseases in some instances, require what might be described as special diets but in fact are only slight modifications of ordinary ones. In fact, even the gastric diet is dying out since a group of British research workers found that ulcer cases recovered more quickly on a normal diet (including sardines) than on a milk one. Dietetic peculiarities form part of certain religious creeds as in Mohammedanism and Judaism and one is usually told that, e.g. the prohibition of pork in both these religions had its origin as a hygienic precaution in areas and at times when 'measly pork' could cause tape-worm infestation. This is not true, for prohibition of pork is only one of many food prohibitions in Judaism (e.g. all the blood must be removed from meat after killing, milk must not be taken with meat, etc.) and the real reasons are to be sought in the unconscious mind as revealed by psycho-analytic theory which would see vegetarianism and the eating of kosher meat as reactions against latent aggression or 'bloodthirstiness' and the prohibition against 'seething a kid in its mother's milk' as a primitive incest taboo, just as the over-valuation of food is a substitute for love. Thus a great many food peculiarities must be understood in primitive emotional terms rather than in terms of the rationalisations given to ac-count for or justify them. At a time when some of us are worrying about overeating it is worth while remembering that 500 million people in the world are suffering from acute mal-nutrition and 1,000 millions from varying degrees of it.

Femur: the thigh-bone and the largest and strongest bone in the body which at its upper end fits into the ball and socket joint of the acetabulum of the pelvis and at the lower end meets the tibia and patella or knee-cap at the knee-joint. The femur is often broken by comparatively slight injuries in old age when the bones have become brittle but requires considerable force to cause a fracture during the earlier years of adult life.

Fenestration: the fenestration procedure or Lempert opera-tion is one of the great contributions to modern surgery for it enables many people to hear who would formerly have been reduced to lip-reading or the use of hearing aids. Unfortun-ately the method does not help those whose deafness is due to damage to the auditory nerve or to a chronic middle ear in-fection with a perforated ear-drum and its use is limited to the sufferer from conduction deafness whose condition is due to ankylosis of the ossicles (*see* Ear) and notably of the stapes which has become rigid and fixed to such a degree that it cannot transmit the vibrations of the ear-drum to the opening in the inner ear and the fluid or perilymph within. The fenes-tration operation creates a new opening into the inner ear to enable the vibrations from the drum to be carried directly to the inner ear, and in order to do this the drum has to be moved so that it lies in contact with and directly over the new opening. This is a delicate procedure which requires great sur-gical skill but with a competent surgeon over 75% of patients show a marked improvement in their hearing. The operation is usually carried out under local anaesthesia and may be fol-lowed by slight dizziness and noises in the head which, how-ever, usually pass off in a week or two.

Ferments: (*see* Enzymes).

Fern-Root: male-fern or filix mas root is used in the form of an extract to expel tapeworms (*see* Worms). It is usually given as an emulsion or in a capsule.

Festinant Gait: the type of gait found in paralysis agitans or in Parkinsonism following encephalitis lethargica (q.v.). It is characterised by a tendency to move quickly as if the legs were trying to catch up with head and shoulders (*see* Parkinson's Disease).

Fever: a condition of the body characterised by a temperature above the normal and accompanied by disturbances of normal functions. The normal temperature is usually given as 98·4 degrees Fahrenheit, but since the body temperature varies throughout the day anything between 98·4 (or lower) and 99·5 may be taken as, for all practical purposes, normal. Thus the temperature rises after a large meal, during hot weather when it is less easy for the body to get rid of heat, after prolonged or violent exercise, and in any case it is at its highest norm between the hours of 4–9 p.m., and at its lowest between the hours of 1.30–7 a.m. In women, the temperature even varies with the menstrual cycle, notably just prior to ovulation (the fertile period) and the method of taking daily temperature readings is used in contraceptive practice to calculate the safe period or, in those who suffer from sterility, to calculate the time when fertilisation is most likely to occur. A raised temperature is usually, but by no means always, a sign of bacterial or virus infection; it may, e.g. be raised very considerably in heat-stroke, in certain types of brain injury or disease, and, especially in children, from nervous shock. The body temperature is controlled by a centre in the brain which ensures that there will exist a balance between heat-production and heat-loss, but in bacterial invasion both these processes are affected, heat-production being greatly stimulated by the breakdown of tissues and their increased oxidation whilst heat-loss is correspondingly diminished owing to disturbance of the functional activity of the heat-eliminating organs and particularly the skin. A fever is usually ushered in by a rigor which may vary from mere sensations of chilliness to violent shivering in which the whole body trembles uncontrollably and the teeth chatter. Although this is often termed the cold stage of a fever because the skin feels cold and clammy, it is in fact accompanied by raised temperature within the body and it is during this stage that convulsions frequently occur in young children. When the temperature becomes established the hot stage has arrived in which the skin is hot and dry and there is a feeling of lassitude, aching muscles, headache, and thirst; the urine is scanty, there may be constipation, nausea and vomiting, and the pulse and respirations are speeded up. This is finally succeeded by profuse sweating, a copious flow of concentrated urine, and general relief of the symptoms which, if it takes place rapidly, is known as the 'crisis' (e.g. in lobar pneumonia) or more gradually when it is known as 'lysis.' A high temperature is often accompanied by delirium and, even when this is not apparent, the patient's mental state is likely to be somewhat confused with a loss of awareness of the passage of time, nightmares, etc. Death during a fever may occur suddenly on slight exertion which the weakened heart is unable to bear, or it may terminate in the so-called 'typhoid state' when the patient gradually sinks into a weakened condition, becomes delirious, and finally comatose. Numerous types of temperature curve are seen when regular readings are marked on a chart and these often give valuable information about the nature of the infection, e.g. prior to the discovery of antibiotics and the sulpha drugs the curve of lobar pneumonia was characterised by a rising temperature reaching its peak after about a week when the condition was resolved in non-fatal cases by sudden crisis and return to normal. The temperature in diphtheria, miliary tuberculosis and typhoid fever is sometimes only slightly raised, whereas children with quite mild infections may have a high fever with convulsions and delirium, so it follows that the degree of fever is not always a reliable guide to the severity of the disease. The commonest type of temperature curve is the *continuous* type in which the temperature rises more or less rapidly, remains at about the same level for some days or even a couple of weeks, and then comes down to normal by either crisis or lysis; to this type belongs most of the common fevers of childhood. In *relapsing* fever the same things happens, and the temperature remains normal for about a week only to be followed by a further bout of fever which, after another latent period, may occur two or three times. *Remittent* fever occurs in typhoid when the temperature, although never coming down to normal, shows morning and evening variations, with a higher evening temperature and a lower morning one. This type of chart is typical of many tropical diseases and sometimes in wasting diseases. *Intermittent* fevers such as malaria show periodic attacks of fever at specific intervals with normal temperature in between; quotidian fever occurs every twenty-four hours, tertian fever every forty-eight hours, and quartan every seventy-two.

It will be seen from the above that the use of the clinical thermometer at home is strictly limited, firstly because the really valuable information is obtained from a regular series of readings from which the trend of the curve can be noted, and secondly because there is little value in a single reading which the user is rarely able to interpret. The degree of fever within wide limits gives no indication of the severity of the disease since a high temperature may mean quite a trivial disease and a low temperature or none at all does not mean that all is well. A patient may be very ill without any fever. Furthermore, the habit of constantly bringing out the thermometer whenever a child complains of feeling unwell is to be deprecated since its sole result is likely to be that he becomes neurotic about his health. If someone who 'feels a cold coming on' takes his temperature – what information has he gained from the observation that his temperature is 100 degrees? Absolutely none at all; for half an hour before it might have been 102 degrees or this might be his temperature half an hour later. If it is normal, it still tells him nothing since it does not stop him from feeling ill nor guarantee that he will not feel worse in an hour or so. A doctor using a clinical thermometer is not basing his diagnosis on its reading but merely using it to confirm what he has learned from other sources, e.g. if a generalised rash is present then a raised temperature makes a diagnosis of scarlet fever more probable whilst a normal temperature (taken together with other indications) might suggest an allergic rash. In the latter case he would think twice before diagnosing scarlet fever as a certainty although probably continuing to treat the condition as the more serious illness whilst (in view of the possibility that the patient is allergic) taking care with the type of drug he prescribes. True, a child who has been irritable and moody will be treated with more respect if it can be shown that he has a fever which may reasonably be supposed to be the cause of his irritability, but the absence of a fever does not justify us in treating him as if nothing were wrong and he is merely bad-tempered. The presence of a fever is always significant but its absence does not imply the opposite. Fever is a symptom and its treatment is that of its cause which is discussed under the names of the various fevers.

Fibrillation: a term applied to tremor in muscles when they are stimulated as found in the body muscles in certain nervous diseases and in the heart in auricular or ventricular fibrillation. In the latter case the auricles or ventricles quiver constantly instead of contracting fully so that beats reach the pulse only irregularly. This is the commonest and most serious cause of an irregular pulse (*see* Heart).

Fibrin: (see Coagulation).

Fibrin Foam: a preparation for arresting bleeding which has the advantage of being absorbable by the tissues and therefore does not need to be removed after the bleeding has stopped. It is a spongy material which is soaked in a solution of thrombin immediately before use. Also used for this purpose are oxycellulose gauze which supplies a large surface where clotting can take place and calcium alginate which is obtained from seaweed. Such haemostatics are a great boon especially in operations on the brain and blood-vessels and in diseases of the blood where the clotting-power is diminished.

Fibrinogen: (*see* Coagulation).

Fibocystic Disease: a disease characterised by softening of bones with the formation of fibrous tissue and the development of non-malignant tumours and cysts which replace bone. It may be generalised when it is known as von Recklinghausen's disease or generalised osteitis fibrosa or localised to one or two bones. In the former type the cause is a benign tumour of the parathyroid glands the removal of which cures the disease resulting from an excess of parathyroid hormone in the blood, in the latter case no parathyroid tumour is found and the blood calcium and phosphatase are not raised as in the generalised type. The symptoms are pain in the back, pelvis, or limbs, tenderness on pressure, and occasionally spontaneous fracture. The localised disease occurs usually in adolescents, the generalised mostly in women over the age of twenty. Symptoms of tetany may occur (q.v.) and, prior to operation a diet rich in calcium should be given. Fibrocystic disease should be suspected when a fracture occurs with little or no violence or when several fractures have occurred more easily than seems normal.

Fibroid: a non-malignant tumour consisting of muscular and fibrous tissue enclosed within a capsule which occurs in the womb, most usually in the main part or body but in about 8% of cases in the cervix or neck. It is commonest in childless women and rarely becomes malignant; most fibroids of the body of the womb are multiple whilst those of the cervix are often single. The symptoms are due to the mechanical effect of the swellings in causing congestion of the womb or pressure on surrounding areas and frequently there are no symptoms at all or only those due to congestion such as flooding during the periods (menorrhagia) or bleeding in between the periods (metrorrhagia). Pressure may cause pain, although this is unusual, or more commonly attacks of retention of urine, varicose veins, swelling of the ankles, and piles, all of which are caused by pressure on the abdominal veins. There may be some discharge if sloughing has occurred and sterility or miscarriage is common. The treatment for fibroids is removal by operation and in some cases, especially if the patient has passed the child-bearing age and there are many fibroids, removal of the whole womb (hysterectomy). Radiotherapy is not often indicated except in the case of small single tumours or when the patient is suffering from some general disease which makes operation inadvisable. The cause of fibroids is not known but in view of the fact that they occur more often in childless women it is not improbable that some imbalance of the sex-hormones is responsible.

Fibroma: a usually small and non-malignant tumour occurring in fibrous tissue. The fibroid tumours of the womb (see above) are composed of both fibrous and muscle tissue hence are described as fibromyomata and, unlike the common fibromata of others parts of the body, may grow to a great size.

Fibrosis: the formation of fibrous or scar tissue in place of normal tissue which has been destroyed by injury, infection, or deficient blood supply (*see* Fibrous Tissue).

Fibrous Tissue: is of two types, white and yellow, the former being very plentiful in the body, tough, and unyielding when put upon the stretch, the latter highly elastic, much less plentiful, but equally strong. White fibrous tissue is composed of thin stringy fibres of a substance known as 'collagen' which are produced by star-shaped cells lying between the fibres. It is found in the ligaments of the body, the sinews, binding the muscle fibres together in all the larger muscles, and in scar tissue and the deeper layers of the skin; in the case of scar tissue, it has the tendency to contract over a period of time sometimes leading to deformity. Yellow fibrous tissue is composed of elastic fibres of a substance known as 'elastin' and is found in the walls of arteries and in those ligaments (e.g. at the back of the neck) where some degree of elasticity is desirable. A cheloid is an overgrowth of scar tissue in an old wound or burn.

Fibula: the splint-bone of the leg which is situated behind and to the outer side of the tibia or shin-bone. Its upper end articulates with the tibia, the lower end with the astragalus where it forms the outer projection of the ankle or external malleolus which is sometimes fractured in accidents (Pott's Fracture, named after the surgeon Percival Pott who first described it, and often mistaken for a simple sprain and therefore missed).

Filariasis: the name of a group of tropical diseases caused by minute Nematode worms or filariae which produce amongst other symptoms the swelling of the legs known as elephantiasis (q.v.).

Fingers: consist of three bones or phalanges joined together by hinge joints and strong ligaments with the exception of the thumb which has only two phalanges. The movements of flexion (bending) and extension (straightening) are carried out by powerful muscles in the forearm which pass as tendons, two in front and two behind, to each finger. These tendons are covered by synovial sheaths which contain fluid to enable the muscles to work without friction and they are inserted in the base of the middle and end phalanges back and front. On the side of each finger are two small arteries and two small nerves which are of particular importance in view of the great sensitivity of the finger-tips; these are branches of the radial and ulnar arteries and nerves of the forearm. The ulnar nerve supplies only the little finger and the adjoining half of the next finger, all the rest being supplied by the radial nerve. At the tip of each finger is the nail (*see* Nail, Diseases of) whilst at the other end it is joined to the metacarpal bones of the hand, one to each finger. The diseases most commonly affecting the fingers, apart from injuries, are those connected with their blood-supply as in Raynaud's disease or chilblains, arthritis (usually rheumatoid arthritis), neuritis, skin dieases, and in the nail, ringworm.

Fissure: a crack or small narrow ulcer occurring most commonly at the corners of the mouth or on the mucous membrane of the anus. Fissures give trouble because they are in parts which are frequently stretched and often take a long time to heal both for this reason and because they are constantly in contact with faeces or saliva which are likely to be infected. Fissures at the corners of the mouth are kept going by movement and because of the natural tendency to keep touching them with the tip of the tongue; in many cases the cause of the fissure is an infection of the mouth itself but cold weather may have some effect since they are more frequent in winter-time. Fissure of the anus is often extremely painful especially on moving the bowels and this causes a tendency to constipation through fear of pain when the bowels act. Since the constipation aggravates the condition a vicious circle is set up. Fissures are usually treated by cauterisation with a caustic stick but it is necessary to exclude infection of the mouth and, in fissures of the anus, to ensure that the motions are kept soft by the use of mild purgatives. Sometimes the mere injection of a local anaesthetic by making normal motions possible cures the fissure.

Fistula: an abnormal channel between a natural cavity and the surface of the body or between two natural cavities, e.g. between the intestines and the skin surface or between the bladder and the intestines. This may arise from errors of development as when a child is born with a channel from the thyroid gland to the surface; from a blocked duct as when, a salivary duct being blocked, a fistula develops which discharges saliva on to the cheek; from injury, as when a torn urethra causes a fistula which discharges urine through the tissues to the skin, or fistula of bowel or bladder following difficult childbirth; from disease, as when a fistula arises between the bowel and bladder from an abscess or tumour in the pelvis. One of the commonest types is fistula in ano, i.e. a fistula between the lower part of the rectum and the skin

209

surrounding the anus caused by an abscess in the region, sometimes tuberculous but more usually of the ordinary type. In most cases the fistula heals when the normal channel is restored, but fistula in ano is more difficult to deal with as it is kept constantly infected by the faeces which pass through. In this case a minor operation is necessary and care is taken afterwards to ensure that closure takes places from the deepest part first.

Fits: (*see* Convulsions).

Flat Foot: an acquired deformity of the foot in which both arches are impaired, more particularly the longitudinal one. The arch of the foot, which is normally seen in a wet footprint as an empty space between the areas marked out by the base of the toes and the heel bounded only by the outer edge of the foot, is flattened so that the whole print looks broader and the empty space no longer exists. The longitudinal arch is supported by the two tibial muscles on the inner side and two peroneal muscles on the outer side which cause it to be hollow from before back as the transverse arch causes the foot to be hollow from side to side; when the latter weakens, the broadening-out of the foot seen clearly in a print results. A person who is flat-footed tends to walk with the toes turned out planting the feet flat on the ground with each step, there is pain along the inner border of the sole and sometimes beneath the ankle on the outer side, walking becomes fatiguing, and it becomes difficult to maintain any job which entails standing or much walking. The causes of flat-foot are (1) general debility or overweight with lack of tone in the muscles, (2) long hours of standing, hence its commonness in policemen, waiters, and nurses, (3) sometimes it occurs following an injury, e.g. a Pott's Fracture of the ankle. The treatment is building up the general health, exercises (walking on tiptoe, raising and lowering the body on tip-toe, walking on the outer edge of the foot, balancing on the outer edge of the foot), supports of the type sold in shops dealing in such appliances which may take the form either of a steel arch or a sponge rubber pad, manipulation, and operation. Supports relieve the symptoms almost immediately but are not usually to be recommended since they not only prevent the arch from becoming stronger by taking away its normal function but even stretch further the already lax tendons and ligaments of the sole thus increasing the degree of flat-foot. Manipulation endeavours to set the foot in the correct position which is maintained for a month or so in plaster and in operative treatment part of the bone may be removed from the inner side to shorten the instep and make a new arch. The results of operation and manipulation are sometimes disappointing and there is no doubt that, in the early stages, the best treatment is improvement of the general health and exercise. Although these points sometimes escape the specialist in orthopaedics, it is worth while noting (a) that many people have flat-foot without any symptoms, (b) that others become obsessed with the condition and use it, in effect, as a neurotic symptom to evade unpleasant duties (e.g the 'excused boots' character well-known to the army of former days), (c) that flat-foot can be a very considerable disability to those whose work involving standing may be imperilled by the condition.

Flatulence: gas in the stomach or intestines which may become evident in distension of the abdomen, unpleasant rumblings inside, a feeling of fullness and discomfort, or the passing of wind by belching or from the anus. The vast majority of cases of flatulence, i.e. all cases of flatus in the stomach and many cases of flatus in the bowels, are a self-inflicted injury caused by the neurotic habit of swallowing air which is absorbed in increasing quantities as the patient tries to bring up the air he has already swallowed. Although dyspepsia is the predisposing cause of this annoying habit (annoying not only to the patient but to those around him since many sufferers from flatulence seem to dramatise their disability), it is obvious that unless the patient makes a determined effort not to bring up any wind his condition will remain. Dyspepsia should therefore be treated but the main emphasis placed on breaking the habit. Flatus in the intestines may come from the stomach but sometimes results from decomposition of foods within the bowel; this is particularly the case in diseases of the liver or gall-bladder when the flow of bile is impeded. This type of flatulence should be investigated medically in view of the fact that it may be a symptom of some more serious disease, but it is usually helped by cutting down starchy foods and taking a light and easily-digested diet with tablets containing bile-salts or dehydrochloric acid.

Flavine: or acriflavine (q.v.).

Flexibilitas Cerea: waxy flexibility is an abnormal state in

211

which the patient's limbs remain in whatever position they are moved by the observer. It is a symptom of catatonic schizophrenia.

Flooding: the common name for excessive bleeding in women whether during the menstrual period, when it is described as menorrhagia, or between the periods, when it is known as metrorrhagia. It may indicate a miscarriage, glandular upset (especially at the change of life), or some local disease in the womb (e.g. fibroids) (*see* Menstruation).

Flukes: (*see* Infection).

Fluorescin: an orange-coloured powder used in watery solution to detect ulcers or injuries on the cornea of the eye which it stains bright yellow-green.

Fluorine: one of the halogen series of elements, i.e. belonging to the same group as chlorine and bromine, which is one of the normal constituents of bones and teeth. Its main interest today is in connection with the controversy about adding fluorine to public water-supplies in which it is lacking in order to prevent dental caries. It has been shown that those who have habitually used water with a concentration of 1 part per million of fluorine are more free from dental decay than those whose water-supply is fluorine-free. Opponents of this scheme contend (1) that as a matter of public morality no one has a right to add materials to the water-supply which all have to use whether they approve or not, (2) that fluorine has not been proved to have the stated effect beyond all doubt, that it may stain the teeth, and that in larger amounts it is known to be poisonous. Those who support it point out, (1) that in fact many chemicals are already added to the drinking supply in order to purify it and kill any organisms present and adding fluorine is no different in principle from this, (2) that there is little or no doubt that fluorine prevents decay and in the amounts used it is neither likely to stain the teeth nor to harm the general health. The latest report shows that in those drinking fluoridated water all their lives the incidence of caries is 66% less than elsewhere.

Foetus: the unborn child, particularly from the stage when it becomes recognisable as belonging to the species of its parents; prior to this it is usually called the embryo. The ovum or egg is fertilised in the Fallopian tube (q.v.) and in the first week of fertilisation passes into the cavity of the womb where within a further two weeks it is about ½-inch long. By the fourth week the embryo becomes curved like a comma and buds appear which will become the ears and the limbs and in the following week the eyes appear and the segments of the limbs are defined. At the end of two months the embryo has a definitely human appearance with a nose, separate fingers, and the tail which has hitherto been prominent is reduced to a rudiment; its length is then just over an inch. In the third month the limbs are clearly human, the finger and toe-nails appear, and sex can be distinguished. In the fourth month the foetus is from four to six inches long, hair has appeared, and the legs have become proportionately longer. In the sixth month the foetus is about a foot long, eyelashes and eyebrows appear and a month later the eyes open and the foetus is capable of being born alive. The following two months see the child becoming plumper and the skin is rosy pink when before it was a dull white. At birth it should weigh from 6½–7½ pounds and be about 20 inches long. Before birth the foetus is dependent upon the mother's blood for its food and oxygen; this takes place through the placenta, a fleshy pad attached to the wall of the womb where interchange of products between mother and foetus takes place although there is no direct connection. The foetus is connected to the placenta by the umbilical cord which passes between the placenta and the umbilicus of the foetus. After birth the umbilical cord becomes atrophied.

Folic Acid: one of the more-recently discovered constituents of the vitamin B group which gets its name from the frequency with which it is found in foliage, e.g. the leaves of green plants such as spinach and grass. It is also found in liver, kidney, and yeast and has been synthesised. Folic acid is used in the treatment of megaloblastic anaemias (*see* Anaemia), especially those with a nutritional origin although in pernicious anaemia liver extract is essential. Apparently folic acid is not a complete substitute for liver extract or vitamin B12 since, although it relieves the blood symptoms of pernicious anaemia, it does not prevent the onset of nervous symptoms due to degeneration of the spinal cord.

Follicular Hormone: the hormone secreted by the follicle of the ovary when the ovum has been discharged.

Fomentation: generally applied to hot, wet, medicated or nonmedicated cloths applied to the body in order to bring blood to the area and absorb discharge. However, a fomentation may be hot and dry or cold with some lotion, e.g. lead lotion in sprains. Few people today make much use of hot boric fomentations for septic sores and in all cases a kaolin poultice is superior since it draws the wound more powerfully and does not turn the skin into a sodden area ripe for reinfection. Turpentine, laudanum, and other types of fomentation have long been discarded with a more rational approach to medicine. Kaolin poultice should be either heated in the tin in a pan of boiling water and then spread on lint or it may be spread on the lint cold and toasted under the grill of an electric or gas cooker. Unless there is much discharge there is no need to change the dressing every time and it can be toasted once more to keep it hot. The only other fomentation in common use is lead lotion applied on lint for sprains and sometimes for skin conditions; its effect is purely a local anaesthetic one. Cold soaks are, of course, used for headaches but are rarely necessary since a headache which does not respond to aspirin or some other analgesic is unlikely to respond to cold water.

Fomites: a term describing all articles which have been in contact with an infected person, e.g. clothes, bedding, toys, books, etc., and which may therefore, at least in theory, spread the disease. The totally different attitude to this problem is discussed under the heading of Antiseptics. Briefly, the risk from such articles is in most cases much less than used to be thought and it is not necessarily believed to be a bad thing to contract the ordinary childhood fevers early in life since they are likely to be caught anyhow and are much more dangerous in adult life. Whereas formerly all bed-clothing, etc., was sterilised by boiling and books and toys were burned, the ordinary case of measles or scarlet fever today is treated little differently so far as this is concerned from any other illness. This, however, does not apply to serious infectious diseases like smallpox or to lice or flea-spread diseases where clothing, etc., may need to be destroyed.

Fontanelle: the gaps in the skull which normally close by the eighteenth month. The largest is the anterior fontanelle at the meeting-point of the frontal or forehead-bone and the two parietal bones of the side of the skull; it is about one square inch in size at birth and the pulsation of the brain can easily be felt through it by the fingers. Delay in closing results from deficiency in vitamin D and indicates rickets or other causes of defective development. In fevers, especially bronchitis and whooping cough, and in minor degree of hydrocephalus the fontanelle is bulging and tense, whilst it sags in fluid deficiency, e.g. from diarrhoea.

Food-poisoning: a very general term applied loosely to the symptoms produced by (*a*) metallic or other inorganic poisons as the arsenic of fruit-sprays, (*b*) poisonous 'foods' such as fungi mistaken for mushrooms, (*c*) bacteria and their toxins. It is now used more correctly for the third group only and such diseases are notifiable. The symptoms of all types of food-poisoning are roughly similar and consist of gastro-enteritis (inflammation of the stomach and intestines) with vomiting and diarrhoea, colic, and a temperature which is more or less raised. Formerly bacterial poisoning was incorrectly described as 'ptomaine poisoning,' but this word is no longer used. The commonest types are those due to staphylocci and those caused by the salmonella group which includes typhoid and paratyphoid fevers and infections with B. Aertrycke, B. Enteritidis, and B. Suipestifer, some of which are harmless to man but harmful to animals and some harmful to both. It is the latter which are often responsible for outbreaks in local communities and they may be spread by the excreta of rats or mice, by infected meat, milk, and occasionally by duck's eggs. Staphylococcal infections are found most frequently in twice-cooked meats or foods requiring much handling, e.g. pies, minced meat, factory-prepared meat products, since septic sores on the worker may cause the food to be infected or tonsillitis or a discharging ear produce the same effect. Dysentery is a separate group (q.v.) and botulism (q.v.), one of the most deadly forms of food-poisoning in which nervous symptoms predominate, is also fortunately one of the rarest. It is caused by infection of badly-canned food. The most important factor in food-poisoning is obviously prevention and it is necessary that strict hygienic precautions should be enforced amongst the workers in food factories and restaurants or canteens; similarly it is unwise to eat twice-cooked foods which may have gone 'off' particularly in summer-time or during hot weather when bacteria have a chance to multiply. In tropical countries special precautions are required in washing vegetables and fruit which are often manured with human excreta. Although most cases of food-poisoning are relatively trivial, all cases should be referred to the doctor because of their infectiousness and their seriousness in young children. It is unnecessary to say at the present time that these conditions are caused by specific germs and their toxins and have nothing to do with the mere fact that food is not fresh although it is in such food that any disease-causing germs present have had a chance to multiply, e.g. we eat cheese and game which has gone 'off' with impunity because they have not been infected with the specific organisms. The treatment of food-poisoning depends on its cause (*see* Diarrhoea, Dysentery).

Foot: the foot is very similar in structure to the hand, the toes being composed of three phalanges with only two in the big toe and the toes join the five metatarsal bones (corresponding to the metacarpal bones of the hand) which, in turn, articulate with the tarsal bones, seven in number, which correspond to the carpal bones of the wrist. The arrangement of the blood-vessels and nerves is similar to that in the hand and fingers (q.v.) the former coming from the anterior and posterior tibial branches of the popliteal artery a continuation of the femoral artery of the thigh, the latter coming from the branches of the anterior and posterior tibial nerves from the sciatic nerve of the thigh. The weight of the foot is borne on three distinct points: the heel, the point where the big toe joins the first metatarsal bone, and the same point at the base of the little toe. The elasticity of the foot is greatest in the longitudinal arch, but the transverse arch is so arranged that only the heads of the first and fifth metatarsals bear the weight. This is altered in flat-foot (q.v.). The main tarsal bones are the astragalus supporting the leg-bones and the calcaneus which forms the heel; the others, smaller in size, are the scaphoid three cuneiform or wedge-shaped bones, and the cuboid bones (*see* Corns, and Bunions; Chilblains; Bone, Diseases of; Gout; Nails; Drop-foot; Flat-foot; Club-foot).

Foramen: natural openings in bone for the passage of blood-vessels or nerves needed in their nutrition; the largest foramen in the body is the foramen magnum through which, at the base of the skull, the spinal cord passes from the brain to the spinal column.

Forgetfulness: (*see* Memory).

Formalin: or formic aldehyde is a gas prepared by the oxidation of methyl alcohol. In solution with water it is used as a 2–10% spray for disinfecting rooms and in 1% solution for hand-washing. Formaldehyde as it is better called is also used in the form of Paraform tablets heated over a flame for room disinfection and in a 1/500 solution as a mouth-wash or gargle. Apart from its use in hardening or preserving specimens, formalin is much less used in medicine than formerly. Room disinfection is anyhow useless.

Formic Acid: found in the stings of certain insects such as ants, bees, and wasps. It has been used in arthritis and other conditions on the naïve assumption that 'natural' products have some mysterious virtue not possessed by synthetic ones and that, since it occurs in creatures which are noted for their activity, a similar result will be produced in those who use it. In fact this form of therapy is used only by unsophisticated people or cranks and what effect it produces is through its counter-irritant action which, put bluntly, means that the sting is sufficiently irritant to distract the attention from the original source of discomfort. A similar result would be produced by burning with a cautery.

Fractures: in theory fractures of bone may occur in any part of the body but in practice they are most commonly found in certain well-defined areas, e.g. the most common fracture of the forearm is a Colles' fracture of its lower end, the most common fracture of the leg is a Potts' fracture in the same area. This is partly due to the varying strength or weakness of bones in different areas, partly to the very similar ways in which people tend to have accidents, e.g. falling on the outstretched hand in the former instance, 'going over on the ankle' in the latter. Numerous different types of fracture are described: a simple fracture occurs when the bones are broken cleanly with little laceration of surrounding tissue and no communication with the skin surface; a greenstick fracture is characteristic of injuries in children when the bones, being soft and not fully calcified, bend rather than break right through; a compound fracture occurs when the fracture communicates with the skin and is obviously in danger of infection; and complete and incomplete fractures are distinguished by the degree of separation of the broken ends – a mere crack needs no further interference whilst a complete fracture with separation of the ends may need to be 'reduced' under an anaesthetic. In comminuted fractures there is much splintering and part of the bone is broken into small pieces and in impacted fractures one part of the bone is telescoped into the other. A depressed fracture of the skull happens when the area of bone affected is pushed inwards below the general level and may press on the brain, thus being a complicated one with damage to nervous or other tissue. When a fracture does not heal in the original position it is said to be malunited, in which case it may have to be broken again and fixed by operation or put in plaster. In early life bones contain a good deal of fibrous tissue and hence are more resilient and more likely to bend than break as noted above, but with increasing age they come to contain increasing amount of calcium and therefore to become more brittle and less easy to heal once a fracture occurs, e.g. a fractured hip in an elderly patient is a dangerous condition because healing without operation would require a long period in bed and this in itself is liable to lead to complications such as pneumonia. Bones are broken most frequently by indirect violence where the force has been applied at some point other than that where the break occurs having been transmitted from the point of impact as in the Colles' fracture of the wrist already mentioned. Direct violence as on the skull or ribs is usually associated with crushing injuries or blows where the bone is broken at the point of impact and, in this case, is likely from the nature of the cause to be complicated or compound. In a few instances a fracture is caused by muscular action (i.e. by the violent and sudden pull of muscles); this is a common cause of fracture of the knee-cap and sometimes happens in throwing at ball-games. Finally, those who are suffering from certain diseases associated with decalcification of the bones or cysts or tumours in bone may have fractures which occur spontaneously with little or no violence; these cases will obviously need further investigation and are to be suspected when a fracture occurs without violence or when a series of fractures occurs with only slight violence. Following a fracture there is a certain amount of bleeding from the blood-vessels which have been torn both within the substance of the bone and its surrounding membrane or periosteum. This forms a clot which surrounds the broken ends and gradually the clot becomes organised through the intervention of white blood-cells from the blood-stream, arteries, veins, and fibrous tissue being formed. This is known as 'soft callus' but with the deposition of calcium salts the fibrous tissue soon begins to harden forming 'hard callus' which initially extends in a ring around the site giving it a bulging appearance. Finally, the excess bone is absorbed leaving the bone as before the injury, unless the ends are not completely in apposition when the bulge may remain to strengthen the area. The use of X-rays has shown that many fractures are never recognised as such, especially when there is no displacement of the pieces of bone, and are simply treated as sprains or bruises, but there are certain signs present in most fractures which enable them to be diagnosed and these include uselessness of the part (particularly when a limb is affected); pain on movement, although variable, is fairly typical since it is usually absent or slight when the part is not disturbed; fracture may be accompanied by the actual sound of breaking, but this is not always reliable since the 'pulling' of a muscle or tendon may produce much the same sound; deformity usually occurs when the ends are displaced, e.g. the limb is shortened, or seems to be in an unnatural position, bent, or in the case of a fractured collar-bone the shoulder droops; on examination there is swelling, movement occurs where it should not, and the ends of the broken bone may be heard or felt grating against each other. The latter is known as crepitus. Compound fractures require first of all to be treated as wounds and ordinarily by the doctor under an anaesthetic; since infection may very easily occur and in such cases can be serious, this is an urgent necessity before the fracture is even looked at. The surgeon will frequently deal with the bone at the same time by fixing it with silver wire or a plate. If the wound is contaminated, scrubbing with antiseptic will be necessary and an injection of anti-tetanic serum may be given. Obviously, when medical help is expected soon, all that is necessary is to splint the bone with some rigid substance such as sticks or rolled-up newspaper in the position which gives least pain and keep the patient comfortable (but not too hot) giving him warm drinks with sugar. Many types of splint are described, but special

219

splints should only be applied by those, e.g. with Red Cross or St John Ambulance training who have some experience. 'Reduction' of a fracture is accomplished by exerting gentle pull on the end of the limb below the break until the ends come into apposition but this is usually done under an anaesthetic and should not be attempted unless no skilled help is going to be available. Fractures of the flat bones, e.g. the skull, cannot usefully be dealt with except by a surgeon. The general first-aid rule in fractures of the limbs is that, provided they are not compound, the clothes should not be removed, movement should be reduced to a minimum, and splints applied in the extended position in the case of the leg or splinted and put in a sling in the case of the arm (exceptions are those in the region of the elbow, when the forearm should be bent at a right-angle to the upper arm by an L-shaped splint, or in a broken collar-bone when it should be slung just under the neck by the wrist). Fractures of other parts, being nearly always the result of direct violence, are likely to be compound and splinting is either unnecessary or impossible as a first-aid measure but the wound must be cleared as soon as possible with Dettol or some other suitable antiseptic and warm water. The antiseptic must not be strong and it must on no account be greasy – in fact, in any sort of major injury or burn oily or greasy applications must be avoided since they are in no way superior to watery solutions, in many ways inferior, and interfere with later treatment by the specialist. Fractures of the hip are common in old people and used to be serious in that they caused shock and necessitated a prolonged period in bed during which pneumonia, bronchitis, or some other complication might arise. Today they are treated by passing a nail into the neck of the femur where it enters the hip-joint (their usual site) through a small opening in the skin and allowing the patient up almost immediately. In cases where this is not possible, the patient may have to be left with the fracture unjoined. When in doubt the best first-aid rule is 'splint them where they lie,' keep fractures of the leg in an extended position, the arm in a sling, and for suspected fractures of the spine keep the patient lying flat on his stomach.

Framboesia: a granulomatous disease (q.v.), also known as yaws, caused by the *treponema pertenue* which cannot be distinguished microscopically from the organism of syphilis, the treponema pallidum. It is found mainly in Africa and the West Indies, but also in South-East Asia and the Pacific islands, and is not a venereal disease being spread through contact when there are abrasions on the skin and probably by flies and insect bites. As in syphilis, the Wassermann reaction (q.v.) is positive and the treatment is with penicillin and arsenical compounds to which it readily responds. The incubation period is at least a month when the onset is insidious with headache, aching in the muscles and bones, and sometimes slight fever. The primary sore is a small boil-like area which soon becomes hard and breaks down to form the raspberry appearance which gives the disease its name (frambosia=raspberry). Others occur in any part of the body, usually painless, but sometimes itchy.

Freckles: small yellow or brown pigmented spots appearing on exposed areas in sunshine in those who are susceptible. They are simply localised areas of sunburn and occur mainly in blonde or red-headed people being found attractive by most men and unattractive by many women who therefore waste much time trying to remove them. Strictly speaking, this cannot be done and once they have formed freckles must be left to fade, but to some extent they can be prevented by the use of sunburn creams and avoidance of exposure. Obviously it is also possible to conceal them with cosmetics or by obtaining a deep sunburn which covers them up (*see* Skin, Sunburn).

Freudian Theory: (*see* Psychoanalysis).

Friar's Balsam: Balsams are substances exuded from the trunks of certain trees and containing resins (which give them their characteristic smell) and benzoic acid. They are mainly used (e.g. balsam of Peru or Tolu) for cough medicines or inhalations and Friar's balsam or compound tincture of benzoin is usually given as a soothing inhalation for colds in the dose of 1 teaspoonful to 1 pint of boiling water.

Friedreich's Ataxia: a hereditary degenerative disease of the nervous system which runs in families and usually arises between the years of 5–15 in either sex. Its earliest symptoms are clumsiness of gait and deformities of the foot but since these are found in other diseases correct diagnosis depends on the specialist. In a few cases the onset may be later in life. As in most other degenerative diseases of the nervous system there is no cure but sometimes the condition ceases to develop of its own accord although the damage already done cannot be un-done and the patient may be bedridden. Exercises and massage are important to keep the muscles in good tone.

Fringe Medicine: a common term used for the methods of people who, sometimes rudely described as 'quacks,' practice medicine usually without orthodox medical qualifications. However the word 'quack' is best reserved for uneducated individuals who peddle remedies on their own, often, or gener-ally, knowing them to be worthless. Those we are concerned with are not like that at all, and there is no reason to doubt that there are as many sincere practitioners of fringe medicine as there are of orthodox medicine. Most of these bodies tend to have the following characteristics: (1) they are usually founded by one man (Hahnemann for homoeopathy, Andrew Still for osteopathy, D. D. Palmer for chiropractic which, more recent in origin than osteopathy, claims to 'adjust the back' and 'correct faulty nutrition'); (2) they are nearly all committed to a 'system,' i.e. most of their theories can be framed in the form 'all disease is caused by . . .' with its corol-lary 'all diseases can be cured by . . .'; (3) unlike scientific medicine, they do not submit their results to scientific criteria of cure.

Now it is only fair in discussing these and other bodies that the writer should state his own feelings openly so that allow-ance can be made for personal prejudices, and his feelings on the present subject can be summarised by saying that, first of all, he has no doubt that many people *feel* better after treat-ment by one or other of these fringe bodies and does not even doubt that some are actually cured in this way. If he had had a severe pain in his foot, he would certainly have considered going to the unqualified 'bone-setter' Sir Herbert Barker (who unfortunately died in 1950), but, since men of this calibre are few and far between, he would not go to an unqualified mani-pulator today. Qualifications are not everything but at least they ensure a certain standard of skill. Furthermore, he is quite sure that if he had the courage to do so he would not only feel better but be much the better for a couple of weeks at one of those naturopath places where people exist for that period on orange juice, massage, and seven-mile walks, or that (like many famous people) he would benefit from a stay at the Bircher-Benner clinic in Zurich on a basic diet of the not unpleasant 'Birchermuesli' and other vegetarian foods. Although a rationalist, he does not doubt that 'miracles' sometimes take place at Lourdes and other centres and, indeed, commends the strict criteria by which the medical commission there defines when a 'miracle' has taken place– which, incidentally, is rather infrequently since, as the authorities themselves have stated: 'God did not create the world to interfere constantly with its laws.' It may also be said that, for a certainty, Chopin (who was suffering from tuberculosis) had his life prolonged by going to a homoeopath rather than an orthodox physician; the homoeopath did not cure him, but at least kept him from being done to death by the horrible methods then in use by orthodox medicine. With the exception of a few outstanding figures, scientific medicine hardly existed until about the middle of the 19th century with the discovery of anaesthetics and antiseptics and drugs which really worked. Even at the beginning of the present century the number of drugs which had a specific effect on disease, i.e. really went to the root of the trouble as quinine in malaria, Ehrlich's Salvarsan in syphilis, or iron in anaemia, could be numbered on the fingers of one hand and there were probably only about a score of drugs in the whole Pharmacopoeia which had any significant effect in alleviating the symptoms of disease.

In America most states permit osteopaths to give drugs and practice surgery and chiropractors work in the Armed Forces; homoeopathy (once practised by numerous orthodox physicians) seems to be dying out both in Britain and America. In this country, on the other hand, a physician would probably get into trouble if he collaborated with any unqualified practitioner. Yet many of these bodies flourish, and we must ask ourselves why. The cynical answers would be (a) that the public is almost infinitely gullible, and (b) that the vast majority of diseases have a large psychological element and that, in any case, although time may not heal all wounds, it helps an awful lot. Most diseases are self-limiting. But the more fundamental answer to the popularity of fringe medicine is, paradoxically, the success of orthodox medicine which has changed the pattern of disease. The great plagues, the specific fevers of childhood, the nutritional diseases, are largely wiped out in technically-advanced countries. People live longer and suffer more often from irreversible conditions which are sometimes concomitants of old age: inoperable cancer, osteo-arthritis, arteriosclerosis. In younger people, the infectious diseases have given way to neuroses and stress diseases, the diseases of malnutrition such as rickets to the diseases caused by eating too much. All these are much more difficult to treat, and the clients of unorthodox medicine are the disgruntled, the neurotic, the incurable who although not necessarily seriously ill want to try something else, the overfed, and the sedentary whose faulty posture leads to vague or positively severe aches and pains. As we have already seen these patients who frankly sometimes bore the average family doctor because they are always in his surgery but reject his advice, can often be really helped by someone who listens, takes their diet and exercise in hand, and gives them the faith to accept a psychological kick in the pants. Tell a business executive that he must diet and, whilst staying at home, he is unlikely to do so on the free advise of his NHS doctor; but tell him of a place in the country where, for the small sum of twenty or thirty guineas a week, he can be starved, rubbed, and take unwonted exercise, and he will think it not only money well-spent but is quite likely to be the better of his stay. (There are, after all, plenty of people in the world who think the treatment they get is worth as much as they pay for it, and the writer recollects a man who, failing to improve on a drug prescribed under the NHS, went to Portugal on holiday and was cured by one for which he paid the equivalent of £8 for a week's supply; the drug, in fact, was the same.)

In spite of all these qualifications, the writer strongly disapproves of fringe medicine for the following reasons: (1) it is simply not true that all disease has a single basic cause and a single basic cure as most of these schools imply. Thus, although D. D. Palmer's son was prepared to state that diphtheria was caused by a dislocation of the sixth dorsal vertebra, it is only those who sit comfortably at home with complaints largely brought on by their own selfish worrying or inertia who are capable of the idiocy of supposing (if indeed they ever think of it) that the millions who die yearly of the infectious tropical diseases in the less-well-developed lands are really suffering from dislocations of the spine, wrong diet, or would respond to homoeopathic remedies. Modern chiropractors, it is true, have progressed so far as to believe that bacteria and viruses actually exist, but the writer, for one, would not be found on their doorstep. (2) Whilst it sometimes happens (as in the case of electro-convulsant therapy in psychiatry) that the orthodox physician does not always know why a particular treatment works, he is always trying to find out why it does. As far as possible, he bases what he does and the results he obtains on scientific criteria of pathology, treatment, or cure (*see* the Introduction on this subject). But no homeopath, no osteopath, no chiropractor, has ever even attempted to demonstrate *that* his theory is true (except by that most fallible criterion of apparent results), or *how* his methods work, by techniques which would satisfy any scientist. (3) Whilst believing that some cures are produced by manipulation, diet, or the 'miracles' of Lourdes, the writer does not accept the official explanation for these cures : every doctor has seen, or at least heard of, cases of 'incurable' cancer which simply disappeared without any treatment, of 'agonising' pains cured by an injection of plain water, or the notorious example of cortisone which initially caused hundreds of rheumatoid arthritis sufferers who had not walked for years to leap from their wheelchairs although we now know that, except in selected cases, cortisone in this condition is no better than aspirin. (4) Whilst no risk is involved in numerous cases who go to naturopaths and the rest for treatment, there is very grave danger for those who have some disease which – diagnosed in time – can be cured by ordinary medicine or surgery. Accurate diagnosis demands all the complicated and expensive techniques only available to the qualified man in touch with a hospital; they are not available to the practitioners of fringe medicine. Such people may sometimes cure, often alleviate, but either way they are frequently guilty by basing their work on absurd theories of what a modern poet has described as 'the worst treason – *doing the right thing for the wrong reason*' (*see* Acupuncture, Homoeopathy, Osteopathy, Diet, Naturopathy).

Frolich's Syndrome: a group of symptoms occurring in pituitary disease which leads to the development of characteristics immortalised by the 'fat boy' in Dickens's *Pickwick Papers*, i.e. a grossly fat child given to overeating, slothful, prone to sleepiness, and sexually and emotionally immature. Treatment depends on the cause which necessitates expert diagnosis (*see* Endocrine Glands, Pituitary Gland). Simple underfunctioning can be dealt with by anterior pituitary hormone injections and dieting, but cases due to a tumour may require X-ray treatment or surgical operation. The condition is sometimes known as Dystrophia Adiposo-Genitalis and Diabetes Insipidus (q.v.) may also be present.

Frostbite: exposure to cold interferes with the vitality of the tissues largely but not entirely by affecting the circulation. The results are seen either in those who, for reasons not fully understood, are hypersensitive to even relatively slight cold and develop such conditions as chilblains, Raynaud's disease, etc., or in normal people who are exposed to extreme degrees of cold for prolonged periods. Into the latter category come frostbite, the 'trench foot' of the first World War, and the 'immersion foot' of the second, both of which were complicated by damp and wet. The first reaction to cold of this degree is contraction of the arteries so that the limb 'goes dead,' and this, if prolonged, leads to gangrene. Removal from the cold in the earlier stages brings about a reaction with flushing and redness which in minor degrees is a welcome sign that circulation is returning but in excess leads even more surely to inflammation and death of the part. Thus the circulation must be restored *gently* by warming against the body of the patient or another person and the treatment usually described in accounts of polar exploration which involves rubbing with snow is generally inadvisable unless no other means of restoring circulation is available, extremes of heat or cold being likely to cause tissue breakdown. The general circulation of the body should be maintained by walking about if possible and hot drinks. Alcohol is usually forbidden, but although frostbite is more likely to attack those who drink a good deal its action in dilating the arteries and stimulating the heart may be helpful as a first-aid measure. The rule is to keep the part mildly warmed avoiding extremes of heat or cold, keep dry, and do not rub. Very cold substances such as carbon dioxide snow (dry ice) used in ice-cream manufacture, etc., produce burns which are treated as ordinary hot ones and, at the other extreme, more moderate degrees of cold are used during surgical operations and other procedures because they reduce the demands of the body cells making prolonged operations simpler and safer. This is known as hypothermia (q.v.).

Fructose: is fruit-sugar, a monosaccharide also known as laevulose found in many fruits which, together with glucose, results from the breakdown of cane-sugar in the stomach (*see* Sugar).

Fruit: most fruits contain at least 80% of water, the amount being less in the starchy fruits such as bananas and the greatest in melons, marrows, cucumbers, pumpkins, etc. The pulp consists mostly of starch and sugar the main other constituents being acids such as citric (notably in the citrus fruits, e.g. orange, grapefruit, lemons, and limes), tartaric, and malic (in apples, etc.), and essential oils or volatile substances which give the characteristic taste. Most fruits contain varying amounts of vitamin C which is high in the citrus fruits (with the exception of limes), blackcurrants, guavas, and rosehips and although acid in themselves their action is to render the blood more alkaline. Dried fruits in which the water has been largely removed such as prunes, raisins and sultanas, dates, figs, dried apples, pears, and apricots, contain large amounts of sugar and starch but correspondingly little vitamin C. Minerals include iron and calcium and most fruits have a slightly laxative action. Some such as rhubarb and strawberries contain oxalic acid and in susceptible people can cause crystals in the urine.

Fuller's Earth: a form of aluminium silicate once mined only near Reigate in Surrey to be used for fulling cloth and wool, i.e. cleansing it of oil and grease. Today it is mined in Florida and used for clarifying cotton-seed and mineral oils for lubrication when it acts as a filter removing impurities. Used alone or with other substances it is employed as a dusting powder although less now than formerly and only after sterilisation as in a very few cases it has caused tetanus owing to spores of the germ being present in the earth.

Fumigation: the process of burning or volatilising substances in order to produce vapours which kill disease germs and vermin. Originally one of the procedures which added a sinister aspect to the infectious fevers when it was used to disinfect the sick-room and fomites or articles which had been in contact with the patient, it is now rarely employed as it is realised that very few germs live long when removed from the human body and that, in any case, it is better that infection should occur early rather than late in life. Its modern use is

227

wholly restricted to disinfection of articles by steam and hot air. Camphor and other resins have no effect whatever on germs and the only justification for their former use was the almost innate human belief that strong or nasty smells and tastes are more potent in driving out illness, germs, bad things, and evil spirits, than odourless and tasteless substances (hence the faith of a large part of the public and especially the neurotic part in 'strong' medicines, i.e. those with a foul taste or smell). Of course this belief based, consciously or unconsciously, on vague notions of devil possession is dying and disinfestation, so far as vermin are concerned, is carried out effectively by D.D.T. and other modern compounds (*see* Infection, Aerosol).

Functional Diseases: in the past this has been used as a term to describe those diseases in which the main element was believed to be neurotic, no organic disease having been found, with the implication that, although structure was normal, function was not. Thus functional dyspepsia was dyspepsia in which no damage to the stomach could be found but undue spasm of the muscles was present due to nervous tension. Formerly this has been an excuse for doing nothing but the realisation that such malfunctioning is just as troublesome to the patient as organic disease, is not synonymous with 'imaginary,' and can lead to structural changes as in the psychosomatic disorders has led to the term being discontinued save amongst those who are entirely mechanically-minded and regard their work as that of a glorified engineer (*see* Psychosomatic Diseases).

Fungus: fungi are relevant to medicine in that (*a*) a few diseases are caused by infection with fungi, e.g. ringworm, actinomycosis, and Madura foot in the tropics; (*b*) many of the antibiotics used to cure these and other diseases are derived from fungi; (*c*) poisoning by fungi used as food in mistake for edible ones occasionally occurs. The real fungus is the mycelium, a matted mass of chain-like cells which in the case of those growing in soil lies beneath the ground, the 'toadstool' or mushroom organ above the ground being simply the spore-bearing part for reproduction. In many fungi, and all those causing infection in man both spore-bearing portion and mycelium are microscopic although they are visible in bulk when they tend to form a circle owing to the limits of growth of the mycelium; thus ringworm like mushrooms and toad-stools grows in circles. The toxin in poisonous fungi is an alkaloid known as muscarine or the substance phallin; such poisoning is rare in Britain where mushrooms are usually cultivated and the other 200 odd edible fungi of a total of 2000 large ones are rarely eaten. Thus in the twenty-five years between 1920 and 1945 only 38 deaths from this cause were recorded. Muscarine is an irritant narcotic which first attacks the gastro-intestinal tract causing diarrhoea and vomiting and subsequently the nerve centres leading to weak heart action, pallor, and unconsciousness or delirium. The treatment is to give an emetic immediately followed by a large dose of castor oil, stimulants for the heart (e.g. alcohol as a first-aid measure), and the doctor will administer atropine which is a direct antidote to muscarine. An antiphallinic serum is also sometimes used. The use of rabbits' stomachs and brains eaten raw is based on the fact that rabbits are immune to poisonous fungi but whether or not this has any effect it is obviously irrelevant in the acute stages and later management is best left to a physician.

Furuncle, Furunculosis: a boil and crops of boils respectively (*see* Boil).

Gait: the way in which a person walks often gives important indications as to the medical or surgical conditions from which he may suffer. Typical are the Chaplinesque gait of severe flat-foot with the toes turned out and the feet placed flat on the ground, the dragging leg following a hemiplegia or stroke, the steppage gait of alcoholic and other forms of neuritis in which foot-drop causes the knees to be raised higher than usual as if walking through heather, the festinant gait of paralysis agitans and Parkinsonism in which short quick steps are taken and the legs seem to be trying to keep up with the top part of the body which is thrust forward. In damage to the knee-joint (e.g. arthritis) the whole leg is held stiff and in hip-joint disease the diseased leg is swung round upon the healthy one, the whole pelvis entering into the movement. When, as in locomotor ataxy, the sensory nerves supplying information from the legs are damaged the heels are placed on the ground with a stamping motion and the eyes kept fixed to the ground; when they are closed or the patient tries to turn he is liable to fall down. Infantile paralysis may produce most of these types of gait depending on the nerves affected which of course are always motor ones. Needless to say, gaits only give suggestions as to what might be wrong and an accurate diagnosis is made on quite other data.

Galactagogues: drugs which increase the supply of milk in nursing mothers in whom the natural stimulus of the child's sucking is not sufficient. The hormone prolactin from the pituitary gland has this action provided the mother is getting a reasonably nutritious diet.

Galactocele: a cyst in the breast due to obstruction of a milkduct.

Gall-Bladder Diseases: the gall-ducts begin as minute channels in the substance of the liver from whose cells they collect bile (q.v.) and these channels uniting like the tributaries of a river finally leave the liver as the right and left hepatic ducts which join and meet the cystic duct from the gall-bladder to form the common bile duct entering the duodenum a few inches from the end of the stomach. Thus, although bile from the hepatic duct is stored in the gall-bladder, blockage of the cystic duct does not prevent some from coming direct from the liver into the small intestine, the gall-bladder being a dead end. Like other fleshy organs, the gall-bladder does not show in X-rays but can be made visible by the use of radio-opaque drugs such as pheniodol which taken by mouth are excreted in the bile so that the bladder and any stones it may contain are shown up. This procedure is known as cholecystography. The function of the gall-bladder is to receive and concentrate bile and store it until is is needed, e.g. after a meal, especially with a high fat content, when it contracts to force the concentrated bile into the intestine together with the more dilute bile direct from the liver where it helps in the digestion of fats. *Cholecystitis* is an inflammation of the gall-bladder caused by an infection which may spread from the liver itself or upwards from the intestine and it is predisposed to by anything which encourages stagnation of bile. Since movement of bile depends partly on the movements of respiration lack of exercise may have this effect and the condition tends, as the saying is, to occur in women who are 'fat, fair, and forty' (frequently they are fertile as well). But it is estimated that about 25% of all women and 10% of all men living in civilised modern communities develop the condition with accompanying gall-stones before the age of 60. It must be remembered, however, that thin men are not immune and that the mere existence of gall-stones does not necessarily produce any symptoms for many people with a gall-bladder full of stones are quite unaware of the fact and apparently little the worse. More commonly one or other of the following symptoms are likely to arise: indigestion following foods which are fatty, fried or greasy, raw fruits with skins, vegetables such as turnips, cabbages or greens, sprouts, radishes, and pickles; feelings of nausea, heartburn, overfullness and flatulence; attacks of pain often severe, knife-like or colicy, in the upper right abdomen sometimes passing to the right shoulder-blade at the back. The indigestion tends to be rather indeterminate, the feeling of bloatedness typical, the times vague unlike the clock-like regularity of peptic ulcer which occurs at more or less the same time after meals, the location to the right side instead of in the middle of the abdomen or to the left as in peptic ulcer or stomach pains and duodenal ones. The acute attacks of biliary colic due to contraction of the cystic duct usually in the presence of a stone are unmistakable (although occasionally mimicked by some forms of appendicitis); they may have one of three endings according as the stone falls back into the gall-bladder when the attack will subside, gets caught in the cystic duct when infection and pain will necessitate an operation, or moves down the common bile-duct either to pass into the intestine with relief of the attack or be caught there when, the flow of all bile being impeded, jaundice appears and an immediate operation is necessary to remove the gall-bladder and open the common bile-duct to remove the stone. Gall-stones may be large, even the size of a hen's egg, and single, or there may be several hundred small stones like bird-seed, but there is little relationship between the size and the amount of distress caused, a small one caught in the duct often giving more trouble than the largest one in the bladder. These stones are formed when there is an upset in the chemistry of the body which causes cholesterol and fats to be inadequately dealt with so that they precipitate out often as a result of earlier infections since 'gall-stones are the tomb-stones of infection.' The treatment of an acute attack, apart from drugs given to relax spasm such as atropine and pain-killing drugs such as morphia, is to give sulpha drugs or antibiotics to deal with the infection, rest the patient in bed, and give a diet rich in proteins and carbohydrates but low in fat with plenty of bland liquids. Patients who have many such attacks or a severe acute attack may require operation in addition to the types of case already mentioned and it is important to realise that no medical treatment can do other than relieve the acute condition. The operation known as cholecystectomy is not a dangerous one and its after-effects are excellent but without operation serious results may follow from the toxic effects of bile obstruction, gangrene of the bladder, or a stone passing into the common bile-duct which makes operation imperative. No drugs dissolve stones and dietary or medical treatment is only palliative in the vast majority of cases. The condition of having gall-stones is known as cholelithiasis; cholecystitis or inflammation of the bladder must be regarded as either caused by stones or a precursor to their formation.

Galls: are excrescences produced in plants and trees by puncture and laying of eggs within by parasitic insects; they are better known as 'oak apples' or 'witches' brooms' and the commonly-used one is the oak-apple produced on *quercus infectoria* by the insect *cynips gallae tinctoriae*. Containing tannic and gallic acids, galls were used as astringents particularly in the form of an ointment with or without opium for applying to bleeding piles although one may doubt their ability to do more than provide temporary relief.

Galvanism: named after Luigi Galvini (1737–98) who spent much of his life in researches on the effects of electricity on animal muscle. Galvanism was a method of alleviation of pain and treatment by the application of electrical currents. Its scope is much limited today as indeed is the use of physiotherapy in general, being mainly used for muscular stimulation on tissues which due to disease of the nerves might otherwise waste or for the relief of rheumatic pains. Nobody now believes that the mere passage of electricity in itself produces any specific effect and the decreasing category of diseases of unknown origin for which (as in the neuroses) it was once used has made it of little interest to the physician although still popular amongst cranks and quacks or in the more scientifically backward areas.

Gamgee Tissue: surgical dressings composed of a thick layer of cotton-wool between two layers of absorbent gauze introduced many years ago by Sampson Gamgee, a Birmingham surgeon.

Gamma Globulin: or G.C. is the name for the protein part of the blood whose molecules can be changed into antibodies by disease-producing organisms. It was produced by the fractional separation of blood-protein by the American Professor E. J. Cohn during the last war and its use depends upon the fact that most people have had measles and many acted as host to the virus of poliomyelitis without necessarily having suffered from the disease. Mixed blood donated by a sufficiently large number of adults will contain antibodies against these diseases in the G.G. fraction which can be used in passive immunisation provided that it is given before the disease has manifested itself. The immunity, unlike that produced actively by the individual's own tissues, is temporary and only lasts for about five weeks but is capable of preventing the disease it contacts or modifying its severity considerably. It is of little value once the disease has begun.

Gammexane: the proprietary name for an insecticide (benzene hexachloride) comparable to D.D.T. and active against a large range of insect pests.

Ganglion: a word referring to two different entities: (1) a clump of nerve-cells in the course of a nerve or net-work of nerve-fibres (e.g. the Gasserian ganglion on the fifth or trigeminal nerve in the skull, the ciliary, geniculate, stellate ganglia, etc.); (2) an enlargement on the sheath of a tendon containing fluid and usually situated in front or, or behind, the wrist. The latter is a minor complaint which, first noticeable when it is about the size of a pea, may either remain in the same state for many years or grow to quite a large size extending down into the palm. Apart from inconvenience there are no symptoms and the ganglion can be burst by a sudden blow from a heavy book or steady pressure from both thumbs. Because of its liability to return surgical scraping out or the injection of sclerosing fluid may be necessary. In some cases a ganglion may be tuberculous in origin when it is necessary to remove the sheath completely. Unlike other swellings in this area a ganglion is mobile and soft and can be pushed from side to side between the fingers of the examiner.

Gangrene: the death of a fairly large area of tissue as in a superficial area where ulceration has taken place or internally when an area is affected by necrosis due to interruption of its blood-supply. The dead portion is known as a slough when the soft tissues are affected or a sequestrum where a piece of bone has died, but to the layman the most typical form of gangrene is when a whole part of a limb becomes demarcated off from the rest, usually in old people with arteriosclerosis or in diabetics, turning first dark dusky blue and subsequently black. Then, if left alone, it will drop off by itself. The portion affected may be a toe and later, because of the poor state of the circulation and perhaps some local infection in the nail-bed, the condition may spread to other toes and even the whole foot. In such cases amputation will be required and this must be at a level where circulation is still reasonably good and there is some chance of the process being stopped – often above the knee. General debility, lack of exercise, chronic kidney disease with arteriosclerosis, injury, and infection in the presence of diabetes, are all predisposing factors and black sloughing areas may also occur in bed-sores in those who are bedridden. In dry gangrene the part becomes mummified but more frequently wet gangrene with putrefaction of the tissues occurs; in the former type the part shows a sharp line of demarcation and will finally drop off but in the latter infection occurs, there is much discharge and swelling, and the temperature is raised with the risk of generalised septicaemia or blood-poisoning. The doctor's aim will be to protect the dry type and leave the course to nature pending a further consideration of the case, but in the moist type antibiotics or sulpha drugs and keeping the part dry in order to delimit it and convert it into the dry variety will be used. If this does not suffice a high amputation may be required in order to save the patient's life.

Gas gangrene is a wound infection caused by the Clostridium welchii, a specific bacillus which, together with others, produces gas in the tissues causing them to swell and give a crackling impression when touched. It spreads rapidly and is anaerobic (i.e. can only live in the absence of oxygen) being common in warfare on muddy and rich soils which contain the germ and is usually treated with oxidising agents (e.g. hydrogen peroxide) and gas-gangrene antitoxin. Nowadays the outlook is greatly improved with penicillin and drastic surgery performed as soon as possible to prevent spread.

Gantrisan: a proprietary brand of sulphafurazole, a useful sulpha drug with low toxicity.

Gargles: various substances which are brought into contact with the back of the throat without swallowing; they are usually employed for such conditions as tonsillitis, pharyngitis, and in general 'sore throats.' Their action is to clean the mouth and throat of mucus and discharge, to increase the blood-supply to the throat by reason of their warmth or the chemicals they contain, and, if antiseptics are used, to kill some of the infecting organisms. But gargles are of strictly limited value since the solution is in actual contact with the membranes for too short a period to produce much effect and the germs, by the time gargling is thought necessary, are too deeply imbedded in the tissues to be reached. However the local anaesthetic effect of aspirin makes soluble aspirin a useful gargle to relieve discomfort (10 grains or two tablets in a glass of warm water which can be subsequently swallowed) and a strong salt solution will cleanse the throat of clinging mucus. Neither as gargles or mouthwashes are strong antiseptics frequently repeated generally advisable, but potassium chlorate (12 grains in a glass of warm water), potassium permanganate (a few crystals similarly used sufficient to make a pink solution which can be seen through), glycerine with borax and boric acid or with thymol, and most of the reputable proprietary gargles are helpful. As already indicated their main function is to add to the patient's comfort by cleaning the throat and relieving irritation rather than by actually curing.

Gas-poisoning: to the gases used in industry for domestic purposes one must add today those usable in warfare, but in general gases produce their effect: (1) by merely irritating the mucous membranes of the eyes, nose, and throat as in the tear gases; (2) by paralysing nerve-endings as in the nerve gases; (3) by irritating and inflaming the bronchial tubes and lungs or stomach as with chlorine and phosgene; (4) by producing generalised effects; e.g. by combining with the haemoglobin of the blood in such a way as to make it useless for carrying oxygen as in the case of carbon monoxide in coal-gas. In non-fatal cases the after-effects usually pass off completely and the men who complained of the after-effects of chlorine poisoning after the first war were in most instances suffering from chronic bronchitis largely unrelated to the effects of gassing. For treatment in emergency *see* Coal-Gas.

Gastralgia: means pain in the stomach from whatever cause as neuralgia means pain in a nerve of a non-specific type.

Gastrectomy: the surgical operation for removal of the whole or part of the stomach. The amount removed will depend upon the reason for which the operation is being carried out and naturally the outlook will also depend upon whether or not the condition was malignant but, with this proviso, the results of gastrectomy are excellent. In a partial gastrectomy the remainder of the stomach is stitched to the small intestine and in a few months the patient will be able to eat normally without any serious disability, his general health and expectation of life being unaffected except for the better. Indications, apart from gastric carcinoma, are chronic ulcers which refuse to respond to medical treatment, repeated bleeding from ulcers, scarring leading to obstruction, perforation or threatened perforation of an ulcer; in general, gastrectomy is now preferred to the operation of gastrojejunostomy in the surgical treatment of ulcer cases. It is important to remember that well over 90% of ulcer cases never require operation at all (*see* Stomach, Diseases of, Gastroenterostomy).

Gastric: relating to the stomach. It is therefore incorrect to use the phrase 'a gastric stomach' which is a pleonasm (the use of more words than is necessary to make sense) and meaningless to boot since the significance of a diseased stomach is not given by words implying 'a stomachy stomach.'

Gastritis: inflammation of the stomach (*see* Stomach, Diseases of).

Gastro-enteritis: inflammation of the stomach and intestines usually due to infection (*see* Diarrhoea, Dysentery).

Gastro-enterostomy: or gastro-jejunostomy is an operation carried out in some cases of peptic ulcer and primarily designed to reduce the acidity of the stomach by connecting the jejunum with the lower part of the stomach so that the alkaline intestinal juices neutralise stomach acid. Since its results are not always reliable the tendency today is to prefer partial gastrectomy with complete removal of the acid-producing area of the stomach.

Gastroptosis: (*see* Visceroptosis).

Gastroscope: an instrument passed into the stomach for viewing its interior by means of a tube introduced down the throat with a tiny light bulb and mirrors; photographs may also be taken in this way.

Gastrostomy: an operation on the stomach whereby, when the oesophagus is blocked by a tumour or damaged by corrosives, an opening is made between the stomach and the abdominal wall through which the patient may be fed. In days when such dangerous corrosive poisons as lye or caustic soda and the mineral acids were more used domestically than today it was not uncommon for them to be swallowed by children or would-be suicides making a gastrostomy necessary in order that the individual could be fed. The operation is less performed now owing to the reduced frequency of this type of accident and the introduction of X-ray therapy for tumours or the operation of *oesophagectomy* in which, if the damaged or diseased area be not too great, it is removed and the two ends stitched together. Even when a large area is affected, it is possible to bring the stomach into the chest, stitching it to the upper part of the oesophagus.

Gaucher's Disease: a rare chronic disease which runs in families and is accompanied by enlargement of the liver and spleen, particularly the latter. The lymph glands are also enlarged, there is pigmentation of the skin in exposed areas, and sometimes spontaneous fractures of bones; even slight injuries lead to haemorrhage beneath the skin with obvious bruising. The immediate cause of these symptoms is the deposition of large fatty cells in the tissues of the bone-marrow, liver, spleen, and glands, this being accompanied by severe anaemia with a relative reduction of white cells in the blood, but the basic cause is unknown although it appears to be an inborn defect in metabolism. Splenectomy (removal of the spleen) is sometimes advocated although there is controversy as to its value, but splenic puncture is necessary in order to establish the diagnosis. Strictly speaking this is a blood disease but *see* Spleen.

Gaultheria: oil of wintergreen, largely composed of methyl salicylate and used as a rub for joint and muscle pains.

Gelatin: a colourless transparent substance used in making jellies and medically as a base for suppositories, etc. It is made from the collagen of connective tissue and, although a

237

protein, has relative little nutritive value. Gelatine is made by boiling down bones and meat and clear soups or stock largely consist of it, hence being less nourishing than is often thought. In the manufacture of jellies, gums, and pastilles vegetable materials such as agar are increasingly used. Calves'-foot jelly used as an invalid food at one time is easily digested but not very high in food value.

Gelsemium: the root of the yellow jasmine containing gelsemine a very poisonous alkaloid. Rarely used now except in the treatment of migraine and neuralgia it is unreliable because of its unpredictable effects and its toxicity except in very small doses.

General Paralysis of the Insane: or G.P.I. is a form of syphilis of the nervous system beginning 10 to 20 years after the initial infection and leading to mental deterioration and death if untreated. The onset of symptoms is often insidious beginning with tremor of the tongue and muscles of the face, deteriorating memory, slurring and stammering speech especially over such phrases as are used by the police to test for drunkenness ('British constitution,' 'The Leith Police dismisseth us,' 'hippopotamus,' etc.), and easily aroused emotions – these, however, are found in many organic brain disorders and even in the ordinary changes of old age. More usually noticed are the mental changes which include the emotional instability already mentioned which causes the individual to laugh or weep too readily, a general attitude which is overconfident and overoptimistic often taking the form of grandiose delusions of wealth which involve him in debt or in absurd actions such as buying a number of expensive cars or getting mixed up in foolish financial schemes which betray his lack of judgement. On the other hand, some cases become depressed and self-condemning, bemoaning early sins of a relatively trivial nature. Conclusive signs are the finding of a positive Wassermann reaction for syphilis in the blood, exaggerated knee-jerks and other reflexes and, absent or diminished reaction of the pupil to light whilst retaining the reaction to accommodation (Argyll-Robertson pupil). In the final stages of a disease which is manifest for only 2–3 years dementia increases, coherent speech is lost, and the patient is bed-ridden with loss of control of bowels and bladder and totally paralysed, death often resulting from some intercurrent disease although always inevitable without treatment. Treatment, which is usually given in a mental hospital owing to the patient's psychological state, has been revolutionised by the use of malarial therapy or other forms of hyperthermia (fever) in which a high temperature is produced which in the case of deliberately induced malaria is brought to an end by suitable doses of quinine; this may be given with penicillin injections or penicillin may be used alone or in combination with arsenical preparations such as tryparsamide. The results are excellent so far as stopping the disease process is concerned but damage already done cannot be repaired. G.P.I. is also known as dementia paralytica; syphilis of the spinal chord is tabes dorsalis locomotor ataxia. Not all cases of chronic syphilis attack the brain and the disease is rapidly dying out in this country because of better and earlier diagnosis and the tendency of people generally to treat the venereal diseases more rationally and seek cure as soon as they first manifest themselves (*see* Syphilis, Locomotor Ataxia).

Gentian: the root of the yellow gentian used as a bitter to stimulate appetite and in such alcoholic aperitifs as 'Entzianwasser' on the Continent.

Gentian Violet: an aniline dye used by bacteriologists to make bacteria visible under the microscope by staining (e.g. in Gram's stain), as a skin antiseptic in impetigo and other cantagious diseases, in the treatment of burns where, in addition to its antiseptic properties, it forms a strong pliable film over the wound, and internally in the treatment of threadworms. Its main drawback is the deep violet staining which soils clothing, is unsightly on exposed parts, and difficult to remove; for this reason it is gradually being replaced by other and more effective remedies.

Genu Valgum: knock-knee.

Genu Varum: bow legs.

Geriatrics: the branch of medicine that deals with the diseases of old age and studies its problems. The term originates with Dr I. L. Nascher of New York who in 1909 was the first to employ it and to emphasise that something constructive could be done about such problems instead of merely accepting them as inevitable. However little was done by medicine until after the last war when, with an increasing number of old people in her population, and social issues arising therefrom, Britain began to take geriatrics more seriously. The problem of the old is essentially one of industrial society in which families tend to become small and children and the old, being unproductive, are regarded as financial liabilities.

The physical and mental changes associated with age come on gradually and at times which depend upon the individual, some being hale and hearty in their nineties whilst others are old already in the fifties. Broadly speaking these are due to changes in the tissues of the brain associated with narrowing and hardening of the arteries which leads to an inadequate blood-supply. The memory for recent events becomes poor whilst that for long-past events is retained; the emotions are superficial and easily aroused so that the individual tends to be sentimental and tearful; and traits which have always been present such as suspiciousness become exaggerated. In more severe cases there is a lack of attention to social conventions and the patient may be dirty, untidy, and incontinent in the control of bowels and bladder. These qualities are exaggerated in those who live alone and get inadequate nourishment. Whilst mentioning the basic physical changes in the body it is important to emphasise that much of the disability of old age is socially conditioned since those who live solitary lives lose interest in themselves and their general attitude changes for the worse. Much is being done in the way of clubs and other communal activities to restore an interest in life to such cases and geriatric specialists have been appointed in most districts (*see* comments on 'institutional neurosis' under Iatrogenic Disease).

German Measles: rubella or (in German) Rötheln, is a mild infectious disease common in children and caused by a virus. In the young it is of little importance apart from the similarity of the rash to measles and scarlet fever. Sometimes the rash, which takes the form of minute pink spots less blotchy and less purplish than in that of measles and unlike the uniform redness of scarlatina, is the first and only sign of infection but more often it is preceded by shivering, fever rarely above 100 degrees, slight sneezing and coughing, or headache. The glands in the neck may be enlarged but the course of the illness is only 2–3 days, complications are unknown, and the sole treatment necessary is rest (not necessarily in bed) and isolation for three weeks. Intramuscular injection of Gamma Globulin within seven days of exposure affords complete protection or attentuates the disease. 'Fourth disease' is a subvariety of rubella which is of little moment save to those who take pleasure in alarming themselves and others by the invention of new disease categories which are almost totally irrelevant. In pregnant women rubella must be regarded as altogether more serious for the unborn child since it is now known that infection during the early months of pregnancy is associated with an unduly high percentage of congenital defects in the infant especially in relation to the eyes, deafness and malformation of the heart (*see* comments under Incubation Period).

Germanin: also known as Suramin, Antrypol, and Bayer 205 is a derivative of urea introduced by the German firm of Bayer and used in the treatment of tropical diseases caused by trypanosomes (*see* Infection), notably sleeping sickness carried by the African tsetse fly. Owing to its ability to produce nephritis, optic atrophy, and other side-effects it has to be used with care.

Germs: (*see* Infection, Bacteria).

Gestation: pregnancy.

Giddiness: (*see* Vertigo).

Gin: an alcoholic drink made from rye or barley with the addition of juniper berries and hops and formerly used medically as a diuretic (q.v.) Its alcoholic content is the same as that of whisky or brandy and the idea once held that it is more likely than other alcoholic drinks to cause cirrhosis of the liver is quite unfounded (*see* Alcohol, Cirrhosis).

Ginger: is prepared from the roots of an East Indian and Caribbean plant for use both as a sweet and condiment or medically as a carminative to stimulate the digestive juices and relieve flatulence. White ginger is the root after scraping, black ginger is merely scalded.

Gingivitis: inflammation of the gums (*see* Teeth).

Glanders: a contagious disease of horses, donkeys, mules, and also cats, guinea-pigs and dogs, which is communicable to man (although rather rarely) through abrasions on the skin or by the eye, mouth, and nose. The cause is the bacillus mallei present in the saliva and nasal discharge of infected animals. A small boil appears on the spot first infected and if this is on the hand the lymph vessels running up the arm soon appear as angry red lines following which the germ enters the general circulation and two or three weeks after contact the temperature rises with vomiting, involvement of the lungs, pustules and ulcers over the surface of the body, pains in the joints, and growing weakness. The acute form of the disease is likely to be fatal within two weeks but chronic infections may last for months, sometimes abating, sometimes becoming more acute, but usually ending in death. Treatment by vaccines is helpful in some cases and the antibiotics are now available and seem to be effective. Diagnosis is made by the use of mallein prepared from the glanders bacilli and used in the same way as tuberculin to detect tuberculosis. In stables it is extremely difficult to diagnose and many of the animals are likely to die and new arrivals be infected before the disease is even suspected. Affected animals must be destroyed and their stables disinfected. The term glanders is sometimes used specifically for the nasal form of the infection, the term 'farcy' being used of the skin eruptions and the underlying nodules.

Glands: a word used to describe several different types of structure within the body: (1) the large glands such as the liver, kidney, and pancreas which produce a secretion (i.e. some substance to be used by the organism, e.g. bile from the liver, the pancreatic enzymes from the pancreas) and discharge it through a duct to the area where it is needed, or an excretion (e.g. bile which is, in part, a waste product or urine the waste excreted by the kidney); (2) the small glands which secrete digestive ferments (e.g. the salivary glands and the glands lining the gastro-intestinal tract) or those which protect and lubricate the skin (the sebaceous glands); (3) the endocrine glands, which secrete substances upon which the whole functioning of the body and mind depend, directly into the bloodstream, hence often described as the ductless glands (e.g. the pituitary, thyroid, suprarenal, and sex glands); (4) the lymph glands. It is with the latter we are concerned here, the others being dealt with under their respective headings.

Lymph glands are found throughout the body but particularly at junctions, e.g. there are superficial glands behind the knee and in front of the elbow, under the arm-pit and at the angle of the jaw, in the groin and behind the ears; deep glands lie in the region where the mesentery or cellophane-like cover supporting the intestines is attached to the back of the abdominal cavity, at the junction of the lungs and bronchi, and in many other areas. Together they form the lymphatic system being joined together by lymphatic vessels which finally join to form the thoracic duct which pours lymph into the bloodstream at the point where the internal jugular vein meets the subclavian at the root of the neck on the left side; a smaller duct collecting lymph from the right arm and the right side of the chest and neck enters the venous system on the right side at the same point. Lymphatic vessels and glands have three main functions: (1) the lacteals in the intestinal walls collect certain foodstuffs during digestion which, passing through the mesenteric glands are poured into the blood-stream via the thoracic duct; (2) the glands are the site where the lymphocytes, one type of white blood corpuscle, are formed; (3) they act as a filter preventing infection from entering the blood-stream. This is the most evident function of the lymph glands since, as everyone knows, they become swollen in the presence of infection in the region and if overwhelmed may break down and suppurate. Hence in a serious infection of the hand the red lines of the lymphatics can be seen running up the arm and the glands in the armpit become swollen and tender; in foot or leg infections a similar change occurs in the groin; and in lung infections the glands at the roots where the bronchi leave the lung to join the windpipe are affected, and in tuberculous disease, may slowly become calcified with the deposition of chalk making them visible in an X-ray to indicate a former battle with the germs. The swellings around the neck in cases of sore throat or ear disease and even where there are lice on the scalp are familiar and enlarged glands of this sort anywhere in the body are described as 'adenitis' which can only be dealt with by seeking and dealing with the source of infection. The glands themselves are best left alone unless they become liable to break down and suppurate when they must be deal with as an abscess (q.v.) Enlarged glands occur in other diseases.

Glandular Fever: or infectious mononucleosis is a fever occurring in epidemics amongst children and young adults the main features of which are a sudden rise in temperature after an incubation period of 5–15 days followed in a day or two by enlargement of the glands of the neck and elsewhere. The enlargement is not great and may not occur until the second week or later; occasionally there is a rash. In the blood the white cells are increased and particularly the lymphocytes, a change which may remain for many months after the disease has recovered and lead to its being mistaken on routine examination for a serious blood disorder such as leukaemia although glandular fever is never fatal and quite a minor illness. In cases of doubt the Paul-Bunnell reaction in which the patient's serum causes sheep's blood corpuscles to clump together and break down may be used to confirm the diagnosis. Only aspirin need be given in treatment.

Glauber's Salt: is sodium sulphate which is used as a purgative in much the same way as Epsom salts. Since it acts by drawing fluid from the tissues into the intestine it is not habit-forming, non-irritant, and like magnesium sulphate useful in stimulating the flow of bile on the rare occasions when aperients are necessary.

Glaucoma: a disease of the eye in which, usually after middle-age, the pressure of the fluids within increases ultimately leading to blindness. The name meaning greenish-grey arises from the changed colour of the lens of the eye in this condition where local congestion or an increase in its size with age causes the iris to be pushed forward thus blocking the canal of Schlemm at its junction with the cornea whence the fluids usually escape. The tension within the eye results in the severe headaches typical of the acute attacks and ultimately by pressure destroys the ends of the optic nerve. In many cases this may be a gradual process with few symptoms, but more frequently there are acute attacks usually at night with severe pain on the affected side often accompanied by nausea and vomiting. Whilst the tension is rising coloured haloes are seen around lights, vision is dimmed, and the eyelids swollen with marked redness of the eye. The doctor will note that a light shone into the eye shows a greenish coloration and that the eyeball feels hard when touched through the eyelids. Although sometimes occurring at birth or in early childhood, glaucoma affects approximately 2% of all people after the age of 40 and, if untreated, is likely to spread to the other eye. Medical treatment during the acute stage is to use pilocarpine or eserine eyedrops which, by contracting the pupil, will widen the escape angle of the eye in order to allow the fluid to drain off but if this does not reduce the tension within one or two days immediate operation is necessary to save the sight. Acute glaucoma is treated by the operation of iridectomy in which a small section of the iris is removed under local or general anaesthesia thus permitting the fluid to escape. In chronic glaucoma a filtration procedure may be carried out with the object of establishing a new drainage path for the fluid. Normal vision is regained in approximately 90–95% of cases when an acute attack is dealt with in time but in the case of chronic disease some prefer medical treatment as the surgical results are less certain.

Gleet: the slight watery discharge characteristic of chronic gonorrhoea.

Glioma: a tumour in the brain or spinal cord composed of neuroglia, the connective tissue supporting the nerve-cells proper and their fibres.

Globulin: a group of proteins insoluble in water and alcohol but soluble in weak salt solution (*see* also Gamma Globulin).

Globus Hystericus: the sensation of being unable to swallow or choking as if a 'lump in the throat' existed, characteristic of certain neuroses and caused by anxiety.

Glomerulonephritis: a form of nephritis in which the glomeruli are mainly affected (*see* Nephritis).

Glossitis: inflammation of the tongue (q.v.).

Glossopharyngeal Nerve: the ninth cranial nerve which is the nerve of sensation for the posterior third of the tongue (taste), the whole of the upper part of the throat and middle ear, and the secretory nerve of the parotid gland. It also supplies motor impulses to one of the muscles in the throat.

Glottis: the opening at the upper end of the larynx or voice-box which is opened and closed by the leaf-like structure known as the epiglottis.

Glucagon: a hormone which increases the amount of glucose in the blood being secreted by the alpha cells of the pancreas in the Islets of Langerhans; its significance so far is mainly theoretical.

Glucose: or grape-sugar is found in most fruits, in honey, and is the main form into which all other sugars and starches are reduced by digestion in the body. With the exception of alcohol it is the only natural food immediately absorbed by the stomach without being digested. It is therefore useful as an energy-producing substance in those who are too weak to digest heavier meals and is sometimes given in such cases either as an enema or intravenously. Since proportionately more energy is used up during fevers and the appetite may at the same time be lost, mildly effervescent lemon-flavoured glucose drinks are very useful in such conditions, being clean to the taste and acceptable when others are not. But it is sheer rubbish to suggest as is often done that normal people when tired require glucose since the great bulk of fatigue (q.v.) is a psychological state allied to boredom which has nothing to do with energy lack but rather with the lack of will to apply it. The housewife who (if one is to believe advertisements) sits down in the mid-morning to a glass of glucose lemonade would do equally well with a cup of tea or coffee and in all probability is more helped by the break and relaxation than either.

Glutamic Acid: one of the amino-acids, the building stones of proteins. It has been used in the treatment of epilepsy and, on the Continent in the treatment of neuroses on the false theory that neurotic nerves need to be 'fed.' There is no evidence that glutamic acid has any therapeutic action worth mention.

Gluteal: the region of the buttocks, applied as an adjective to the muscles, nerves, and blood-vessels therein.

Gluten: the protein part of wheat flour which becomes sticky in consistency (c.f. the word 'glutinous') on the addition of water. Since it can be separated from the starchy carbohydrate part of flour gluten is used in making diabetic bread and rolls which can also be included in reducing diets for the overweight.

Glycerin: also glycerine and glycerol, is an alcohol widely used in medicine for various purposes, e.g. because of its property of absorbing water it is used with other substances in dressing septic wounds, as a throat paint with tannic acid, in inflammation of the gums, as a base for skin lotions to prevent chapping, or in laryngitis. It is occasionally used as a purgative in doses of 1–2 teaspoonfuls and, because of its pleasantly sweet taste, is added to many medicines and with gelatine forms the base of many pastilles.

Glycerophosphates: formerly much used in 'Nerve tonics' because of the false assumption that, since glycerophosphoric acid is a constituent of nerve tissue, and the neuroses were allegedly due to under-nourishment of such cells, glycerophosphates would feed them. In fact neuroses have nothing to do with the state of nourishment of the nerve cells and glycerophosphates are excreted from the body unchanged.

Glycogen: or animal starch is the form in which glucose, as the end-product of carbohydrate digestion, is stored in the liver. It is also found in muscles being broken down into glucose when required.

Glycosuria: the presence of sugar in the urine (*see* Urine, Diabetes).

Goitre: abnormalties of the thyroid gland which surrounds the front and sides of the windpipe in the lower part of the neck are usually associated with swelling and hence were one of the earliest forms of disease described by the ancient Chinese and Indians as well as the Greeks of classical times. Such disease takes one of four main forms: (1) absence or under-activity of the gland in which there is *cretinism* at birth or *myxoedema* in adult life; (2) *colloid goitre* in which there is a diffuse and even swelling without bodily disturbance other than that due to pressure; (3) *hyperthyroidism* or *toxic goitre* in which there is either a diffuse generalised swelling or a localised lump and the body functions are speeded up, the eyes sometimes being protuberant; (4) *nodular goitre* without bodily disturbance in which numerous lumps about the size of a pea may be felt or several large ones which can reach the size of a grape-fruit. Cretinism leads to a form of idiocy and dwarfism which can now be completely avoided by the early use of thyroid extracts taken throughout life and myxoedema, occurring usually after middle age, can be similarly treated (*see* Myxoedema). Colloid goitre, now much less frequently seen than formerly, is most common in adolescents and young adults living in areas where the iodine supply of water and food is inadequate, iodine being necessary to the formation of the thyroxin. This is commonest in limestone areas as certain parts of Switzerland and Derbyshire in England hence the old name of 'Derbyshire neck;' the condition is avoided by the administration of iodine added to water, table salt, or chocolate as a prophylactic measure The over-activity of the gland which is typical of toxic goitre and often found in young women, although not exclusively so, is evidently a result of glandular imbalance since the thyroid like all the other endocrine glands normally works in harmony with the whole endocrine system, a harmony which is easily disturbed by such crises as puberty, childbirth, and the change of life. It is related to severe nervous stress, although whether as cause or effect is as yet undecided, and leads to the typical picture of a young adult who is tense and restless, irritable, losing weight, prone to sweating, tremor of the hands, and attacks of palpitation, and often shows prominence of the eyes which may be very marked in the later stages. Such cases were formerly treated only by surgical removal of all but 5–10% of the gland, the remaining tissue rapidly regenerating after operation or thyroid extract being given if necessary. But many may now be treated medically by the administration of the drug thiouracil or by radioactive iodine, the latter being also given in certain cases of cancer of the gland. However, these methods are valueless in the most commonly found goitres which are the non-toxic, nodular, or colloid types where operation is still required. In general, and subject to the specialist's advice, the following are ordinarily indications for operative treatment: (a) when medical treatment fails to cure an overactive gland; (b) when the goitre presses on the windpipe causing discomfort or persistent hoarseness; (c) when one or more isolated lumps are present. Operation is advisable in the latter case since such nodules may become toxic, or increase in size and press on the surrounding structures, or in 7–10% of cases become malignant. Removal of the thyroid is not dangerous, and nodules once removed will not come back although in about 5% of cases where the whole gland is over-active some recurrence of symptoms may take place which is usually controlled by the use of radioactive iodine. The risks of not having an operation which has been advised are that the heart will sooner or later be damaged by the strain put upon it, that pressure effects may become serious necessitating later surgery, and that cancer may occur. Few operations lead to more satisfactory results and the unpleasant symptoms usually go in a few days; even cancer of the thyroid is cured in a very high percentage of cases. The scar is insignificant and only a thin pale line is visible at the base of the neck afterwards. (For radioactive iodine *see* Isotopes, for thiouracil *see* Thiorea.)

Gold: gold salts were formerly used in the treatment of tuberculosis in the form of sodium aurothiosulphate (Sanocrysin, Crisalbine, Solganal B Oleosum), sodium aurothiomalate (Myocrisin, Allochrysine), or calcium aurothiomalate (Collosol Auro-calcium). This has largely been given up but they are still used in suitable cases of rheumatoid arthritis where minute doses produce a reaction in the affected tissues which leads to scarring and healing. The drug is given either intramuscularly or intravenously and side-effects include abdominal pain with vomiting, diarrhoea and jaundice, skin eruptions with itching, albumen in the urine, and rarely blood diseases.

Golden Ointment: yellow mercuric oxide ointment commonly used for inflammation of the eyelids.

Gonad: the male or female sex glands.

Gonadotrophic Hormone: the hormone from the anterior lobe of the pituitary gland which stimulates the activity of the sex glands thereby producing the same effect as the sex hormones.

Gonorrhoea: one of the venereal diseases spread by sexual intercourse with an infected person, although eye disease may reach the infant from an infected mother, or vaginitis the young female child from infected towels or clothes. The infecting agent is the diplococcus (*see* Bacteria) Neisseria gonorrhoea which, in men, produces a thick yellow discharge from the urethra at the end of the penis after an incubation period of 2–10 days. Later, if the disease is untreated, the discharge becomes clear and sticky and there is pain on passing water or the associated organs (testicles, bladder, prostate gland at the base of the bladder) may become inflamed and painful. Still later complications are scarring of the urethra so that urination becomes difficult or impossible (stricture), arthritis of the knee, ankle, wrist or elbow, usually supposed by the patient to be 'rheumatism,' and septicaemia with inflammation of the heart-valves (endocarditis), or abcesses in various parts of the body. In women, there is yellow vaginal discharge, pain on passing water and inflammation of the glands at the entry to the vagina; the chronic infection may pass to the womb, Fallopian tubes, and ovaries leading to frequent miscarriages, sterility, and, less frequently, peritonitis which may be fatal. The eye disease of infants or ophthalmia neonatorum is much less frequent since the use of silver nitrate eye drops on all new-born babies became general, but, neglected, is one of the commonest causes of blindness. The treatment of early gonorrhoea has been revolutionised by the discovery of the sulpha drugs and penicillin; the latter drug being capable (often in a single injection) of wiping out this

249

ancient and devastating affliction of the human race. It need hardly be pointed out that early treatment is absolutely essential and no false modesty should prevent those who fear they have become infected from seeking advice, although a great many people who report with urethral discharge are suffering from a non-specific urethritis resulting from inoculation by foreign but not disease-producing germs through intercourse combined with a guilty conscience. The discharge from acute gonorrhoea is thick, creamy, and plentiful, that from non-specific urethritis, thin, colourless, and scanty; nevertheless, *all* abnormal discharges should be investigated and the specialist's conclusions accepted since it is quite common for those who are not naturally promiscuous to become neurotic about a non-venereal discharge although, in fact, there is no dubiety whatever about the results of diagnosis in the hands of an expert (*see* Venereal Disease).

Goulard's Water: lead and opium lotion, used in the treatment of sprains and bruises and applied on a piece of lint soaked in the solution.

Gout: a disease in which there seems to be a strong hereditary tendency characterised by swelling and pain in certain joints (the big toe, fingers, thumbs, knees, wrists or elbows) and an excess of uric acid in the blood. Middle-aged men are usually affected, but women and younger people are not immune. Typically the attack comes on without warning and often on waking in the morning when the big toe is found to be swollen, red hot, tense, shiny, and exquisitely painful; predisposing causes are heredity and an excess of rich food and alcohol but an attack may be precipitated by damp, tiredness, chill, or an overlarge meal the night before. Gout is a disorder of nucleo-protein metabolism and therefore foods containing such substances and fats should be avoided, e.g. sweetbreads, liver, kidney, meat soups and extracts, brains, sardines, herring, pork and veal. Alcohol, if taken, should be limited to light, dry, wines and port, sherry, spirits, and beer should be avoided. The uric acid excretion in the urine falls before and rises during, the attack for a few days. Subsequent attacks may occur and ultimately give rise to a state of chronic gout with some crippling of the hands and feet. In treatment the affected joint may be covered with lint soaked in lead and opium lotion, the food intake reduced during an attack, and plenty of bland fluids taken whilst the doctor will probably prescribe colchicum and cinchophen (Atophan) which usually cut the attack short – some, however, prefer not to use cinchophen which can cause liver disease. Butazolidin (phenylbutazone) salicylates, and cortisone preparations are also sometimes used, especially in the chronic stages. Deposits of uric acid are likely to form around the joints in chronic cases when they are known as 'gouty tophi' but it is important to realise that the deposition of crystals in the joints is characteristic of gout alone and the manufacturers of proprietary medicines who seem to infer that 'rheumatics' in general has something to do with 'crystals in the blood' which have to be 'dissolved away' are talking nonsense (*see* Colchicum, Cinchophen, Rheumatism).

Graft: the term applied to a small piece of tissue removed from a person, animal, or plant and implanted in another or the same organism in order to make good some defect or (in the case of plants) to build a composite individual plant. In modern surgery the commonest types of graft are skin, bone, and blood-vessel in that order. *Skin grafts* have the purpose of covering areas which have been exposed by burns, accidents, or surgical removal for some other purpose; since grafts from one person to another are generally unsuccessful for reasons to be mentioned later, and the only successful ones of this type take place between identical twins, they have been largely abandoned and the skin used is taken from another part of the patient's own body in one of four ways: (1) *Pinch grafts*, used for covering small areas are round pieces of the superficial layer of skin about a quarter of an inch in diameter often taken from the thigh and placed as island over the affected part where they take root and grow together to cover it; (2) *split-thickness grafts* are sheets of skin removed by a special instrument known as a dermatome consisting of a razor-sharp knife attached to a drum which can measure accurately and slice a graft of about four by eight inches containing both the superficial and part of the deep layer of skin of the thigh, abdomen, or back, usually to put on large burned areas where the skin is completely destroyed; (3) *full-thickness grafts* contain all the layers of the skin except the basal fatty one and are used in parts subject to friction or pulling where (2) would not be suitable, such

251

grafts are cut exactly to size and stitched into place, the donor area being also closed by stitches; (4) *pedicle grafts* are those in which one part containing the full thickness of the skin is attached to the area to be covered whilst its other end remains attached by a pedicle containing the necessary blood-vessels and nerves to its original site until the graft has taken, when the connection can be severed. In this way pieces of flesh can be 'leap-frogged' from one part of the body to another, e.g. a piece of the abdomen is attached at one end to the arm or hand and, when it becomes firmly attached, cut free of the abdomen and attached to the face whilst retaining its pedicle with the arm until it takes there also and may become an artificial nose when its connection with the arm is severed. In *blood-vessel grafts* which were devised during the last war and as a result of animal experimentation portions of a vein from the superficial tissues of the arm or a segment of an artery from a Blood Vessel Bank are used to replace a segment of a vital artery which has been destroyed. They are also occasionally used in such conditions as poor circulation due to arteriosclerosis, Buerger's disease, or Raynaud's disease, and the operation of free vein graft has been employed in coronary artery disorders whereby a strip of superficial vein from the arm is attached at one end to the aorta or main artery of the body and at the other to the main venous channel of the coronary circulation to the heart muscle. The blood then runs in the reverse direction through the veins (which are not subject to arteriosclerosis) and out through the arteries. The operation is still in the experimental stage but results appear to be good. *Bone grafts* are usually taken from the patient himself (autogenous graft) from the wing of the ilium above the hip area or from the fractured bone above the affected part; occasionally they are obtained from a Bone Bank (homogenous graft), e.g. a part of rib removed at a chest operation or a piece of bone taken from an amputated leg or a dead body at a post-mortem examination. They are used in cases where healing of a fracture refuses to take place normally or where some loss of bone has occurred between the fractured ends and in spinal fusion operations to permanently stiffen a part of the spinal column where displacement of the vertebrae has occurred, e.g. in spondylolisthesis or severe and progressive curvature of the spine. The once familiar sight of hunchbacks is rare today since medical treatment of tuberculosis of the spine followed by spinal fusion operations have been employed. In more recent times attempts have been made to transplant whole organs, but the great difficulty has been the fact that, just as the body's immunity reactions act to destroy the invading cells of bacteria, so they also destroy any cells from non-identical organs. Such grafts therefore could only take when removed from an identical twin and several such operations have been performed successfully. But research has shown that embryos tolerate and do not kill alien cells and, further, that radiation can induce embryolike tolerence in adults when the correct dosage is administered; by this means in the historic case of the Riteris brothers in America a kidney was successfully transplanted for the first time from one non-identical twin to another. More recently in Britain this technique has been used to graft a kidney from a totally unrelated person.

Gram's Stain: a method of differential staining of bacteria devised in 1884 by J. H. C. Gram who showed that, when treated by a dye such as gentian violet and subsequently with iodine, some bacteria fix the dye whilst others do not. Thus the pneumococcus is Gram-positive whilst the somewhat similar gonococcus which does not fix the dye is Gram-negative and the two may be easily distinguished.

Grand Mal: (*see* Epilepsy).

Granulation Tissue: the new tissue, red and velvety in appearance, which grows over any raw surface as a prelude to healing. When excessive it may need to be pared down or cauterised with copper sulphate. Tumours (in the strictly medical sense which merely means a swelling) of granulation tissue are found in tuberculosis and syphilis, being known as granulomata.

Graves' Disease: exophthalmic toxic goitre or Basedow's disease (*see* Goitre).

Gravid: pregnant.

Greenstick Fracture: the type of fracture found in the long bones of young children and usually due to indirect violence where the bone does not break completely but rather bends owing to the smaller amount of calcium in its structure (*see* Fracture).

Gregory's Mixture: or powder is pulvis rhei compositus, a mixture of rhubarb, heavy and light magnesium carbonates, and ginger once used in doses of 10–60 grains as an antacid and purgative for digestive upsets.

Grey Powder: a powder containing mercury and chalk once used for infantile diarrhoea but generally discontinued because of its proneness to cause mercurial poisoning.

Grinder's Disease: a disease of the lungs caused by inhaling particles of metal and once common amongst knife-grinders in Sheffield.

Gripes: the colic of infants (*see* Colic).

Grippe: a popular name, especially in France and the U.S.A., for influenza.

Groin: an area which includes the upper part of the thigh and the lower part of the abdomen; the groove across it covers the inguinal (Poupart's) ligament and its main abnormalities are hernia and enlarged lymph glands once known as 'buboes.'

Growing Pains: pains occuring in children during the course of development, usually in the legs and back. These may be due to a variety of causes such as physical strain or exhaustion, disease of the bones, or a manifestation of rheumatism. Skilled advice should always be sought, although they are unlikely to be serious.

Growth: a popular term for tumours, cysts, cancer, and other sorts of swelling (*see* under the appropriate headings).

Guinea-worm: (*see* Infection).

Gullet: the oesophagus connecting the throat with the stomach (*see* Throat).

Gumboil: an abscess at the root of a decayed tooth recognised by pain and swelling on the exterior of the face. In the early stages it may be relieved by painting the gum with tincture of iodine, packing any cavity with cotton-wool soaked in oil of cloves, hot mouth-washes, aspirin, and hot applications to the cheek. Antibiotics may be prescribed if necessary but the dentist should be seen once the swelling has begun to subside as the tooth may have to be removed.

Gumma: a hard swelling usually in the skin or connective tissue but sometimes in internal organs such as the liver or brain; it is caused by syphilis and sometimes gives rise to symptoms due to pressure or interference with the function of the organ where it is situated (*see* Syphilis).

Gums, Diseases of: (*see* Mouth and Teeth).

Gynaecology: the branch of medicine dealing with the diseases of women.

Gynaecomastia: abnormal enlargement of the male breast as in diseases of the pituitary or sex glands cirrhosis of the liver, and deliberate or accidental administration of female sex-hormones.

Habits: a loose term for any settled tendency or practice applied in its medical connotation to (*a*) habit spasms and tics, (*b*) drug addiction, (q.v.), and (*c*) sex practices such as masturbation (*see* Masturbation, Sexual Problems).

Haematemesis: vomiting of blood, a symptom which should always be brought to the attention of the doctor as soon as possible. Small amounts of blood often come from the back of the throat during the exertion of vomiting or may be swallowed and vomited later when it has come from the throat or nose; in the latter case it is likely to be dark in colour due to partial digestion. Gastritis following the intake of irritating foods, or strong alcohol sometimes results in similar amounts of blood being vomited, but larger amounts arise from gastric or duedenal ulcer in which case the vomit may have a coffee-grounds appearance due to changed blood. A considerable haematemesis is almost always the result of an ulcer which has broken into a blood-vessel or ruptured portal varices – the varicose veins which arise in cases of cirrhosis of the liver at the end of the oesophagus and the opening of the stomach due to congestion of the portal circulation. Such haemorrhages are severe and often fatal requiring to be treated with the greatest urgency. Less commonly bleeding accompanies certain fevers, blood diseases, and tabes dorsalis.

Haematocele: a cavity containing blood as when an injury or a ruptured aneurism (q.v.) causes blood to flow into a natural cavity or amongst loose connective tissue.

Haematocolpos: the retention of menstrual blood in the vagina by a hymen which completely closes the entrance. A small and painless incision immediately frees the accumulation.

Haematology: the branch of medicine dealing with diseases of the blood.

Haematoma: a collection of blood under the skin or beneath

255

the meninges covering the brain (subdural haematoma) resulting from any injury or operation and sometimes from childbirth when it may appear upon the child's head.

Haematothorax: an effusion of blood into the pleural cavity of the chest.

Haematuria: the presence of blood cells in the urine which may come from any part of the urinary tract and be serious or relatively trivial in significance. Some indication of the site of the bleeding may be obtained from the appearance of the urine which is dull brown or smoky in appearance when the blood comes from the kidneys as in acute or subacute nephritis, high blood-pressure, or some cases of pyelitis and stone in the pelvis of the kidney. Blood from the bladder may come from inflammation as in cystitis or from a stone in this area in both of which cases it is likely to be mixed with pus, but bright red blood in fair amounts is nearly always the result of a papilloma or wart in the wall of the bladder. A fractured pelvis or inflammation of the urethra, purpura and other blood diseases, bilharzia in the tropics, prostatic enlargement, scurvy, and malignant scarlet fever or smallpox, are other causes. Rarely, haematuria occurs periodically without any discoverable disease being present and is probably due to congestion of the kidneys. All such cases require speedy investigation in order to discover the site of bleeding; this may or may not necessitate a cystoscopic examination (q.v.).

Haemochromatosis: or bronzed diabetes is a disease characterised by the symptoms of diabetes (including glycosuria) combined with bronzing of the skin cirrhosis of the liver, fibrosis and enlargement of the pancreas and spleen, and abnormal deposits of the pigment melanin (haemosiderin) in the skin with haemosiderin and haemofuscin (which is iron-free) deposits in the internal organs, heart, and muscles. The symptoms are a deep bronzing of the skin, enlarged liver, and glycosuria with thirst and loss of weight occurring in men more often than women who are over the age of 40. The condition is probably due to an inborn defect of iron metabolism and the long-term outlook is not good.

Haemocytometer: a microscope slide marked into squares for counting the concentration of red and white cells in the blood.

Haemoglobin: the colouring material of the blood composed

256

of a protein known as globin and the iron pigment haemin. It exists in two normal forms, oxyhaemoglobin which is the oxygenated arterial haemoglobin as it leaves the lungs and simple haemoglobin which is the substance after it has given up its oxygen to the tissues of the body and returns through the veins. Although a complex substance, haemoglobin has the same structural formula as the chlorophyll or green colouring matter of plants save that the latter contains magnesium in place of iron.

Haemoglobinuria: the presence of blood pigments, especially methlaemoglobin, but not of red cells, in the urine due to intravascular haemolysis (breakdown of the cells in the bloodstream). This may be due to chemicals such as potassium chlorate, arsine, certain sulpha drugs of the earlier types, quinine, and nitrites; to infections such as syphilis, malaria (blackwater fever), and yellow fever; to mismatched blood transfusions; and it may occur in crushing injuries or after extensive burns. Attacks of haemoglobinuria in otherwise normal people occur after exposure to cold or violent muscular exercise; in this case there is a haemolysin (blood-dissolving substance) circulating in the blood which at low temperatures attaches itself to the red cells causing them to break down. The presence of blood-pigments in the urine and their nature is determined by examination with the spectroscope.

Haemolysis: (*see above*) breakdown of the red blood cells and release of their pigments is produced by the substances already mentioned and occurs particularly rapidly after the bite of venomous snakes, the venom containing a haemolysin.

Haemolytic Disease of the Newborn: (*see* Icterus Gravis Neonatorum).

Haemophilia: a hereditary disease confined to members of the male sex, known as 'bleeders' in whom uncontrollable bleeding may follow even the slightest injury or wound. It is now believed to be due to the influence of a recessive gene (*see* Heredity) carried in that part of the large female X chromosome which has no counterpart in the smaller male or Y chromosome; thus it is carried by the female but only appears in the male, its frequency in Britain being about 1 in 35,000 persons. As is well known, Queen Victoria carried the gene which was handed on to her daughter the Czarina of Russia in whose son the disease became manifest with fateful consequences for the future of the world. The coagulation defect is caused by the absence of antihaemophilic globulin which is necessary to the first stage of clotting (*see* Coagulation) having some connection with the activation of thromboplastin. When normal serum is given to a sufferer from haemophilia the power to coagulate is temporarily restored to the blood, but this benefit, although useful in emergency, only lasts for 2–5 days; a highly concentrated anti-haemophilic globulin plasma has been prepared from animals which is effective in much smaller quantities but this, too, has only temporary results. All treatments are therefore palliative and depend upon avoiding injuries since even a cut finger may cause the patient to bleed to death in a couple of days and the administration of anti-haemophilic globulin when bleeding occurs; the wound itself may be encouraged to clot by the application of oxidised cellulose (oxycel), gelatin products (gelfoam), or calcium alginate gauze. The general outlook, however, is not good. There are other rare diseases, also hereditary, in which similar bleeding occurs due to another upset in the coagulation mechanism than that just described and with a different hereditary transmission from haemophilia. These are known collectively as parahaemophilia and the missing coagulation factors have been described as factors V, VI, and VIII although their exact nature is not known. Factor VI is also known as the Christmas factor since its absence in a patient of that name was first described by an investigator (q.v.). Special identity cards giving the patient's name and blood-group and the name, address, and telephone number of his doctor have been issued to sufferers from haemophilia and Christmas disease by the Ministry of Health and the Department of Health for Scotland in order to ensure that no time is wasted in case of emergency.

Haemoptysis: the spitting up of blood from the chest (i.e. from the larynx, trachea, bronchi, or lungs). True haemoptysis may be due to pulmonary tuberculosis, valvular disease of the heart or heart failure (especially mitral stenosis and left ventricular failure), bronchiectasis, pulmonary infarction (i.e. a clot of blood in the lungs), pneumonia, tumours of the bronchi or lungs, abscess or gangrene, wounds, and some of the less common infections. It may also occur in blood diseases (e.g. purpura, pernicious anaemia, leukaemia), in deficiency of vitamins K. P, or C, measles, high blood-pressure, and emphysema. Spurious haemoptysis is blood coming from the throat, gums, or nose and this is on the whole more frequent than the genuine type although all suspected bleeding must, of course, be investigated.

Haemorrhage: bleeding. Haemorrhage may be external or internal, arterial, venous, or capillary. In a cut artery the blood is bright red and jets out synchronically with the beat of the heart; venous blood is dark and flows in a constant steady stream, whilst oozing from capillaries is intermediate in colour. The main points in controlling severe bleeding are to make the patient rest, keeping him moderately warm but not hot, and avoiding all stimulants since anything which stimulates the heart will also increase bleeding. Movement should be avoided. In internal bleeding no food or drink must be given and only small sips of iced water. External bleeding from wounds or injuries can be dealt with by a tourniquet when the limbs are affected, and this must be frequently loosened otherwise the part of the limb from which the blood is cut off will be seriously damaged. A tourniquet must always be visible and the patient must not be given into other hands without pointing out that it has been applied. Pressure should be put on the bleeding area and in venous bleeding this should be on the side away from the heart, the limb being raised; in arterial bleeding pressure should be on the side nearest the heart. The pressure-points familiar to the first-aider are better derived from some knowledge of anatomy and how the circulation works than learned by rote. Various types of internal haemorrhage dealt with elsewhere are Epistaxis or bleeding from the nose (*see* under Nose), Haematemesis or vomiting blood. Haemoptysis or spitting blood, Haematuria or blood in the urine, and Melaena or blood in the motions (*see* also Coagulation and Haemophilia).

Haemorrhoids: (*see* Piles).

Haemostatics: substances which control the flow of blood in haemorrhage, also (although infrequently used in this sense) instruments which have this function as tourniquets or artery forceps. Haemostatic substances are sometimes described as styptics and the most commonly available are heat and cold since, although warmth increases bleeding by dilating the capillaries, water just hot or cold enough to be uncomfortable to the hand contracts them. On the whole heat is more effective than cold in this respect. Adrenaline, perchloride of iron, and witch-hazel, are effective in slight or capillary bleeding but, of course useless in haemorrhage from one of the larger vessels. Dressings suitable for controlling more serious bleeding are mentioned under Haemophilia, Fibrin Foam.

Hair: there are many misconceptions about hair perhaps because it falls into the no-man's-land between medicine and cosmetics. Only a few can be noted here, but it must be realised that hair is a dead structure which is kept glossy by the secretion of the sebaceous glands and therefore it is untrue that cut hair loses some property which can be prevented from escaping by singeing, and, so far as one knows, hair cannot be fed for such nourishment as the scalp requires comes to it from the blood-stream. There is no 'correct' number of times to wash the hair during the week since this depends on aesthetic considerations and individual variations in the natural oiliness of the scalp; women may shampoo their hair once weekly or once every two weeks, and some men wash it daily but this would be a mistake if the scalp is naturally dry unless oil is added afterwards. Washing the hair has nothing to do with physiological functions although many women believe that it should not be done during the menstrual periods, a totally fallacious belief. Nor are there any hair tonics which prevent falling hair although it is not impossible that stimulant lotions which act by improving the blood-supply to the scalp may delay loss of hair which, by and large, is controlled by heredity and the endocrine glands. Where baldness (q.v.) is due to disease it is obviously possible to do something about it but most men will become as bald and as grey (or otherwise) as their fathers and at the same age no matter what they do. The fact that men often become bald whilst women rarely do has been attributed by the lunatic fringe to numerous factors, e.g. that women keep their hair long, or brush it more frequently, but the fact is most probably that large amounts of male sex-hormone in the blood tend to cause baldness whilst the female sex-hormone prevents it; both types of hormone are found in either sex and there is some foundation for the belief that baldness is in some measure associated with virility and preponderance of the male hormone. Eunuchs do not go bald. The main point to be made, however, is that most forms of 'scalp treatment' are a waste of money since they do nothing whatever for normal hair and diseased hair requires proper medical diagnosis and treatment by a skin specialist (*see* Baldness, Superfluous Hair).

Halibut-Liver Oil: a particularly rich source of vitamin A (30,000 I.U. per gramme) and vitamin D (2,500 I.U. per gramme). It is obtainable as oil or in capsules and is a more convenient means of giving the vitamins than the old-fashioned cod-liver oil which is less concentrated.

Halitosis: (*see* Breath, Bad).

Hallucinations: are not to be confused with *illusions* or *delusions*. An *illusion* is an error of sense perception in which a person misinterprets something that he actually experiences (e.g. mistaking a piece of clothing hanging on a door for a ghost) whilst a *delusion* is a faulty belief peculiar to the individual himself and not shared by others of the same social group (e.g. a man who believes himself to be Napoleon shares his belief with no one whilst one who believes that the British people are descended from the lost ten tribes may be wrong but his belief is shared by others of the British Israelite sect and a similar belief is held by the Mormons who believe that the Red Indians are the missing tribes). It is the social acceptability of a belief not its truth which is the criterion of its normality and a delusion is a false belief private to the individual. Hallucinations are false sense perceptions in which the individual experiences something which others agree is simply not 'there' and, unlike an illusion, is not simply a misinterpretation of what really is there; they are often backed by delusions and, in fact, it might well be said that a delusion is father to a hallucination in that the person frequently experiences what he expects to experience. Hallucinations may be visual, auditory, or related to the senses of smell or touch, those connected with hearing or smell being usually purely psychological in nature whilst those of sight, touch, and sometimes smell may have an organic basis. Ordinarily hallucinations have been regarded as symptomatic of insanity, but there can be no doubt that trance states in hysteria may bring them about as can drugs, alcohol (especially the visual hallucinations of delirium tremens), brain disease, the trances of mediums and witch-doctors, and religious ecstacy. Schizophrenia is the classical cause of auditory hallucinations, but it is certain that simple or deeply religious people experience similar phenomena without any mental or physical illness being present although these are disapproved of in our predominantly materialistic and rationalistic culture which does not accept the metaphysical views upon which they are based. The significance of hallucinations must be judged (a) in the context of the individual's ordinary beliefs and cultural level, and (b) in relation to the rest of his behaviour (see Mental Illness).

Hallux: the big toe.

Hammer-Toe: (see Corns and Bunions).

Hand: the ability of man to oppose the thumb to the other fingers so that small objects can be grasped is one of the distinguishing features of the human race and related to the hand's extreme delicacy and intricacy as an instrument. Thus when the brain, on which the hand is represented over a much larger area than in other animals, becomes diseased loss of the finer movements of the hand is one of the first signs that all is not well. The hand possesses twenty-seven bones: eight carpals in the wrist roughly arranged in two rows of four each; five metacarpals in the palm; and fourteen phalanges in the fingers, the thumb containing only two and the rest three. From the muscles of the forearm twelve tendons run in front of the wrist passing under a ligament and enclosed in a complex synovial sheath to be attached to the fingers where they bring about flexion; at the back of the wrist a similar number of tendons cause extension. The turning of the palm downwards is termed pronation while supination, which again is most highly developed in man, is the turning of the palm upwards and these movements are brought about by the pronator and supinator muscles assisted by the biceps. Because supination is the more powerful movement this has determined the thread direction in such instruments as corkscrews and screwdrivers. Forming the ball of the thumb and little finger and filling in the spaces between the metacarpal bones are the short muscles whose function is to separate and bring the fingers together and to bend the hand at the knuckles. The blood-supply comes from the ulnar and radial arteries, the former passing down the inner side of the arm, the latter down the same side as the thumb; both form arches deep in the tissues of the palm from which branches run down both sides of each finger. The ulnar nerve supplies the skin with sensation over the little finger and the inner half of the next one, the radial nerve the back of the remaining fingers and the median nerve the front.

Few parts of the body tell so much about the individual as his hand; ignoring as superstition the theories of the palmist and treating with reserve beliefs that the shape of the hand is related to the personality so that long sensitive fingers are associated with artistic tendencies (as in the chimpanzee?) or short stubby ones with practical virtues, it is nevertheless true that we can infer a great deal about a man from his hands, e.g. his care, or lack of care, his work (especially in the case of craftsmen), his general sensitivity or lack of it, etc. From the medical point of view the doctor will note their shape and size sometimes finding the large hand of acromegaly (q.v.), the claw hand of ulnar paralysis, the wasting of the muscular pads at the bases of the thumb and little finger which signify progressive muscular atrophy, the main d'accoucheur (midwives' hand) with the thumb and fingers held in a cone as with tetany, paralysis agitans, and other nervous diseases, the clubbed fingers of chronic heart and lung disease, the nodules of gout, the swollen joints of rheumatoid arthritis, and so on. Then there is the tremor of the alcoholic (sometimes accompanied by wrist-drop) and the different types of tremor associated with organic deterioration or mere nervousness; the purplish discoloration of the palm in cirrhosis of the liver; the whitish or bluish fingers of Raynaud's disease and other circulatory conditions; the loss of the sense of pain in syringomyelia (often indicated by old scars from unheeded cigarette-burns or cuts); and many other signs too numerous to mention. But it need hardly be said that no diagnosis would be made on the basis of any one of these signs or symptoms taken in isolation. They are suggestive rather than conclusive.

Hanging: in general, and apart from judicial hanging, this is done with suicidal intent although cases are not unknown where murder has been carried out by suspension, death ordinarily being due to strangulation. Since this is a relatively slow means of dying an individual found hanging should be cut down immediately, his body being supported whilst this is being done, the noose must be loosened and removed, and artificial respiration applied at once. If a doctor is present in time injections to stimulate the heart-beat will be given and efforts at resuscitation carried on for some time until it is certain that life is extinct or recovery begins. In judicial hanging the method has been different since the late Mr Hangman Berry devised his scientific formula for calculating a drop which would neither cause death by slow strangulation nor, as all too frequently happened, pull the condemned man's head completely off – an unaesthetic sight at the best of times. Functioning at the turn of the century Mr Berry, who took his profession so seriously that he used to hand the condemned evangelical tracts suitable to their condition, showed that the best results were obtained by a drop of six feet on an average varying inversely with the weight of the body. Such a drop would dislocate the neck without undue mutilation or, medically speaking, cause the odontoid process at the base of the skull to break through its ligament and crush the vital centres in the medulla. But accidents will happen and it was necessary for Sir Bernard Spilsbury to amend the formula and recommend an increase of three inches in the drop. Since those who accept capital punishment in spite of the fact that it has been abolished by most civilised countries where the murder rate has subsequently gone down, are hardly likely to listen to reasoned argument, nor is this the place for it, we may leave further discussion to the moralists.

Hare-Lip: (*see* Palate).

Hashimoto's Disease: a disease characterised by a diffuse enlargement of the thyroid gland resulting from an increase of fibrous tissue and infiltration of lymphocytes rather than an increase of colloid material as in the commoner type of goitre. The patient, usually a middle-aged woman, has a general enlargement of the gland, but initially there are no symptoms elsewhere and no signs of thyrotoxicosis, although the condition usually ends in myxoedema caused by lack of thyroid hormone. (*See* Myxoedema).

Hay Fever: an allergic disease characterised by irritation of the mucous membranes of the eyes, nose, and air passages brought about by the pollen of various grasses and plants and therefore seasonal in incidence, coming on regularly at the same time each year. As explained elsewhere (*see* Allergy) all proteins when they get inside the body unchanged act as anti-gens, i.e. they stimulate the formation of anti-bodies against them, and normally this takes place in the blood-stream. But if, as in allergic subjects, antibody formation is slow and inadequate the antigen diffuses into the body cells where a re-action takes place with the formation of the poisonous sub-stance histamine. All allergic diseases therefore are ultimately forms of histamine poisoning and hay-fever is the type affect-ing predominantly the eyes and nose, just as asthma affects the bronchial tubes and certain types of allergic dermatitis the skin. Most cases of hay-fever occur in summer and spring when the antigen is grass-pollen, but some occur in autumn when the pollen of ragweeds is the usual cause. The tendency to allergy seems to be inherited but not necessarily the specific form taken by the disease, so it is quite common in a family to find one member suffering from hay-fever and another from asthma or occasional skin rashes. Such subjects are more often men than women and tend to be sensitive and highly-strung; structural defects are sometimes found in the nose by en-thusiastic ear, nose and throat specialists but the same defects often exist in the absence of hay-fever; and, not unnaturally, the condition usually improves following a period of rain or at the seaside. Treatment may take the form of a course of vaccine prepared from pollen which must be given throughout the preceding winter each year or the use of antihistamine drugs which must be taken throughout the season. A change of environment to escape the pollen is not open to everyone and is rarely necessary with the new drugs; the nose is best left severely alone so far as operative measures are concerned but sprays containing hydrocortisone are often helpful. Suit-able antihistamines (to be prescribed by the doctor) are Anthi-san, Antistin, Ancolan, Benadryl, Histantin, Phenergan, and Thephorin; such drugs have different effects on different indi-viduals and if one does not help or has unpleasant side effects another should be tried.

Hazeline: or Witch-Hazel is prepared from the leaves or bark of Hamamelis virginiana and used as an astringent extract or ointment for the eye, skin, and anus. It is soothing and stops minor bleeding and discharge.

Headache: is one of the commonest symptoms in medicine and it is a fair estimate that at least 90% of all headaches have no organic basis so far as structural defects are concerned. This does not, of course, mean that nothing at all is happening in the body but rather that what does happen is temporary and of emotional origin, the most frequent emotions being anxiety or suppressed anger and resentment. In such cases the immediate cause of pain is in all probability a spasm of the sheet of muscle passing over the scalp from the eyebrows to the back of the neck or of the other muscles in the neck region; this is an evolutionary relic of a type of reaction seen in the lower animals, (cf. the angry or suspicious dog or ape whose hair stands on end over the back of the neck as the muscles tense for action). Some kinds of headache appear to be caused by dilation of the arteries in the brain or tension upon the membranes covering it; for the brain itself has no capacity to feel pain and can, in fact, be operated on or touched with impunity whilst the patient is fully conscious. In migraine (q.v.) the headache is probably of this type, as may also be the very severe headaches in brain tumour or other space-occupying diseases within the skull. Congestion inside the spaces of the skull such as the sinuses causes severe pain and even mild congestion within the nose makes most people feel 'headachy.' Possibly eye defects can produce headaches by congestion although it is unlikely that all the many people with headaches who seem to think that this is an immediate indication for having their eyes tested are right – even if they rarely leave their oculist without a new pair of glasses – but some of the more serious eye diseases such as glaucoma (q.v.) cause very severe pain. Other causes frequently given for headaches are dental sepis, constipation, indigestion, kidney disease, 'rheumatism,' and high blood-pressure, but there is not the slightest reason to believe that any of these directly lead to headaches, although worry about them very well may. The idea that high blood-pressure and headaches are inevitably associated together dies hard, but the fact is that the vast majority of cases of hypertension have no symptoms at all and the condition is found accidentally; *people* who know that their blood-pressure is raised often have headaches but this is largely due to anxiety. For practical purposes it is important to note how the patient describes his pain: the nervous headache is often described as 'terrible' and likened to 'red-hot needles' and so on because it is really a dramatisation of the individual's quite real problems. Furthermore it is 'all over' the head and in this way quite unlike the physically-caused headache which is sharply localised to a particular part, keeps the patient still rather than restless and talkative, and is usually associated with other symptoms. Severe localised headache accompanied by vomiting attacks and a slow pulse always requires immediate attention as these are signs of raised pressure inside the skull. In migraine the headache is frequently preceded by vomiting and there are eye symptoms which are described elsewhere. The headaches of sinusitis may be at any point of the forehead or face depending upon which sinuses are affected (*see* Sinusitis); they may be just above the eyes at the base of the nose, in the corner of the eyes, over the cheeks, and so on, and there is usually a history of nasal discharge and 'catarrh.' Teeth have been held responsible for many things but rarely convincingly although toothache from a molar or premolar tooth is sometimes referred to the side of the head, and since constipation does not 'poison the blood-stream' it cannot cause headache, although here again worry about it can. The treatment of headache is the treatment of its cause (*see* Hypertension, Neurosis, Migraine, Sinusitis).

Health: the basic principles of a healthy life are well-known: care of the teeth (q.v.); a well-balanced diet with adequate supplies of vitamins and minerals in addition to suitable amounts of carbohydrates, proteins, and fats; adequate exercise; cleanliness, and fresh air; freedom from undue anxiety and nervous tension, and the rest. However, a look at these requirements in the light of modern knowledge must result in their being somewhat modified. It is true that a well-balanced and well-digested diet is important but this is obtained in different parts of the world in widely differing ways: the vegetarians with their relatively low protein diet, the Eskimos with their high fat diet, hunting tribes with their almost wholly meat diet, and Latins with a diet high in carbohydrate and vegetable oils. All seem to be equally suitable although it has recently been suggested that diets rich in cholesterol, i.e. animal fats, eggs, liver, kidneys, etc., make one prone to coronary thrombosis. What seems much more likely is that over-eating is harmful and there is some correlation between longevity and a slim build. The correlation between coronary disease and lack of exercise leads one to believe that a moderate amount of exercise is important to the ordinary individual although many invalids who are totally immobilised live long lives; violent exercise as in athletes correlates in no way at all with either subsequent health or with long life. Apart from keeping free from infection it would seem that the main function of bathing is cosmetic and, indeed, very few infections enter the body through the skin, most of those in temperate climates being air-borne or taken in the food or in water. Some diseases (e.g. poliomyelitis) in fact are more prone to attack the healthy than the weakling but there can be no doubt of the connection between bad housing and insanitary surroundings and such diseases as bronchitis, rheumatism, tonsilitis and adenoids, and upper respiratory tract infections. Climate has been discussed under that heading and when climate is separated from the conditions associated with specific climatic conditions it will be seen that climate in itself plays a relatively small part in the maintenance of health or the production of disease. Thus malaria used to be common in England and its presence in tropical climates is in a sense incidental for when the disease is wiped out as it will be during the present century the climates will have remained virtually unchanged. Similarly smoking and foreign substances in the atmosphere are associated with bronchitis and lung cancer but these are unconnected with the climate in itself. There are few doctors today who believe that cold and damp in themselves produce illness but there can be little doubt that the incidence of colds and sinus diseases is closely related to sudden changes of temperature when we leave our overheated rooms to go into the cold air outside or vice versa. Addiction to alcohol is an important factor in causing disease both directly and indirectly (*see* Alcoholism), yet the moderate drinker lives longer than the total abstainer and there is not the slightest evidence that puritanical attitudes in life lead to longevity and a healthy life. Constipation is also dealt with elsewhere and, except as a symptom of other diseases, is of little significance. Even the presence of serious disease does not necessarily shorten life and most doctors know of patients with chronic bronchitis or bronchial asthma and enlarged hearts who live to a ripe old age in spite of their troubles and indeed one of the most striking experiences of medical practice is how these cases live on whilst apparently healthy patients are carried away in their prime. We must reconcile ourselves to the fact that a great part of longevity and health is, in a technically advanced society such as ours, based on constitution and inheritance and is not to be wooed by crank diets and taking care.

Hearing: (*see* Ear, Deafness).

Heart: the heart is more or less conical in shape and lies enclosed in its fibrous sac or pericardium between the two lungs in the chest. The apex beat is normally felt about 1½ inches below the left nipple and any gross deviation from this in the outward direction is an indication that the heart is enlarged. Each half is composed of two chambers, an auricle and a ventricle, and between these are placed valves to ensure that the blood flows only in one direction; those on the left side are called the mitral valves because the two flaps resemble a bishop's mitre, those on the right are known as the tricuspid valves because they have three flaps. There are also valves at the origin of the two great arteries, the pulmonary which leads out of the right ventricle to pass to the lungs and the aortic opening from the left ventricle into the aorta. In this way blood is kept from flowing back into the chamber from which it has just been pumped out and when the valves are defective from disease the sound of the blood passing through a narrowed valve (stenosis) or leaking back through an inadequate one (incompetence) is heard by the doctor through his stethoscope (*see* Valvular Disease). When either of these conditions occur enlargement or dilation of one of the chambers will occur as it thickens to force blood through a narrowed valve or becomes too full through receiving both its normal complement of blood and more which has regurgitated from the part above the diseased valve; thickening of the chamber with enlargement is one of the ways in which a heart compensates for a valvular defect dilation, a sign of its failure. The valves and the rest of the inside of the heart are lined with endocardium and disease of the valves is often known as endocarditis. In most cases this is the result of old infections, particularly rheumatic fever, scarlet fever, and diphtheria, but sometimes there develops an acute infection of the valves accompanied by fever which is called bacterial endocarditis. The muscle of the heart is the myocardium and this, of course, has to have its own blood-supply which comes from the coronary vessels arising from the aorta just above the aortic valve; when these become blocked a very serious condition arises since the part of the heart affected cannot get its blood-supply. The severe pain occurring in this condition known as coronary thrombosis if the vessel is blocked or angina pectoris if the vessels have gone into spasm, is a form of cramp similar in nature to that experienced elsewhere in the body. The nervous supply to the heart comes from three sources (like that of most other internal organs): there is a supply from the sympathetic nerves coming in this case from the ganglia (cervical ganglia) in the neck and one from the parasympathetic system through the vagus nerve. The first of these speeds up the heart-beat whilst the other slows it down but in addition to these the heart has nerves coming from ganglia in its own substance. The function of the latter is to ensure that the beat of the heart is synchronised because the auricles and ventricles are largely separate, there being common superficial muscle fibres for both auricles and both ventricles and separate deep fibres for each chamber. Fibre bundles (the bundle of His) connect auricle to ventricle and transmit the impulse from one to the other so if these bundles are damaged the ventricles contract very slowly at their own natural rate, the condition being described as 'heart block' or Stokes' Adams' syndrome. It will be seen that most damage is done to the heart by infectious diseases which usually attack the endocardium but may cause deterioration of the muscle and infection of the pericardium. But occasionally bacterial or other poisons affect the heart and finally old age causes its muscle to degenerate and weaken both directly and by narrowing of the arteries.

Heartburn: a burning pain in the region of the heart and up the back of the throat caused by excess acid in the stomach and relieved by alkalies.

Heart Diseases: these may be classified in various ways according to the part affected or their cause. Thus *pericarditis* is inflammation of the cellophane-like covering of the heart, usually complicates some other disease such as rheumatic fever, scarlet fever, diphtheria, etc., and is recognised by pain over the heart with fever and difficulty in breathing. In *myocarditis* the actual muscle of the heart is affected or its blood-vessels and so we have coronary thrombosis (q.v.) and angina pectoris (q.v.), both due to faults in the blood-supply and accompanied by severe pain in the chest passing down the left arm and coming on quite suddenly. General disease may cause the heart muscle to atrophy or become fatty and poor blood-supply may cause it to become fibrosed (see Myocarditis) whilst too much work against a high pressure causes it to become enlarged and finally to fail (see Hypertension). *Endocarditis* is an inflammation of the delicate lining of the inside of the heart which also forms the valves and may be acute or chronic. The acute type is that usually known as bacterial endocarditis in which germs are actually growing on the heart valves, requiring treatment with antibiotics, the chronic type is that most commonly described as *valvular disease* and is described under that heading. Disorders of the heart-beat such as a too rapid pulse or a too slow one or an irregular beat are usually classified as diseases of the neuromyocardium, i.e. they are fundamentally caused by interference with the nerves which control the beat as in heart-block, auricular fibrillation, certain kinds of rapid pulse (tachycardia) or slow pulse (brady-cardia) (q.v.). The failing heart is discussed with valvular disease. In addition to all these must be mentioned the cardiac neuroses such as Effort Syndrome (q.v.) which are mainly of psychological origin. For congenital heart disease see Heart Surgery. The *symptoms* of heart disease, curiously enough, are not very frequently such as one would directly relate to the heart. Thus pain over the heart, palpitation, and discomfort in this region in the vast majority of cases are caused by gastric upsets (heartburn), pressure caused by flatulence since the stomach is separated from the apex of the heart only by the diaphragm, and nervous tension which is by far the common-est cause of palpitation. The exceptions to this rule are the pain caused by pericarditis in the early stages – although in this case the patient is usually incapacitated by some other disease – coronary thrombosis, and angina pectoris. In these two diseases the pain is severe and tends to pass down the left arm or shoulder; coronary thrombosis often happens whilst the individual is resting or asleep since that is when the blood in the coronary vessels is most likely to clot, but in angina the pain is brought on by exertion bringing about spasm which passes off when the exertion is stopped. Although it is often claimed that palpitation can be caused by local sepsis,

271

excessive smoking, etc. (*see* Tachycardia), there can be little doubt that the most important factor is nervous tension. The worried patient often seen in general practice holding his hand over his heart and thinking that he is going to drop dead at any moment prompts questions directed to his home and business worries rather than to his heart, whilst *as a generalisation* the patient who really has heart disease is often unworried and unaware of the connection between his symptoms and his heart. These are likely to be: breathlessness, tiredness, swelling of the ankles which is worse at night-time, headache and giddiness, sometimes fainting attacks, bronchitis and spitting of blood, 'sleep-starts' when he wakes up suddenly at night unable to get his breath. Obviously all of these are caused by inadequate oxygenation of the blood due to the impaired circulation or to congestion in particular areas.

Heart Surgery: although it is not difficult to reach the heart surgically and the organ itself is tough, being merely a muscular pump with the sole function of driving blood round the body, surgeons long hesitated to intervene from fear of haemorrhage or a sudden stoppage of the beat through upsetting the delicate balance of cardiac nervous control. It is only in the last twenty years that intervention has been attempted save as a last resort and it is not surprising that some of the first successes were in the field of congenital heart disease in children since many of these patients, if running a serious risk from the operation, were doomed to certain death in a few years without it. More recently still new developments in surgical technique have made heart operations increasingly safe, e.g. the mechanical heart to which the patient's circulation can be connected whilst the surgeon operates in a field freed from the risk of haemorrhage, clear of blood, and freed too from the necessity to hasten through his work. Essentially the mechanical heart, one model of which was devised by Charles Lindberg the air pioneer in collaboration with the biologist and physician Alexis Carrel, is simply a pump which takes in venous blood, aerates it by passage in a thin film over glass plates, and subsequently pumps it back into the arterial system; another method formerly employed was the connecting up of one of the child's parents to act as a pump in the same way—provided, of course, that his or her blood is of the same group as that of the child. Congenital heart defects are caused by faulty development and often by the failure of structures which are useful and necessary to the foetus in the womb to disappear. The part played by infection of the mother in early pregnancy with German measles and of dangerous drugs (thalidomide) are mentioned elsewhere but the subject is a complex one and here it must suffice to describe briefly five of the main types of congenital defect (*see* Drugs, their Dangers).

(1) *Patent ductus arteriosus:* as the lungs of the child in the womb are useless whilst it is receiving its oxygenated blood through the placenta from its mother, a small duct exists between the pulmonary artery (which later will carry blood to the lungs for oxygen) and the aorta in order to shunt it away. If this duct persists after birth not enough blood reaches the lungs and the child becomes underdeveloped, short of breath, very liable to catch whatever infections are about, and sooner or later heart failure will arise as the heart is overworked in its futile attempt to get sufficient blood through the lungs. All that is required in this case is that the duct should be tied off and severed, an operation which is successful in practically every case, provided that other abnormalities do not exist.

(2) *Septal defects:* defects in the walls between the chambers of the heart ('hole in the heart') may be between the two auricles or the two ventricles, and, although the harm done depends upon the size of the hole it is apparent that it is caused by the mixing of venous blood from the right side of the heart which has been deprived of its oxygen by passage through the body with arterial blood which has just been oxygenated by passage through the lungs. Some holes are small and cause no symptoms but operation is necessary when a large hole makes the patient so seriously disabled that he or she is unlikely to live for any length of time. Such operations are serious, and when the hole is between the ventricles not at present very satisfactory or safe, but a similar defect between the auricles can be more readily dealt with.

Tetralogy of Fallot or 'blue baby' gets its name from the blue appearance of these infants at birth and the fact that four (Greek *tetra*) defects are usually present. Here again the symptoms are caused by insufficient oxygenation of the blood and the modern operation transposes and transplants some of the great blood-vessels of the heart so that it flows back to the

273

lungs for oxygenation, e.g. transplantation of the subclavian artery into the pulmonary just before it enters the lungs or joining the aorta to the pulmonary artery. The relief of shortness of breath and the blue colour of the skin or cyanosis follows immediately after a successful operation and the expectation of life is increased. Without operation life would be short and wretched.

Pulmonary Stenosis is a congenital defect in which there is a narrow pulmonary valve, an underdeveloped pulmonary artery, or a partition of muscle within the right auricle which interferes with normal blood flow through the lungs. The patient is unable to lead any active life, breathless, and unlikely to live for long without operation. Here the right ventricle is opened and the abnormal partition cut or narrowed valve widened. Most cases are highly successful.

Coarctation of the Aorta: narrowing of the aorta as it leaves the heart is a birth deformity which leads to high bloodpressure, absent pulses in the legs, and the development of collateral circulations over the upper part of the body, i.e. the blood-vessels elsewhere enlarge in order to compensate for the defect. Life is unlikely to be prolonged beyond the fortieth year and death frequently results from cerebral haemorrhage (stroke), heart failure, rupture of the aorta, or some acute infection. The operative treatment involves removal of the narrowed part of the aorta and stitching together the ends either directly or with an intervening graft from a bloodvessel elsewhere in the body or from a bank (*see* Grafts). The mortality rate for this operation is decreasing and results are good in about 75–80% of cases. Congenital heart defects account for only about 1–2% of all heart cases but surgery is increasingly used for acquired disease in adults. Thus stenosis or narrowing of the aortic or mitral valves is treated in some cases by valvotomy when the valve is dilated either by the surgeon's finger thrust through an incision in the right auricle or the aorta (depending on which valve is affected) or, when this is inadequate, a special knife known as a valvotome is attached to the finger and the stenosed tissues divided. In this way stenosis is transformed into incompetence which is much less serious. Commonly nowadays diseased valves are removed and replaced by plastic ones and plastic tubes are also used to replace diseased portions of the larger blood-vessels. Another important advance is in the treatment of heart-block where the impulses arise normally in the upper chambers of the heart but fail to be transmitted along the conducting tissue to the ventricles. In this case the heart-beat may be as low as 25 per minute instead of 70 or so and it is necessary to introduce an artificial pace-maker. A thin nylon tube containing the conducting material is threaded through the veins from a suitable part of the body until the end reaches the inside of the heart and to the other end is attached a small transistorised battery which is then sewn under the skin of the abdomen or elsewhere. The battery takes over the control of the heart and gives it 70 shocks a minute bringing the condition back to normal.

Heat-Cramps, Heatstroke, Sunstroke: until fairly recently it was usual to distinguish between heatstroke and sunstroke, the former being produced by excessive heat whether in the tropics or in a steel foundry in northern Europe, the latter being produced by the rays of the sun especially upon the head or spine. In fact, no such state as sunstroke exists if by this it is implied that the rays of the sun *in themselves* and apart from a hot climate can cause any damage other than sunburn of the skin. The only useful function of solar topees is to keep the scalp from being burned by the sun or keep its light out of the eyes and any other broad-brimmed hat would do just as well but spine-pads have no use whatever. 'Sunstroke' and heatstroke are the same entity and result from a hot atmosphere, particularly one which is also damp, in which excess heat cannot escape from the body. In the early stages there is excessive sweating leading to salt loss and therefore to painful cramps and concentration of the blood which disturbs the circulation and brings about ultimately a condition resembling surgical shock. In the later stages the whole heat-regulating system breaks down, sweat is inhibited, and delirium and coma herald a fatal end in serious cases. In the mild case there is only slight or severe headache, sweating, cramps, and irritability and fatigue. The treatment consists in removal to a cool place, giving large amounts of normal salt solution (1 teaspoonful to a pint of water) either by mouth or intravenously, and in severe cases the naked body should be wrapped in a wet sheet soaked in water and kept fanned until the temperature falls to about 102 degrees. Delirium, cessation of sweating, and a temperature above 105–7 degrees are bad

275

signs. Some people seem to be more liable to heat stroke than others but beyond ordinary sensible precautions experience during the war showed that much of the traditional rigmarole about midday suns, special clothing other than that which commonsense suggests, and the rest is unnecessary as, indeed, a glance at the local inhabitants might have suggested or even a glimpse at our own past. The 'light nourishing diet' formerly advised looks rather silly in face of the hot bulky curries of India and the light airy clothes in face of those of our forbears like the explorer Mungo Park who at the end of the 18th century sought the source of the Niger comfortably dressed in his everyday Scottish suit and top-hat. Today the main menace is from the too lightly clad brigade of sun-worshippers with neither knowledge nor experience of hot countries who get badly sun-burned and develop headaches to pester their more sensible relatives, their employers, and their doctors in the belief that they have 'sunstroke' (*see* Sunburn).

Hebephrenia: a state of rapid deterioration of the mind with lack of social interest and self-centred delusions arising in early adult life which forms one of the sub-divisions of schizophrenia.

Heberden's Nodes: small hard lumps appearing at the last joint of the fingers in some cases of rheumatoid arthritis.

Heliotherapy: treatment by the sun's rays or ultra-violet rays produced by a special lamp. Formerly much used for medical purposes the method has fallen into relative disuse and its only common function is to provoke a skin reaction in certain diseases of the skin (*see* Light Treatment).

Helminths: a name for parasitic worms (*see* Worms).

Hemeralopia: a state of day-blindness in which the individual can see better in the half-light of approaching darkness than in full daylight.

Hemianaesthesia: loss of the sense of touch down one side of the body.

Hemianopia: also known as hemianopsia or hemiopia means loss of half of the field of vision due to some lesion within the skull which can be localised in part by the area of sight affected. This may be in the middle of the field of vision only, the left and right sides being clearly visible, or the central field may be clear whilst the sides are invisible, or the whole field may be obscured save the farthest out parts.

Hemiatrophy: wasting of one side of the body or the half of a part of the body such as the face resulting either during the course of development or as a consequence of some nerve disease.

Hemicrania: headache limited to one side of the head.

Hemiplegia: paralysis of one side of the body as after a stroke.

Hemlock: the name given to a group of plants two of which are found in Britain – the water hemlock or cowbane (Cicuta virosa) and the common hemlock (Conium malculatum). Both contain the deadly poison coniine, the latter being the plant from whose juice Socrates died as this was the official method of execution in the Athens of his day. Its effects are well exemplified in the account given by Plato, for Socrates after drinking was told to walk about until his legs felt heavy (motor paralysis) and later, when his foot was pressed, he could not feel (sensory paralysis). Death finally occurs from paralysis of the respiratory system. The effect of coniine in diminishing muscular contractions was once valued by doctors and the drug was used to treat chorea, whooping-cough, and epilepsy. Its use is now extinct.

Heparin: a substance obtained from liver, muscle, and lung which prevents coagulation of the blood by neutralising thrombin (*see* Coagulation). It is used to avoid clotting in such diseases as coronary thrombosis which are characterised by this and being inactive by mouth it is usually given by intravenous injection. Proprietary forms of heparin are Liquemin and Pularin. The same precautions are necessary as with other anticoagulant drugs.

Hepatitis: inflammation of the liver usually in the form of *infective epidemic hepatitis* caused by a virus which has jaundice as its most obvious symptom. The incubation period is about a month and jaundice usually makes its appearance after the first week and may last for two or three weeks more although, as after most forms of jaundice, depression and poor appetite may linger for some time. The patient should be isolated for a fortnight and put to bed with a light diet, plenty of fluids with glucose, and as little fat as possible. Since there is usually an associated inflammation of the stomach (gastritis) alkalies may be necessary and Epsom salts which stimulate the flow of bile may be used if the patient is constipated. Alcohol must be avoided. The disease is not a dangerous one but can be a considerable nuisance if allowed to spread, the infection probably occurring by droplet infection from coughing and sneezing. Infective hepatitis amongst allied troops seriously hindered the Italian campaign in the last war. Rarely it may lead to cirrhosis (q.v.).

Heredity: this vast subject which forms the theme of the science of genetics can only be dealt with summarily here. The scientific study of heredity was initiated by the Austrian monk Gregor Mendel (1822–84) who, although one of the greatest of scientific geniuses, died virtually unknown, his work being made generally known only after his death. Mendel's most important experiments were carried out on the common garden pea in which it is a relatively simple matter to distinguish several inherited characters and to cross-fertilise one plant with another. Thus some seeds are round, others wrinkled; some are green, others yellow; some plants are tall, others dwarf. By deliberately fertilising one plant with another, Mendel was able to show how such characteristics are handed on. It might be supposed that traits of this type mingle to produce others which are a compromise between the two, e.g. that the offspring of a tall and a dwarf parent would be medium-sized, and so it sometimes turns out in a state of nature where few characters are present in the pure form. But Mendel was able to show that when the two pure lines are crossed the offspring are hybrid talls because the characteristic of tallness is dominant and when these are interbred the third generation are in the proportion of one pure tall to one pure dwarf and two hybrid talls. The pure lines when mated with each other breed true, only producing talls or dwarfs; but when the hybrids (who all *appear* tall) breed the above proportions appear. These facts are shown in the accompanying diagram.

(1) Tall crossed with dwarf

(2) Tall Hybrid

(3) 1 Tall (pure)   2 Tall Hybrid   1 Dwarf (pure)

The reason for these proportions although not known to Mendel is apparent when we consider the processes of cell-division and reproduction. Every living cell (with rare exceptions such as the human red blood cell) contains a central nucleus which controls cell metabolism and carries the material which is the agent of heredity in the form of the chromosomes; ordinarily these are in a confused network which resembles a roughly crumpled skein of wool, but when cell division is about to occur this breaks up into numbers of separate chromosomes. These are rod, comma, or globular-shaped bodies along which are strung the minute genes which are the actual carriers of the units of heredity. The cell narrows at the middle and the chromosomes divide equally down the centre of each so that when the narrowing becomes a distinct 'waist' and then a dumb-bell shape just before the two new cells separate each part will contain exactly the same genes as the other. This process is known as mitosis and obviously there is little possibility of variation for the two cells which have separated in this way contain identical hereditary material. But the mechanism of evolution and progress is divergence and it is this factor which is introduced by sexual reproduction when two cells unite each with a different hereditary content. Before this can happen however the number of chromosomes must be halved in the sex-cells – otherwise the chromosome number would be doubling each time mating occurred. So in the development of the sex-cells or gametes the chromosomes, instead of dividing down the middle, go half to one cell and half to another, e.g. the human body cells each contain 48 chromosomes but the germ cells only 24, the rest coming at fertilisation from another individual of the opposite sex. Now let us consider once more Mendel's tall and short pea plants and it will be seen that each pure-bred tall pea and each pure-bred dwarf one carries in every body cell two units (or genes) for tallness or dwarfness so that when they divide to form the sex-cells all will contain only factors for tallness or dwarfness. The hybrid types, on the other hand, have body cells which contain one gene for tallness and one dwarf gene and when they divide to form sex-cells some will carry only tall characteristics and others only dwarf ones. When two hybrids are crossed the possibilities for the offspring are: tall unites with tall, tall unites with dwarf, dwarf unites with tall, dwarf unites with dwarf. So there will be a proportion of two hybrids who appear tall but are not pure-bred, and one each of pure tall and dwarf stock; in short, three will appear tall and one dwarf.

Most characters have a variation which is, in a sense, its opposite like tallness and shortness, blue eyes and brown eyes, and the one which imposes its appearance on the hybrids is known as the dominant gene the other being the recessive one. According to the theory of Weissmann the genes are totally unaffected by any events in the life of the individual who carries them and changes in the genetic constitution of a species is brought about by natural selection which weeds out the useless traits by causing those who carry them to die out earlier than those with useful variations as Darwin pointed out, e.g. in a wood near London a certain kind of moth had a wing coloration which perfectly fitted in with the light grey bark of the trees on which they usually rested and so it was invisible to prowling birds. But gradually the smoke of the growing city blackened the trunks of the trees and the light-coloured moths were easily seen and picked off by their enemies; some, however, had chance variations of wing-colour which were nearer in tint to the blackened trunks and these not only survived but increased since they naturally produced a higher proportion of dark-winged offspring. Today no light-winged moths survive. This is natural selection which only involves the carrying on of useful variations *already present* and their multiplication in a favourable environment. The other main mechanism of evolution is mutation in which the genes are radically changed by factors which, on the whole, are not fully known. X-rays and atomic radiation can produce them, but such mutations are in the majority of instances harmful, only a minority being useful and progressive. From this it follows that the parent's way of life has little bearing on the inherited traits of their offspring and if, for example, children of neurotic parents or alcoholics followed the example of their parents it might be supposed (by a minority) that this was because both shared the same heredity or (by a majority) that they had *learned* the behaviour in question in the course of upbringing. Lamarck's theory which, roughly speaking implies that giraffes acquired long necks by constant stretching to reach the more tender leaves at the tree-tops and handed this acquired trait on to their offspring is thoroughly discredited, although the Soviet geneticist Lysenko made himself notorious by maintaining something of the sort. Acquired traits are not inherited but it is certain that influences within the mother's womb can affect the developing child, e.g. German measles and glandular changes and, indeed, perhaps the larger number of cases of mental defect (q.v.) are not inherited with the germplasm but arise in this way.

What implications have these discoveries for general medicine? The answer must be: on the whole, extraordinarily little. A number of diseases are inherited (e.g. certain forms of idiocy, haemophilia, Huntington's chorea) in a fairly definite way but with most the issue is far less clear. For instance the fact that obsessional neurosis is more frequent in the children of obsessional parents is more suggestive of training than heredity and many other diseases in which there is a familial incidence are extremely complex problems even more so because with human beings moral issues are also involved. Epilepsy, for instance, seems commoner in the families of epileptic parents but it would be an overconfident physician who would recommend a man not to marry a woman whose aunt had suffered from epilepsy or even a man who had a history of epilepsy himself. In general there is a very small minority of cases where the question of heredity is so clearcut that those with the defect would be well-advised not to have children and most diseases do not come into this category (see Eugenics, Haemophilia, Sex).

Hermaphrodite: everybody is born either male or female since this trait is handed on with the sex chromosomes which rigidly determine sex at the moment of conception. But there are some children in whom, perhaps under glandular influences, it is difficult in early life to tell since the sexual organs show characteristics of both sexes. Adults do not change sex but there are some people who have a pathological urge to do so and alter their appearance, sometimes with the help of surgery and hormones, to that of the other sex – but this does not make them belong to it. Sex-change does not and cannot occur in human beings.

Hernia: the protrusion of any organ in whole or in part from the compartment containing it. The human body is composed of a number of distinct compartments, e.g. the head, neck, chest, abdomen, limbs, etc., through which the important blood-vessels and nerves must nevertheless pass and hernias ordinarily develop at these points of exit and entry especially when the relatively complex arrangements to allow this without interfering with the fairly rigid isolation of each compartment have failed to develop properly. Thus hernias are commonest at the groin where the large vessels pass from the abdomen into the thigh or in the region where the spermatic cord leaves the abdominal cavity; other areas sometimes affected are the umbilical region in the infant and sometimes the adult and the diaphragm where the oesphagus enters the abdomen. Less common are the bulgings which may occur almost anywhere when the muscles or bone are injured or grow weak, e.g. in a serious injury to the skull the brain may herniate or to the chest the lungs. However by far the most common type is hernia of the bowel the common name for which is 'rupture.' A fairly large number of infants are born with hernias in the groin, umbilicus, or diaphragm due to faults of development but most are acquired later in life at the same sites aided by weakness of the muscle, lack of exercise, overweight, sudden strains either at work or from persistent cough, straining at stool, and pregnancy. Some of these ruptures are small and all that escapes is the peritoneal lining of the abdominal cavity but others are large and permit a quite extensive protrusion of internal organs such as the large or small bowel. The protruding organ is covered by the peritoneal sac which is pushed forward with it and the skin. When this has happened there are various further possibilities: (1) it may be possible to 'reduce' the hernia, i.e. it can be easily pushed back into place although it comes out once more when the patient stands up unless he wears a truss; (2) it may become adherent to its new surroundings and therefore irreducible; (3) it may become obstructed when a portion of bowel within becomes blocked with faeces which are unable to move leading to the symptoms of intestinal obstruction; (4) it may be strangulated, the circulation of blood in the intestinal loop being blocked by the edge of the hernial opening and this creates an immediate emergency since the bowel will become gangrenous and the patient, if untreated, die in a few days. The danger of any kind of hernia, no matter how little it troubles the patient initially, is that it may become strangulated in this way, perhaps when surgical aid is not at hand. Since the inguinal canal is the site where the testicle in man passes out from the abdomen just before birth to its final position in the scrotum and the other predisposing factors of strain in lifting, etc., are more usual in men than women hernia is in general commoner in the male sex, although femoral hernia is more frequent in women than men. *Inguinal hernia* in the groin is the commonest type and most frequent in men for the reason already given; the inguinal canal is always more or less open being kept so by the presence of the spermatic cord along which the hernia may pass to the scrotum in some cases. The canal ends just above the pubic bone in the front and near the middle of the pelvis where a bulge will be seen on standing and, if the patient coughs, the vibration is transmitted to the swelling. Such a hernia may be direct or indirect, the former protruding more or less directly forward through a tear in the abdominal wall almost in the middle line, the latter following the course of the inguinal canal. *Femoral hernia*, commoner in women, is into the crural canal which is smaller in size and separated from the inguinal one by the inner end of the inguinal ligament (the line seen on the skin which separates the abdomen from the thigh). The space lies to the inner side of the femoral vessels passing from the abdomen to the thigh, and it is along these that the sac extends downwards.

A large proportion of the umbilical hernias in infants heal of their own accord before the second year, but when this does not happen an operation is required. The hernia of this type occurring after pregnancy in adult women should always be surgically dealt with. Incisional hernias on the site of an old operation scar may similarly need treatment and so may epigastric hernias in the upper abdomen where the rupture in the midline is thought to be due to a defect from birth in the abdominal wall. The least common ruptures are gluteal and lumbar ones at the back of the abdominal wall where a bulge is seen. Diaphragmatic hernias are more often diagnosed nowadays when X-rays are so frequently taken and occur when the stomach or intestine pushes through a weak area in the diaphragm into the chest. Sometimes the stomach may end up almost entirely in the chest cavity.

Unless there is some pressing reason to the contrary, all hernias should be surgically dealt with by replacing the organ which has herniated back where it belongs, removing the bulging sac of peritoneum, and repairing and reinforcing the torn or weakened muscle fibres. The only really valid

283

contraindication is when the patient is old or weak and the tissues so debilitated that a repair would be unlikely to succeed. Occasionally when previous attempts at repair have failed any further attempts may be advised against. But it must be remembered by those who wear trusses, however comfortable, (a) that any truss weakens the abdominal wall and therefore makes later surgical treatment less likely to succeed, and (b) that the longer an operable rupture is untreated the greater are the chances of strangulation. Finally, no hernias are hereditary, many hernias are congenital (i.e. present from birth), and only a few are *solely* caused by injury. More than 90% of operations lead to permanent cure and four out of five recurrent hernias can be cured by a second operation the few which are not being in people after the age of 60 or so who are also debilitated in some way. Return to work is in a month for those who are light workers and two months for heavy manual workers but the latter should avoid really heavy manual work for at least four months.

Heroin: or diamorphine hydrochloride is now rarely used in this country owing to its extreme tendency to cause addiction and the possibility of seriously depressing the respiratory centre especially in those with disease of the lungs. It is certainly the most potent inhibitor of cough known but newer drugs are taking its place.

Herpes: a virus infection affecting the nerves, in this case the sensory cells in the ganglia of the posterior roots of the spinal cord, i.e. the point where the nerves carrying sensations pass into the cord just behind that at which the motor fibres pass out. Thus herpes or 'shingles' is to the sensory nerves what poliomyelitis is to the motor ones although with consequences to the individual which if unpleasant are much less severe. The virus is either related to, or identical with, that of chickenpox and it is not uncommon for an adult in a house where a child is suffering from chickenpox to develop shingles. Like poliomyelitis, the disease is localised attacking only one, two, or occasionally three roots and nearly always on one side of the body. Coming in at the throat, the virus is carried in the blood to the posterior root ganglia and the patient begins to complain of severe pain in the area supplied with no other symptoms until the infection travelling down the nerve fibres reaches the skin where a series of blisters appears often showing very clearly the belt-like distribution of the affected nerve. At this time the virus can be obtained from the fluid within the blisters. Shingles or herpes zoster is entirely different from herpes simplex or 'cold sore,' the blisters which sometimes appear at points where the skin and mucous membrane meet, e.g. the lips, the edge of the nostrils, or the conjunctiva of the eye, usually after another mild infection such as a bad cold although herpes simplex of the lips was once almost invariable in lobar pneumonia, now fortunately a rare disease. Shingles unlike 'cold sore' very rarely occurs more than once and a single attack, like chickenpox, confers permanent immunity; it clears up in one or two weeks when the blisters form scabs which dry up and fall off, but sometimes in older people the itching may persist for many months. There is no specific treatment for either type of herpes and all that need be done is to relieve the discomfort caused by the rash, e.g. by painting with collodion (New Skin), or the use of hydrocortisone or other antipruritic ointments if recommended by the physician.

Hesperidin: is contained in vitamin P obtained from lemon juice and Hungarian red peppers. It is believed to control the permeability of the capillaries and is therefore given in diseases where there is increased capillary fragility, e.g. purpura, or haemorrhages into the eye.

Hexamethonium: proprietary names Vegolysen and Vegolysen T (H. tartrate) is one of the methonium compounds or quaternary ammonium substances which act by producing a block in the ganglia of the autonomic nervous system thus causing a lowering of blood-pressure which is used in the treatment of cases of hypertension (*see* Hypertension, Methonium).

Hexamine: (Urotropine, Methanamine, Metramine) is made by the action of ammonia on formalin and in acid fluids liberates formaldehyde as an antiseptic. Hence it is used in urinary infections such as pyelitis and cystitis – inflammations of the pelvis of the kidney and the bladder – in which case the urine must be kept acid by giving simultaneously but separately acid phosphate of sodium; in cholecystitis for which it is also sometimes used, the urine must be kept alkaline during treatment.

Hexobarbitone: a drug given in tablet form (Cyclonal) to induce sleep or as a mild hypnotic when sleep has been

285

interrupted; Evipan tablets are similarly used. Cyclobarbitone sodium is used as an intravenous anaesthetic to make the patient unconscious for surgical operation. Hexobarbitone is the British Pharmacopoeia name for N-methyl-cyclohexenyl-methybarbituric acid, being one of the barbiturates (q.v.).

Hexoestrol: a synthetic ovarian hormone related to stilboestrol and with the same actions although less potent and less likely to lead to nausea. Its chemical name is dihydrostilboestrol (*see* Stilboestrol).

Hexylresorcinol: a drug, usually given in capsules, for the treatment of roundworms and threadworms. Proprietary names: Caprokol, Crystoids, Sucrets, and S.T.37.

Hiatus Hernia: diaphragmatic hernia in which the stomach passes into the chest, either partially or almost completely by way of the opening ordinarily occupied by the oesophagus or gullet (*see* Hernia).

Hiccup: a spasmodic indrawing of air into the chest ending in a click due to the sudden closure of the vocal chords. It is caused by irritation of the nerves supplying the diaphragm usually from indigestion but occasionally occurring towards the end of fatal diseases, e.g. uraemia, typhoid fever. There are many 'cures' amongst which are the drinking of large amounts of cold water, holding the breath, drinking peppermint water or spirits, alkalies, and, perhaps the most effective, inhaling carbon dioxide. The latter can be done by breathing in and out of a paper bag held over the nose and mouth. When hiccup lasts any length of time a doctor should be consulted.

Hip-joint: a ball and socket joint formed by the ball-shaped end of the femur or thigh-bone and the acetabulum or cup-shaped hollow in the side of the pelvis. Because of its capsule of fibrous tissue and the strong ligaments surrounding it, dislocation is not very common except in congenital dislocation of the hip in infants which may be on both sides and is easily recognised by delay in walking, dipping gait, and shortening of the leg. This should be treated as soon as possible (*see* Joints, Fractures).

Hippus: rhythmic contractions of the pupil at a regular rate which is found in certain functional nervous diseases, e.g. allegedly in hysteria.

Hirschsprung's Disease: or megacolon is a disease of children in which the colon is much dilated from birth owing to the absence of certain nerve fibres which are necessary in order to permit the area where the bowel joins the rectum to relax normally. Hence there is spasm which may persist throughout life. The most obvious symptom is prolonged constipation and the bowels may not open for 1–2 weeks or more but this may alternate with attacks of diarrhoea and swelling of the abdomen with gas which is easily seen on observation. Occasionally the distension is so great as to cause breathlessness from pressure on the diaphragm and swelling (oedema) of the genital area and legs through interference with the circulation. Treatment is directed at the spasm of the pelvirectal sphincter (band of muscle at the beginning of the rectum) which is removed completely, the two cut ends being joined together. This procedure is followed by complete cure in more than 90% of cases. Formerly the operation of sympathectomy was applied to the lumbar ganglia which bring about spasm or similar results were obtained by repeated spinal anaesthesia but this, on the whole, being replaced by the operation described except in minor cases which can be dealt with by suitable drugs and dieting. Megacolon is found more often in boys than girls.

Hirsuties: or hypertrichosis is the growth of superfluous hair in women with distribution of the male type both on the face and body. It is sometimes associated with disorders of the suprarenal glands above the kidneys (*see* Superfluous Hair, Suprarenal Glands).

Histamine: a substance found normally in the body and obtainable by the action of certain bacteria on the aminoacid histidine; it is normally destroyed by the enzyme histaminase. When injected it stimulates the secretion of gastric juice but in sufficient amounts leads to the condition of surgical shock with dilation of the capillaries and a fall in bloodpressure. In surgical shock following accidents and injuries the symptoms are produced by the liberation of histamine from the body cells in which it is ordinarily locked up and similar results are produced in the allergic diseases (q.v.) which are manifestations of histamine poisoning (or poisoning by a histamine-like substance) similarly released. The anti-histamine drugs (q.v.) are employed to combat these effects. Anaphylactic shock is also caused by histamine (*see* Anaphylaxis).

Histology: the study of the microscopic structure of tissues.

Histoplasmosis: a disease occuring mainly in the United States caused by the fungus known as histoplasma capsulatum and characterised in infants by fever and enlargement of the liver and spleen with anaemia. The lungs, stomach, and intestines are also affected and in older children the disease may resemble tuberculosis of the lungs. In adults it tends to be limited to the skin.

Hives: a popular name for nettle-rash (q.v.) or urticaria.

Hodgkin's Disease: or lymphadenoma is a form of anaemia associated with swelling of the lymph glands throughout the body, enlargement of the spleen, and the absence of any increase in the number of white cells in the blood. Its cause is not known but it has been suggested (*a*) that it is caused by a specific infection and (*b*) that it is basically a cancerous condition. Few authorities now believe in the former theory and in most respects lympadenoma behaves like a cancer. The disease usually starts in the glands on one side of the neck where it is often discovered accidentally but less frequently it may begin in the abdomen or at the root of the lungs; in any case, except in the uncommon acute type, it remains practically symptomless for a considerable time and it may be a year or even more before recurrent attacks of fever and increasing anaemia make their appearance. The lumps in the neck and the swelling of the spleen will then be discovered by the doctor on examination and a gland may have to be removed for miscroscopic examination to confirm the diagnosis. In cases of Hodgkin's disease it will be found to contain fibrous tissue and the typical giant cells. No treatment has yet been discovered to cure this disease which is invariably fatal, but the use of deep X-ray therapy initially causes the enlarged glands to melt away as if by magic, although in spite of treatment they always return and necessitate further therapy. Nitrogen mustard or tetramine may also be used and this acts as a direct cell poison causing the glands to disappear often after a single treatment but, as with X-ray therapy, they inevitably recur and the result is only palliative.

Homatropine: an alkaloid (q.v.) derived from atropine or belladonna used to dilate the pupil before examining the interior of the eye. The effect of the 1% solution passes off

in a few hours but may cause blurring of vision from paralysis of accommodation whilst it lasts.

Homoeopathy: a system of medicine founded by S. C. F.
Hahnemann (1755–1843) at the end of the 18th century. Born
at Meissen in Saxony he studied medicine at Leipzig and
Vienna, finally graduating at Erlangen and settling down as
a physician in Leipzig. Dissatisfied (quite justifiably) with
the state of medicine at that time Hahnemann put forward
in 1796 his new principle of 'the law of similars' to the effect
that diseases should be treated by drugs which produce symptoms similar to them in healthy people (similia similibus
curantur.) This concept, if not of universal application, was
considerably in advance of contemporary medicine since it is
true that many symptoms can be regarded as resulting from
the body's attempt to throw off the disease, e.g. diarrhoea is
clearly an attempt to get rid of irritant matter or disease-
causing germs and prior to the discovery of antibiotics and
sulpha drugs it was more appropriate in many cases to give a
purgative such as castor oil to aid the process rather than
opium to slow it down. But this does not apply to all symptoms and even when it does, diarrhoea, for example, may be
so severe that its original function is lost in the harm it is
doing to the patient by loss of fluids and damage to the intestine; in such cases it must be stopped regardless of the
lesser harm done by the temporary retention of poisonous or
irritant products. Four years later Hahnemann produced his
other principle, that drugs should be given in almost in-
finitesimal doses and, with all respect due to a great man,
this has been accepted by no one save homoeopathists even
when based on the pseudo-scientific theory of dynamisation,
or increase of force with diminution of matter, such dynamisation being allegedly produced by trituration or grinding
to a fine powder and extreme dilution. Although many
eminent physicians have given their approval to homoeopathy
it is remarkable that this theory which could be quite easily
put to the test in animal experiments has never in fact been
so tested and one can only conclude that its practitioners are
aware of the fallacies involved. Tests on the human being are
rarely valid if we are to reply solely upon subjective feelings
of improvement since it is entirely obvious that these are
more likely to depend upon faith and suggestibility than

289

objective results; for, as pointed out elsewhere, the fact that 90% of patients feel better after a certain line of treatment tells us nothing whatever except that that is how 90% of patients felt. How they objectively *are* is quite another matter. Hahnemann's system caused great antagonism and he had to leave Leipzig finally ending up in Paris where he ran a successful practice based on these principles (which, as already admitted, were infinitely superior to the bulk of orthodox medicine at that time). Homoeopathy is practiced by a decreasing number of orthodox physicians and there are a number of excellent homoeopathic hospitals in England which, so far as one is aware, pay comparatively little attention to its original principles and certainly do not use the new specific drugs such as sulphonamides and antibiotics in diluted doses. In contrast with homoeopathy orthodox medicine is described as allopathy or heteropathy, meaning that it treats diseases by giving remedies which produce opposite results from the symptoms. This, however, is a misnomer because modern medicine is based on scientific research unsupported by any one overall theory and the trouble with homoeopathy is precisely that it is a system and nature cannot be confined by any such rigid schemes. It may be taken almost as an axiom that any system which begins with the assumptions: '*every* disease is caused by . . .' or '*every* disease can be cured by . . .' as do osteopathy, Christian Science, homoeopathy, and the rest is bound to be wrong. *Some* diseases, yes, *all* diseases, no.

Homosexuality: (*see* Sex).

Hook-worm: the ankylostoma or uncinaria causing ankylostomiasis (*see* Infection, Ankylostoma).

Hordeolum: a stye in the eye (*see* Blepharitis).

Horehound: a group of perennial herbs found throughout Europe but not very common in Britain where the white or common horehound is infrequently found and black horehound only south of the Forth and Clyde. The dried leaves of the former (Marrubium vulgare) are used for coughs either mixed with sugar or in a fluid extract (1–2 teaspoonfuls) although more often nowadays by herbalists than physicians.

Hormones: or autacoids are substances which, secreted by the ductless or endocrine glands, influence tissues and organs in other parts of the body. Examples are oestrin, thyroxin, insulin, cortisone, etc. (*see* Endocrine Glands and the various glands separately described).

Horner's Syndrome: a group of symptoms resulting from paralysis of the sympathetic nerves in the neck. These are: small pupil, sunken eye, and drooping of the upper eyelid.

Hospital: a place for the reception and treatment of the sick. The word, derived from the Latin hospitalis, and meaning pertaining to a host or guest has also given rise to the words hotel and hostel which now have a different significance. There were hospitals of a sort attached to the temples of ancient Egypt from about 4000 B.C. where patients slept in the hope that the gods would cure them but the temple of Aesculapius at Cos associated with the name of Hippocrates 'the father of medicine' who died about 370 B.C., although originally based on the same principles, became much more sophisticated as under his influence diseases came to be better understood. In the East the Indian emperor Asoka founded a hospital at Surat and the famous sultan Haroun-al-Rachid who died in A.D. 809 built numerous hospitals in Baghdad. Constantinople under the Byzantine empire had the Pantoorator which was far in advance of anything in medieval Europe with specialists in various branches of medicine, women doctors for childbirth, a pharmacy and an almoner's department, disinfection of the patients' clothes on admission and issue of clean clothing and bedding whilst under treatment, and so on. But until the 18th century there was comparatively little provision for the institutional treatment of the sick in Britain where, by 1710, the only general hospitals in London were St Thomas's and St Bartholomew's. But subsequently the number of hospitals slowly increased and during the 19th century numerous dispensaries, some of them founded by religious bodies, were set up to provide some form of out-patient treatment. The important events which made hospitals as we now know them possible were (*a*) the discovery of anaesthetics (q.v.) which put an end to the bloody, agonising, and necessarily brief surgical operations carried out only as a last resort and opened the way to modern surgery; (*b*) Lister's introduction of the antiseptic technique in surgery (1865) which reduced the dangers of sepsis; (*c*) the improvements in the standard of nursing

291

carried out by Florence Nightingale as the result of her experiences during the Crimean war and later introduced by her to St Thomas's nursing school.

Before the introduction of the National Health Service Act in 1948 there were four chief classes of hospital in Britain according to their type of administration: (1) the Voluntary Hospitals supported by public subscription and administered by a board of managers chosen by the subscribers. Originally introduced into Europe from the East in the early 13th century with the support of Pope Innocent III and Louis IX of France, such hospitals were supported by the rich for the benefit of the poor as a form of charity but later the greater part of their revenue came from those who had been, or were likely to be, treated there. In the latter period subscriptions, often collected in the form of a small donation from the weekly wage, had become a sort of insurance against illness or accident of the wage-earner; (2) Council Hospitals supported by the local town and county councils and administered by their local health authority under the supervision of the Ministry of Health were primarily for the treatment of infectious diseases but after 1929 there were also municipal hospitals for the treatment of general medical and surgical complaints. With whole-time resident medical and surgical officers and salaried consultants these were supported by the rates and by recovering the cost of treatment from patients in proportion to what they could afford to pay; (3) State Hospitals run by the Military, Naval, Prison and Pension authorities and run by a staff of officers from the service to which they belonged, were relatively few in number and supported out of Parliamentary grants, whilst (4) *Private Hospitals* were owned and run by private individuals or companies for profit; the smaller ones with ten or twenty patients are known as 'nursing homes.' Of course, hospitals are also classified according to the type of cases with which they deal, as general hospitals taking all types of case (large with 100–1000 beds, intermediate with 50–100 beds, and cottage hospitals with fewer than 50); special hospitals reserved for one type of case as children, maternity cases, cripples, mental patients, eye, or ear, nose and throat patients; teaching hospitals attached to a medical school; and convalescent hospitals. Others were reserved for foreigners, e.g. the German and

French hospitals in London, for cults, e.g. Masonic hospitals and religious bodies, e.g. Jews.

Under the National Health Service Act all hospitals with the exception of teaching hospitals (which have been given a large measure of independence and allowed to keep their own Board of Governors and control their own endowments) and nursing homes passed to the control of Regional Boards appointed by the Minister of Health. The Regional Boards divided the hospitals in their areas into units under the control of Hospital Management Committees. The endowments of the Voluntary hospitals were transferred to a Hospital Endowments Fund to be used for purposes outside the official budget and they were no longer allowed to appeal for funds. All treatment is free or rather paid out of the patients' National Health contributions, but there are blocks of private wards for those who wish to pay for privacy and additional comforts.

Hour-Glass Stomach: the appearance seen in an X-ray of a stomach which is constricted in the middle either as a result of spasm or, more commonly, from the scar-tissue of an old gastric ulcer.

Housemaid's Knee: or pre-patellar bursitis is a swelling of the bursa in front of the knee-cap due, as the name suggests, to excessive pressure from kneeling (*see* Bursae).

Humerus: the single bone of the upper arm, fitting into the ball and socket of the shoulder joint at the upper end and articulating with the radius and ulna of the forearm at the lower.

Humour: a term now only used for the aqueous and vitreous humours of the eyeball, but formerly associated with a theory of the nature of disease originating with the Pythagorean philosophers in the 6th century B.C. but accepted by Hippocrates (400 B.C.) Aristotle (300 B.C.), Galen (A.D. 200), and most other physicians in one form or another up to the end of the 18th century. This ascribed temperaments and diseases to excess or defiency of humours classified as, sanguine (full-blooded), phlegmatic (dull-watery), choleric (fiery, due to yellow bile), and melancholy (depressed, due to black bile). Although as a theory of disease this view is long outdated, the modern analyst and psychologist Erich Fromm uses the terms to classify the various inherited temperaments; for clearly there is some ground for supposing the types of optimist and pessimist, the quick to anger and slow to be moved, to be basic psychological categories of personality.

Huntington's Chorea: an hereditary disease transmitted by both sexes, occurring between the ages of thirty and forty, and characterised by the type of involuntary movements seen in chorea (q.v.) and progressive mental deterioration. Finally the movements become very severe and the patient completely paralysed and demented. The condition is slowly progressive and there is no treatment. Institutional care is usually necessary in the later stages.

Hutchinson's Teeth: the narrowed and notched incisor teeth typical of congenital syphilis and named after the physician Sir Jonathan Hutchinson (d. 1913) of London who first described them.

Hyaluronidase: an enzyme which breaks up hyaluronic acid, the substance which helps to bind the tissue cells together. Because of this property hyaluronidase is able to facilitate the subcutaneous injection of fluids and drugs and, by separating the cells of a tissue, to increase the area of effective local anaesthesia. Proprietary names are Hyalase and Rondase.

Hydatid Cyst: the cyst produced by the immature form of the tapeworm (*see* Worms).

Hydatidiform Mole: a disease of the superficial layer of the chorion, the outer of the two membranes covering the foetus, which becomes overgrown during the first weeks of pregnancy and so increases in size as to grossly enlarge the womb and usually kill the foetus. It is not particularly common and sometimes becomes malignant resulting in a chorionepithelioma. The symptoms are, enlargement of the womb quite out of proportion to the period of pregnancy, pain in the back and loins, and vomiting. The only treatment is to empty the womb usually through the vagina but if the growth is very large sometimes through an opening in the abdomen. Because of the risk of cancer the patient should be kept under observation for a year.

Hydnocarpus Oil: is obtained by crushing the seeds of Hydnocarpus Wightiana and given by subcutaneous or intramuscular injection in the treatment of leprosy. Its action is similar to that of chaulmoogra oil which it is to some extent superseding.

294

Hydrallazine: or Apresoline is used in the treatment of hypertension especially when it persists after the operation of sympathectomy.

Hydrargyrum: mercury.

Hydrocele: a common condition of men in which there is a sac of water fluid surrounding the testicle on one or both sides of the scrotum; it appears at any age without known cause. Hydrocele is more of a nuisance than a serious disease but since it may be of any size from that of a lemon to that of a large melon its painlessness is small consolation for the inconvenience it causes. Treatment of small hydroceles may be by injection of some sclerosing fluid which causes the formation of scar tissue and obliterates the sac but this may have to be repeated and recurrences are quite frequent so operation to remove the whole sac is usually recommended although a few patients prefer to report periodically to have the fluid withdrawn through a needle. The operation is simple and recurrences are rare after surgery.

Hydrocephalus: a condition in which there is an excess of cerebrospinal fluid within the skull which usually leads to abnormal enlargement of the head. It may be congenital from unknown causes or acquired as a sequel to meningitis or a brain tumour which by interference with the circulation of the fluid or its absorption produce the symptoms. An operation may be performed either with the purpose of reducing the formation of fluid or shunting it through a communication between the distended ventricles within the brain and the subarachnoid space without, but although good temporary results have been obtained these are rarely permanent and the more recent methods have not been in use sufficiently long for their effectiveness to be evaluated. Apart from the obvious enlargement of the skull above the eyebrows the symptoms are due to pressure on the brain and include headache, irritability, interference with vision and hearing, and imbecility in the final stages.

Hydrochloric Acid: a gas which dissolved in water forms a strong corrosive acid. In the gastric juice hydrochloric acid is present in a much diluted form (c. 2/1000 parts) and in excess leads to the hyperchlorhydria often associated with peptic ulcer. Its absence is known as achlorhydria and, although this may be symptomless, in other cases it can cause dyspepsia just as readily as excess acid. In such conditions hydrochloric acid is often administered in doses of half to one teaspoonful of the dilute 10% solution or as recommended by the doctor (*see* Achlorhydria, Hyperchlorhydria, Hypochlorhydria).

Hydrochlorothiazide: a new and very potent non-mercurial diuretic (q.v.) used to increase the loss of fluids from the body in congestive heart failure and oedema associated with kidney or liver disease. It is also useful in bringing about an initial loss of weight (fluid loss) in obesity and in the treatment of premenstrual tension which is also characterised by fluid retention. There are numerous proprietary brands, e.g. Hydrosaluric.

Hydrocortisone: the addition of a single hydrogen molecule to cortisone (q.v.) strongly influences its properties, notably by enhancing its anti-rheumatic powers and its local action on the skin, etc. Like cortisone it is mainly employed for its ability to reduce inflammation, e.g. in skin diseases, eye conditions, hay-fever, itching of all sorts, arthritic conditions, allergies, and the rest. Preparations may be in the form of drops, lotions, sprays, ointments and creams, tablets, or for injection into joints and go under various proprietary names as well as the official one, e.g. Hydro-Adreson, Hydrocortisyl, Hydrocortone, Hydrodeltalone, Hydroderm, Hydrodyne, Hydroptic, Hydrospray, etc. In many of these the drug is combined with antibiotics or with aspirin (for use in rheumatic conditions).

Hydrocyanic Acid: is prussic acid (*see* Cyanides).

Hydrogen Peroxide: being decomposed into water and oxygen when brought into contact with the tissues, especially in the presence of dead cells and pus, hydrogen peroxide exercises its effect as an antiseptic by virtue of its feed oxygen. It is mild, safe, ordinarily non-irritant, and is most useful in removing dressings that 'stick,' in disinfecting small amounts of drinking water, in cleansing suppurating wounds where the bubbles formed help to remove discharge and destroy anaerobic organisms, as a mouthwash and in the treatment of inflammations of the gums, in removing wax from the ears, and in stopping bleeding from capillary oozing.

Hydrolyzed Protein: protein which has been pre-digested into its constituent amino-acids by hydrolysis, i.e. by breaking down with water. It may be used as a readily absorbed form of protein in liver and other diseases although it is questionable whether this type of product is often necessary.

Hydronephrosis: a disease in which there is distension and destruction of the kidney at the pelvis where the ureter leaves the organ and within the kidney tissue itself; it is brought about by partial or intermittent blockage of the ureter whether from a stone, a stricture, or a growth. Total obstruction is more likely to lead to atrophy of the kidney. The symptoms are constant or intermittent pain in the loins generally on the right side, nausea and vomiting, and scanty passing of urine with periodic passage of large amounts followed by relief of the pain. A swelling may be seen in the loin of the patient who is most often a woman and X-rays following the injection of radio-opaque fluid up the ureter from the bladder demonstrate the blockage. Occasionally hydronephrosis may be caused by an abnormal branch of the renal artery pressing on the ureter or kinking of the ureter when the pain, resembling renal colic, is known as a Dietl's crisis. The usual treatment for hydronephrosis is removal of the affected kidney (nephrectomy) but in some cases where the damage is not too great and the cause of obstruction can be moved this may be adequate.

Hydropathy: the use of water in treatment whether externally or internally, once extremely popular and carried out at a hydropathic. Although nobody would deny that baths and the rest are both useful and pleasant, few today would be prepared to accord hydropathy the grandiose position it once held. Like many forms of physiotherapy it is most successful in the treatment of conditions which are vague, ill-defined, neurotic, degenerative and hence not responsive to other forms of treatment, or simply non-existent. Natural waters taken internally are purgative or diuretic and more conveniently bought in a tin.

Hydrophobia: (*see* Rabies).

Hydrotherapy: (*see* Hydropathy).

Hyoid Bone: a small U-shaped bone at the base of the tongue which in the front of the neck can be felt about an inch above the Adam's apple or thyroid cartilage. It is usually broken during strangulation and this fact is a valuable sign in a body where most of the tissues have disintegrated that there has been foul play.

Hyoscyamus: a drug prepared from the common henbane which has a potent effect in relieving pain caused by muscular spasm of the involuntary muscles, e.g. in the bladder and ureter or urethra. It may be used as the tincture or in the form of the alkaloid hyoscine obtained from it. In addition to its atropine-like properties in relieving spasm hyoscine is a cerebral depressant used in states of mental excitement such as mania, delirium tremens, or the delirium of fever. It is given in paralysis agitans, in 'twilight sleep,' and combined with morphia prior to surgical operations. Hyoscine is also known as scopolamine and like hyoscyamus can be used to dilate the pupils, to prevent sea-sickness, and is combined with strong purgatives to prevent colic and griping. It has also been given for the latter action in the treatment of duodenal ulcer where it has the additional effect of reducing the secretion of hydrochloric acid.

Hyperacusis: an abnormally acute sense of hearing.

Hyperaemia: the congestion of a part with blood.

Hyperaesthesia: increased sensitivity to sensations as found in certain organic nervous diseases.

Hyperchlorhydria: excess hydrochloric acid in the stomach (*see* Stomach Diseases).

Hyperemesis: excessive vomiting especially the vomiting of pregnancy or hyperemesis gravidarum. This is commonest with the first child and begins usually before the fourth month from one or other of three causes: reflex when there is stimulation from a displaced or too rapidly enlarging womb, toxic when it is an early sign of the toxaemia of pregnancy, and psychological which is much the commonest type. With modern drugs the vast majority of cases can be easily controlled, e.g. Dramamine, Largactil, Stelazine, Sparine, etc.

Hyperglycaemia: excess sugar in the blood as in diabetes (q.v.).

Hyperhidrosis: (Hyperidrosis) excessive sweating (see Perspiration).

Hypermetropia: long-sightedness (*see* Spectacles).

Hypernephroma: the commonest type of malignant tumour in the kidney amongst adults; it consists of tissue similar to that in the cortex of the suprarenal gland but is not derived therefrom.

Hyperpiesis: or hyperpiesia is another word for high blood-pressure or hypertension (q.v.).

Hyperplasia: an abnormal increase in the number of cells in a tissue.

Hyperpyrexia: the raised temperature of fever (q.v.).

Hypertension: high blood-pressure is associated with a number of diseases, e.g. nephritis (q.v.) and other kidney conditions, some disorders of the ductless glands especially the pituitary and suprarenals or to a lesser degree with ovarian disorders at the menopause, hardening of the arteries or arteriosclerosis (*see* Arteries), polycythaemia (q.v.), the toxaemias of pregnancy, and uraemia which is the final stage of kidney disease. But in primary or essential hypertension, by far the commonest type, no such cause has been found although the disease seems to begin with spasm of the smaller arteries which finally necessitates a raised blood-pressure if the blood is to reach the tissues in adequate amounts. The narrowing of the arterioles leads to fibrosis of the tissues which is specially marked in the kidneys and as their tissue is increasingly destroyed the pressure must become ever higher to keep them going. Death may occur in the fifties and sixties age-group from a stroke, heart-failure, or uraemia, but many sufferers live to a ripe old age. The process seems to be connected with the endocrine pattern in general and the suprarenal glands in particular and often seems to run in families, but from the psychological point of view essential hypertension appears to be related to suppressed emotions of anxiety or resentment, the patient often being a man who is over-controlled and basically afraid to let his feelings of anger or frustration rise to the surface. Since emotions and the autonomic nervous system together with the ductless glands are intimately associated so that it might be said that the former are the subjective aspect of the latter, it need occasion no surprise to find that many authorities regard essential hypertension as fundamentally a psychosomatic (q.v.) disorder. In normal stress the blood-pressure rises but in essential hypertension the emotion persists in a latent form and keeps the pressure permanently raised until actual structural changes develop. This is partly speculation but there can be no doubt (*a*) that release of such emotions is followed by lowering of the blood-pressure in the early stages, and (*b*) that, on the physical side, the suprarenal glands, which are associated with the emotions of rage and fear, play a

299

major part in causing the spasm. It is noteworthy that one function of these glands is the production of secondary sexual characters in the male, i.e. masculinisation of the body, and women are much less prone to develop serious degrees of high blood-pressure than men. There are few characteristic symptoms of essential hypertension and the condition is very often found by accident on routine examination, but at a later stage, when symptoms do arise the most frequent are headache (although only a small proportion of all headaches are related to high blood-pressure), giddiness, and noises in the ears (both of these are also common neurotic symptoms). There are few diseases where it is more necessary for the specialist to treat the patient as an individual; for once it is realised that the blood-pressure rises in response to a need to push the blood through narrowed arterioles and that without this blood the organs will become fibrosed it becomes clear that, although there are many ways of lowering the blood-pressure, it is by no means automatically advisable to do so. From what has been said, it is evident that theoretically four ways of treating the condition are possible: (1) psychotherapy directed towards removing the emotional difficulties; (2) dampening down the response of the lower centres of the brain to external stimuli causing anxiety or anger; (3) interrupting the nerves which transmit such impulses to the walls of the arteries; (4) suppressing the secretion of the substance from the kidneys known as renin which raises the pressure. Psychotherapy as a sole method of treatment is unlikely to be helpful and, of course, is not helpful at all when organic changes in the tissues have already taken place; but in all cases the patient's emotional problems and attitude to his disease should be taken into account. Frankness on the part of the doctor is all very well, but nobody who has seen the kind of neurotic sufferer who demands to know his actual blood-pressure and to have frequent readings taken which, perhaps, he carefully copies down in a notebook as if his life were dependent upon every two points or so as it moves up or down, can suppose that it is a good thing to encourage such behaviour. At the best such information conveys very little to the patient and at the worst a rise of a few points which is quite insignificant medically may cause anxiety which raises the pressure even higher. It is true that a systolic pressure which is persistently above 150 mm. of mercury and a diastolic pressure (i.e. the pressure at the point when the heart is relaxing between beats) persistently about 95 mm. is often significant, but it must be taken in conjunction with other factors such as the question as to whether it is really persistent or only high from the anxiety of the examination, the patient's general health in other respects, the level of the diastolic pressure which is, on the whole, the more important as indicating how far the circulatory system is able to relax, and such other matters as personality, weight, age, and employment. Medically, sedatives of the tranquillizer groups are often helpful and specific drugs for lowering the pressure, e.g. hydrallazine, rauwolfia, veratrum, and methonium compounds, are generally used, the choice of drug depending upon the patient's condition. They must never be used indiscriminately since the mere lowering of blood-pressure cannot be taken as an aim in itself. The operation of sympathectomy is sometimes carried out in selected cases and this involves cutting the sympathetic nerve fibres to the abdominal organs to relax the spasm and lower the pressure, but in many cases the pressure returns in a short time to its original figure. Diet is a less significant part of treatment than formerly although the weight must be brought down to the correct figure and salt may be prohibited but this is a matter for the patient's own physician to decide. Meat in the diet has no bearing whatever on the problem of hypertension.

Hyperthermia: the treatment of certain diseases by the artificial induction of fever. This can be done (a) by the intravenous injection of dead bacteria, e.g. T.A.B. vaccine, (b) by the introduction of live parasites into the blood to produce malaria which is terminated when desired by anti-malarial drugs, (c) by the use of an apparatus known as a hypertherm which takes the form either of a Turkish-bath cabinet containing electric light bulbs or a more elaborate machine resembling a radio transmitter in which the body acts as the aerial, (d) formerly by the creation of bacteria-free abscesses when sterile protein or irritant substances were injected. By these means a temperature of 105–6 degrees may be safely induced which is used in the treatment of general paralysis of the insane (G.P.I.), a form of syphilis of the brain, in certain types of arthritis, in some degenerative nervous diseases (e.g. disseminated sclerosis), and prior to more modern methods in such psychoses as schizophrenia. The method is still important in the treatment of G.P.I., but otherwise little used.

Hyperthyroidism: over-action of the thyroid gland as in exophthalmic goitre (*see* Goitre).

Hypertrophy: increase in size of an organ usually as the result of compensation to make up for increased work or stress imposed upon it, e.g. the enlarged heart of athletes, the thickened arteries of high blood-pressure, the enlargement of one kidney when the other has been removed.

Hypno-Analysis: the use of hypnosis (q.v.) or drugs such as pentothal (thiopentone sodium) to abbreviate the process of analysis in psychological illnesses. Such methods are sometimes used (*a*) to allow the patient to get rid of repressed emotions by abreaction as in the war neurosis, or (*b*) to give positive suggestions of health, but hypnoanalysis properly speaking refers solely to *analysis* carried out in these circumstances, i.e. the recovery of repressed material and its neutralising by explanation and understanding rather than by suggestion or the mere release of emotion.

Hypnotics: drugs which indue sleep (*see* Insomnia).

Hypnosis, Hypnotism: a state of artificially-induced trance which causes the individual to be more open to suggestion. It has also been termed mesmerism, animal magnetism, odylic force, and induced somnambulism. Induced trances of one sort or another have been part of the stock-in-trade of the medicine man, witch-doctor, religious devotee, the reputable and not so reputable physician, and many other would-be influencers of mankind from the dawn of human history. Indeed, it is difficult to say where suggestion begins and rational attempts to convince end, e.g. what the politician says by way of logical argument is not independent of his personality nor is the physician's bed-side manner irrelevant to the effectiveness of the remedy he prescribes as many clinical tests have shown. But for practical purposes hypnosis is a deliberately-induced trance in which there is an emotional rapport between the operator and his subject such that he is enabled to produce the desired results with greater facility than otherwise and demonstrate certain phenomena characteristic of the hypnotic state, e.g. anaesthesia of parts of the body, the recovery of forgotten memories, etc. This definition is admittedly inadequate, for it must be remembered that some animals can be hypnotised (and in this case emotional rapport is presumably absent, the main feature being inhibition of some fields of behaviour); that there are various degrees of hypnosis in the sense of increased suggestibility without the production of trance and in this respect the vast majority of people can be hypnotised (hence the fallacy of discussions around this point although only a minority of individuals can be deeply hypnotisd to such a level that complete anaesthesia of a limb or other part is capable of being induced). It should be unnecessary to add that there is nothing whatever mysterious about hypnosis which in its simplest form is simply the inhibition or 'putting to sleep' by monotonous stimuli of a part of the brain much as a clock, no matter how noisy, ceases to be heard after a few minutes in the same room, added to a maintenance of contact by the hypnotist with the uninhibited part. Anybody can induce hypnosis when shown how to do so and although many highly intelligent people use the method, undue confidence, a god-like feeling of superiority, and a measure of stupidity, are undoubtedly a help. Hypnotism has always been at the mercy of the charlatan and humbug and historically its first significant appearance in European society dates from the sensational work of Anton Mesmer who from 1774 onwards was the rage first of Vienna and then of Paris. Mesmer believed in a physical 'animal magnetism' but the physicians who made hypnosis respectable were Braid of Manchester who suggested that hypnosis was merely a form of sleep which could be produced by gazing at a bright light, Professor Elliotson of University College, London, and Esdaile, an army surgeon in India who was able to perform many surgical operations under hypnosis prior to the advent of chloroform. Nobody can be hypnotised against his will and allegedly bad effects produced by music-hall performers on the stage or over the radio are an unconscious self-deception by hysterics looking for some excuse on which to hang their symptoms. Amongst the results brought about by deep hypnosis or hysteria (which for the present purpose can be regarded as a state of self-hypnosis) are: anaesthesia of a part which, however, does not correspond to the anatomical distribution of its nerves; the apparent symptoms of organic illnesses which similarly do not bear expert examination; the recall of long-forgotten events and even their enacting; apparent double personality; the disappearance of symptoms, at least temporarily, hypersensitivity of the senses which may enable the subject to appear capable of telepathy; and less frequently physical phenomena such as bleeding, stigmata, and other pseudo-religious or mystical states.

In medicine hypnosis is used in inducing anaesthesia, e.g. in childbirth, in hypnoanalysis (q.v.) where information about the causation of symptoms may be obtained and used for cure, and occasionally for positive suggestions of health. The latter process is poorly regarded by psychiatrists in general since, on the reasonable assumption that every symptom has a cause, its mere removal without dealing with this cause is likely to lead to nothing more dramatic than another symptom taking its place. Drawbacks to hypnosis are: its unreliability, since not everyone can be deeply hypnotised, its tendency to produce an emotional attachment (transference) between operators and subject which is precisely what most doctors want to avoid lest it should get out of control, and the suggestion (not entirely justified) of hocus-pocus and mystery which is likely to exist in the mind of the subject if not of the operator. Basically any method which is not uniformly reliable is unsatisfactory to the physician and there is no uniformity about the results of hypnosis even if its results are often impressive. The Society of Medical Hypnotists in London is the official body for medical hypnotists in Britain.

Hypocalcaemia: a level of calcium in the blood below the normal 9–11 mg. per 100 c.c.s. Its symptoms are overexcitability of the nervous system as in tetany (q.v.) and inadequate production of hard bone as in rickets. Calcium metabolism is controlled by the parathyroid glands excess secretion of which causes hypocalcaemia; vitamin D controls the distribution of calcium in the blood and bones.

Hypochlorhydria: inadequate secretion of hydrochloric acid in the stomach which may sometimes lead to dyspepsia treated by giving dilute hydrochloric acid by mouth. Total absence is known as achlorhydria (q.v.), but neither state necessarily leads to problems although the latter has a certain diagnostic significance mentioned under this heading.

Hypochlorous Acid: the main active ingredient in such antiseptics as Eusol and Milton, the former being prepared from bleaching powder and boric acid. The Carrel-Dakin treatment of wounds by these substances has been largely given up with the advent of the new sulpha drugs and antibiotics but Milton is a powerful and safe antiseptic for general home purposes.

Hypochondriasis: consists in a fixed belief in the existence of physical disease when no evidence for it exists. The hypochondriac may be suffering from a specific mental illness such as a depressive state, a neurosis, or even schizophrenia, but a large number of cases fit into none of these categories frequently being middle-aged people, usually men, and often with a family history of preoccupation with bodily functions. The complaints usually centre around the abdominal organs e.g. obstruction of the bowels, vague pains therein, or peculiar feelings described in a bizarre way, and nothing said by the physician or demonstrated by special examination will convince the patient more than briefly that nothing organic is wrong. Such cases should always be referred to a psychiatrist as there is often a very considerable risk of suicide.

Hypodermic: under the skin, as hypodermic injections. The main reasons for giving drugs in this way are that by mouth they might be irritant or (as in the case of many hormone preparations) destroyed in the stomach. Also injection produces the effects of the drug more rapidly.

Hypogastric Region: the middle and lower part of the abdomen below the umbilicus and above the pubic region.

Hypoglossal Nerve: the twelfth cranial nerve supplying the muscles of the tongue and others adjacent.

Hypoglycaemia: deficiency of sugar in the blood which occurs rarely in starvation since the body makes all possible attempts to keep the level of blood-sugar constant, e.g. by breakdown of glycogen in the liver. In overdoses of insulin hypoglycaemic shock may occur with tremors, weakness, breathlessness, excitement, and finally unconsciousness; this is often difficult to tell from *hyper*glycaemic shock which may lead to diabetic coma when the sugar level is too high. The main distinguishing points are the absence of sugar in the urine in the former and the acetone in the breath of the latter which gives it a sweetish smell. Hypoglycaemic symptons are readily

305

relieved by sucking a lump of sugar or a glucose sweet which diabetics should always carry.

Hypomania: a state of mental excitement less in degree than that of mania (*see* Mental Illness).

Hypophosphites: the hypophosphites of calcium, iron, etc., like the glycerophosphates, are sometimes given in 'tonics.' Like the latter they have no effect whatever.

Hypophysectomy: surgical removal of the pituitary gland or hypophysis.

Hypoplasia: under-development of an organ.

Hypopyon: an accumulation of pus in the anterior chamber of the eye (*see* Eye).

Hypostasis: a collection of blood within the blood-vessels and fluid within the tissues in the lower parts of the body when a poor circulation is unable to overcome the effects of gravity, e.g. hypostatic congestion of the ankles and feet in heart-failure or the hypostatic congestion of the base of the lungs in those who are enfeebled, old, and bed-ridden which often leads to pneumonia.

Hypothalamus: the region of the forebrain below, and forming the underpart of, the thalamus. It is the controlling centre of the sympathetic and para-sympathetic system (i.e. the autonomic nervous system) which regulate the involuntary behaviour of the internal organs and form the physical basis of the emotions (*see* Nervous System).

Hypothermia: the technique of lowering the body temperature before operation until a state of artificial hibernation has been reached with a resultant reduction of the need for oxygen by the tissues especially in the case of heart and brain operations. In this way the circulation can be cut off for long enough for the surgeon to operate within the heart, and the brain (which under ordinary circumstances is irreparably damaged by deprivation of oxygen for more than three minutes) can be cut off from circulation for up to twelve minutes whilst surgery is carried out. The advantage in time gained by the surgeon is considerable and the method has also been used to reduce the body's needs temporarily during the critical period following a serious brain injury. Two methods are used in inducing hypothermia; in the more common the patient is lowered into a bath with ice-water and ice packs to keep the temperature down, in the second the blood is circulated through a special cooling machine outside the body. By these means the body temperature is lowered from the normal 37 degrees centigrade to about 30 degrees, but more recently the Westminster Hospital in London have reported using an artificial heart with a heat exchanger in the circuit by which means temperatures of 15 degrees centigrade (half-way to freezing-point at 0 degrees) have been maintained for operations lasting up to fifty minutes with the heart completely stopped. The heat exchanger unit surrounds the blood in the circuit with water at 2 degrees to cool and 42 degrees to rewarm, the former process taking about thirty minutes for an adult and much less for a baby.

Therapeutic hypothermia is one thing but we are only quite recently coming to realise the dangers of spontaneous hypothermia, as a killer in the weak, elderly, and old. So serious has this problem become that in 1964 a special committee of the British Medical Association published a memorandum on the subject which pointed out that 'hypothermia in the elderly is a medical emergency' and the large number of cases reported show a mortality of up to 75%. This type of heat loss is found amongst the elderly and poor, the lonely and mentally-confused, who are unable to afford adequate heating, bedding, or clothing. In the case of younger people heat loss would be made up by the production of heat by the body but the mechanism does not work adequately amongst the older age-groups especially in winter.

This emergency has largely been overlooked in the past because those affected do not ordinarily complain of cold in spite of the fact that their temperature may have fallen to 90 degrees F. or less. In addition to age, weakness, and inadequate protection against cold other factors influence hypothermia such as heart disease, pneumonia, certain drugs, and alcohol and the resultant symptoms are a semi-conscious state, mental confusion, slow breathing, and pulse-rate, and low blood-pressure. Although even those parts of the body which have been covered are felt by the physician to be cold this is not, as already mentioned, felt by the patient. In treatment, which is urgent, the important thing is *not* to apply heat to the body since, in the poor state of the circulation, any warming of the skin will carry blood away from the essential organs. The patient should simply be covered to prevent further loss of heat and the temperature allowed to rise of itself. More specific treatment has to be applied by the doctor.

Hysterectomy: the surgical operation of removing the womb. *Subtotal hysterectomy* removes the body but not the cervix (i.e. the portion projecting into the vagina) and is commonly performed for fibroids (q.v.); *total hysterectomy* may be carried out both for malignant tumours and fibroids, the cervix being removed in this case. When other pelvic structures are removed the operation is described as Wertheim's operation and still more radical, when nearly all pelvic structures are removed, is the procedure of *pelvic exenteration*. When the womb is small, the ligaments supporting it lax, and the condition benign, a vaginal hysterectomy may be performed to remove the womb through the vagina instead of through the abdomen as in other types of operation. The question often arises in hysterectomy whether the ovaries should be removed or one or both left, and this ordinarily will depend upon the age of the patient, since removal might be less important to a woman at the change of life than to a young one, and upon the condition of the ovaries and tubes. These considerations are important because loss of both ovaries means not only sterility but loss of their internal secretion with its important physical and psychological effects upon the whole body; these results do not follow if one be left behind. Contrary to general belief hysterectomy does not lead to loss of sexual desire and, in those who have feared further pregnancies, may even lead to happier relations.

Hysteria: a nervous disorder characterised by dissociation (i.e. the apparent cutting-off of one part of the mind from another), a high degree of suggestibility both from the self (autosuggestion) and from others, and a great variety of phenomena which may give the impression at first of organic disease although the condition, which is due to the repression of certain emotions or memories, is wholly psychological in origin (*see* Neuroses).

Hystero-Epilepsy: supposedly a state in which fits occur midway in type between those of hysteria and true epilepsy. Since the fits in the two disorders are very rarely even remotely alike to an expert, there is no reason to think that any such condition exists although epileptics may show hysterical manifestations.

Iatrogenic Disease: a disease unwittingly produced by the doctor, primarily in the sense that his diagnosis may induce a neurosis, e.g. the mere fact of taking the blood-pressure, especially if done repeatedly, can lead to anxiety on the part of the patient and an obsession with the subject even when this is objectively unnecessary. Patent medicine advertisements or medical dictionaries too if read by susceptible people (i.e. those who have a fund of unattached anxiety waiting for an apparently rational hook on which it may be hung) can produce the same result. This is particularly true of matters which stir the individual's guilt-feelings such as sex, mental disorder, and venereal disease which are so frequently and often illogically associated together. Obviously the physician must be careful to avoid the development of such a situation, but it is fair to point out that it is only those already suffering from anxiety or guilt who respond in this way and the main part played by the doctor is that he may present a more 'rational' excuse for worry than would otherwise have been concocted. A much more serious type of iatrogenic illness which has been described recently occurs in those unfortunates who by reason of old age or chronic mental illness are confined to institutions largely because society in the form of their friends and relatives no longer has any use for them. This 'institutional neurosis' takes the form of what seems to be a progressive dementia or deterioration of conduct sometimes mistaken for a physical degeneration of the brain or the result of the disease for which they were admitted, but in fact largely caused by the lack of social contact and the inevitable loss of the personal touch in overcrowded and understaffed hospitals and homes. Old people who, as much or even more than anyone else, need a feeling of belonging and significance – the feeling that somebody cares – rapidly deteriorate in such circumstances and we are just beginning to realise that the so-called demented schizophrenic in our mental hospitals is to a very considerable extent the result not of the disease only but of its 'cure' by institutionalisation.

Ichthammol or Ichthyol: is ammonium ichthyolsulphonate, a dark brown viscous fluid of fishy odour obtained from the distillation of fossilised fish deposits in the Tyrol and subsequent treatment with water and ammonium sulphate. Ichthyol has some antiseptic action and is mildly irritant to the skin being used as a paste or with gylcerine in chronic skin diseases and also as a vaginal tampon with glycerine in cervicitis. It has been given by mouth for numerous diseases but there is no reason to believe that it is in any way effective. Large quantities cause diarrhoea.

Ichthyosis: a congenital affection of the skin due to absence of the secretion of the sebaceous (or grease) and sweat glands. It is accompanied by dryness, roughness and cracks, and produces a condition which to outward appearance resembles the skin of a lizard or coarse fish. Ichthyosis seems to run in families and does not affect the general health, although in winter the skin becomes harder and is more prone to crack. The only treatment in general use is thyroid extract and daily warm baths with starch followed by the application of oil or 50% glycerine in water. Recently remarkable results have followed deep hypnosis in a few cases.

Icterus (Icteric): means jaundice (q.v.).

Icterus Neonatorum Gravis: congenital haemolytic anaemia, erythro-blastosis foetalis, are all terms referring to a congenital haemolytic anaemia (i.e. one characterised by the breakdown of red cells) accompanied by jaundice, often familial in incidence, and until recently usually fatal to the new-born baby in whom it occurs. The cause of the destruction of red cells which results in jaundice and the appearance in the blood of erythroblasts or immature red cells is the immunisation of the mother who is rhesus negative by a rhesus positive foetus (*see* Rh Factor). The mother's anti-Rh agglutinins pass through the placenta and agglutinate the cells of the child. The birth of a child who shows, or begins to show, anaemia, jaundice, or oedema should immediately lead to an investigation to discover whether the mother is Rh negative and the infant Rh positive and if this be the case an immediate transfusion with suitable blood (i.e. group O Rh negative) is necessary if the child is to survive.

Idiocy: Idiocy is legally defined as a form of mental defect in which persons are 'so deeply defective in mind from birth or from an early age as to be unable to guard themselves against common physical dangers.' It is the lowest grade of mental defect – idiocy, imbecility, and feeble-mindedness – and the condition is readily recognisable from a very early age. Physical deformities are common in idiots, and paralysis and convulsive attacks are also frequent (*see* Mental Defect).

Idioglossia: the continued utterance of meaningless sounds as in some mental defectives or demented schizophrenics. In certain religious sects it is regarded as a sign of peculiar holiness often on the assumption that the 'language' spoken is a dead one known to the individual by supernatural means.

Idiopathic: a term applied to diseases to indicate that their cause is unknown, e.g. 'idiopathic epilepsy' is true epilepsy not secondary to some other organic disease.

Idiosyncrasy: a response to a certain drug in a given individual which is different from the normal one. Allergy (q.v.) is an idiosyncrasy of some people to protein substances in food or pollen.

Ileitis: the ileum is the last eleven feet of the small intestine and regional ileitis, which occurs quite frequently in young men and women is a non-specific inflammation accompanied by ulceration, abscess formation, and by the appearance of small perforations and adhesions of the loops of ileum one to another. The symptoms are abdominal colic, irregularity of the bowels, loss of weight, and slight fever. Usually the abdomen is distended and the thickened loops of intestine may often be felt. Occasionally obstruction (q.v.) takes place. When this condition progresses a surgical operation is required which may be either a short-circuiting of the diseased loops so that no food flows through, or a resection (removal) of the diseased parts with implantation of the normal end into the colon.

Ileocaecal Valve: the valve at the junction of the small with the large intestine (i.e. of the ileum with the caecum). It is situated by the caecum and appendix at the right lower corner of the abdomen and permits the flow of the intestinal contents onwards into the large intestine while ordinarily preventing its return.

Ileostomy: an operation in which a loop of ileum is brought out on to the abdominal wall forming an opening through which faeces are discharged. It is carried out, e.g. for ulcerative colitis in order to rest the large bowel and permit healing to take place. Subsequently it may be possible to close the opening and restore continuity of the intestines.

Ileum: the last eleven feet of the small intestine.

Ileus: severe colic due to obstruction of the intestines; in paralytic ileus there is no mechanical obstruction but the same result is produced by paralysis of the gut muscle, sometimes a complication of acute appendicitis.

Ilium: the haunch-bone, the uppermost of the three bones forming the side of the pelvis. Its crest can be felt just below the lower ribs.

Illusion: (*see* Hallucination).

Imbecility: the second most severe degree of mental defect (q.v.) legally defined as occurring in 'persons in whose case there exists from birth or from an early age mental defectiveness not amounting to idiocy, yet so pronounced that they are incapable of managing themselves or their affairs, or, in the case of children, of being taught to do so.'

Imipramine: or Tofranil, a drug used in the treatment of depression.

Immersion Foot: a condition commonly seen in the last war in shipwrecked sailors or airmen who had spent long periods before being rescued and resulting from prolonged immersion of the feet in cold water. This led to constriction of the smaller arteries, coldness and blueness, and finally to ulceration and gangrene (q.v.).

Immunity: (*see* Infection).

Impaction: the jamming of two objects together as an impacted tooth so firmly lodged in its socket that eruption is impossible, an impacted fracture where the two ends of the bone are pushed one into the other, or impacted faeces where the faeces have become hard and dry and lodge in the rectum or colon.

Impetigo: a very contagious skin disease caused by streptococci or staplylococci and once common in school children although much less now than formerly. The sores, usually on the face but capable of spreading elsewhere, are at first small blisters that ooze then dry with the formation of yellow crusts which are quite unmistakable. It is easily spread by the hands from one part of the body to another or by touch or infected towels to another person. No disease is more easily treated provided the right methods are used and spread prevented (this, however, is often none too easy in a small child who wants to keep fingering the sores). All crusts are removed by bathing in hot water after softening with olive oil, and penicillin cream is applied twice or three times daily. If the scalp is affected the hair must be cut short and penicillin used as a spray. Sulphonamide powder or ointment is also useful. Attention must be paid to towels, etc., and if the treatment is not completely successful within a week it is certain that it has not been carried out as instructed.

Impotence: is the inability of the male to perform sexually which may be due either to organic or psychological factors and be temporary or long-lasting. The failure to have an erection can result from such organic conditions as endocrine disease resulting in diminished activity of the testicles or to thyroid or pituitary disturbances. Occasionally there may be local defects such as a tight foreskin or diseases of the central nervous system such as tabes dorsalis and serious general diseases like untreated diabetes or chronic alcoholism may cause impotence. However the vast majority of cases are psychological in origin resulting from feelings of guilt, anxiety, distaste for the sexual act either in general or in a particular case, latent homosexual tendencies, and sheer ignorance. The ability in men to have sexual intercourse satisfactorily is tied up with the higher centres and particularly with self-confidence and self-regard and it frequently happens that failure on one occasion perpetuates itself owing to the fear on each subsequent occasion that all will not be well. Since erection is almost impossible in the presence of conflicting emotions of anxiety and desire, love and fear, impotence results in such circumstances. The comparatively rare organic types can be dealt with by the use of sex hormones (e.g. testosterone propionate) but otherwise treatment must be directed to removing anxiety. Aphrodisiacs to increase sexual excitement (e.g. cantharides or 'Spanish Fly') are both useless and dangerous producing their effect by local irritation of the urethra. Since any such method also irritates the kidneys, often causing blood in the urine, it should never be used. Sexual desire should not be treated as a mechanical procedure to be stimulated by mechanical means and in the absence of desire or affection for the partner nothing is likely to be successful; the impotent male has to conquer the two emotions of anxiety and conceit in the form of a constant wondering whether he is likely to 'succeed' or not. For in this case he is indulging in intercourse filled with concern for himself rather than his partner as should normally be the case. Nearly all men are at some time impotent but if this is to be anxiously regarded as indicating

313

the possibility of future failure the condition will be likely to persist. Desire and introspection cannot exist together and anxiety is the most potent anaphrodisiac.

Incisor: the front four teeth of each jaw whose function is cutting (*see* Teeth).

Incompatibility: in medicine the inclusion of drugs in a prescription which cancel each other out because their biological effects are opposed or because they interact chemically, producing a new and unwanted substance.

Incompetence: in relation to the valves of the heart (e.g. mitral or aortic incompetence) is a condition resulting from endocarditis where the valves will not close completely so that blood pumped out is liable to flow back into the chamber it has just left (*see* Valvular Disease).

Incontinence: the inability to control bladder or bowels found in conditions where they are diseased or injured or, more commonly, when nervous control is lacking from disease in the spinal cord. In psychological conditions such as the dementia of schizophrenia incontinence results from indifference with regression to childish levels of behaviour.

Incoordination: the inability to coordinate movements, e.g. standing with the eyes closed or touching the tip of the nose with the tip of the index finger with the eyes closed, due either to damage to the sensory (kinaesthetic) nerves which inform the brain about the body's position in space or to defects in the motor nerve muscles.

Incubation Period: the period elapsing between infection with the germs of a disease and the appearance of the first symptoms. In any given disease it is relatively constant and a person who has been so exposed is known as a contact. Such contacts should usually be isolated and watched (although during the period of incubation they are not infectious), since e.g. in measles, they may be highly infectious whenever the first symptoms set in and before any rash has developed. In scarlet fever on the other hand risk of infection is greatest during the later stages of the disease. Roughly speaking, incubation periods may be divided into those which are short, lasting 2–5 days (e.g. scarlet fever, diphtheria, influenza, plague and cholera) and the longer ones lasting from 10–15 days (smallpox, measles, chickenpox, typhoid fever, whooping cough). The two main exceptions are German measles (17–18 days) and mumps (21 days). Quarantine periods are ordinarily longer to make allowance for difficulty in recognising the disease in the early stages, but contacts with German measles, mumps, and chickenpox need not be excluded at all so far as children are concerned (but see entry under German measles) and in the case of whooping-cough and measles only infants who have not had the disease need to be excluded for three weeks and two weeks respectively from the date of onset of the last case in the house. In scarlet fever and diphtheria contacts should be kept in quarantine for a week after the beginning of the patient's illness. Of course, many schools make their own arrangements to avoid trouble with parents.

Indian Hemp: (*see* Cannabis Indica).

Indigestion: (*see* Dyspepsia, Stomach Diseases).

Infants and Infant Welfare: it is important to realise that the term 'normal infant' simply means the average and this may be quite misleading in any one case (e.g. so far as weight is concerned infants who are quite healthy may fall considerably short of or greatly exceed the average weight). The figures given here are only rough guides and no attempt should be made to compel one's own child to conform unless there are other signs that its condition is not satisfactory.

Weight: at birth the average infant weighs 7–7½ lbs; the weight is approximately doubled by the fifth month, trebled by the end of the first year, and at the end of the second year the child should weigh about 28 lbs. Apart from the first week when there is a slight initial loss, the weight increases by about 6–8 oz a week but minor variations are of little significance and small infants (since infants vary within the normal as much as their parents) may do quite satisfactorily with a weekly gain of 4–6 oz.

Height: this again varies greatly as does the height of the parents but, broadly speaking, the hereditary factor in height does not make its influence felt until about the 5th year and prior to that height is largely dependent upon nutrition. At birth the average infant is about 20 inches and at the end of the year about 28 inches increasing about 3½ inches a year thereafter until the 5th year when the hereditary factor begins to make itself felt.

Sleep: during the first month an infant sleeps nearly all the time except for feeding and dressing but by the 6th month this has altered gradually to about 12 hours at night, two hours in the morning, and two or three hours in the afternoon. At one year the period of sleep is twelve hours at night, two in the morning and one in the afternoon and at eighteen months a morning sleep of two hours only followed by an afternoon out and early to bed since too much sleep during the day may result in loss of sleep at night. The bed-clothes should be warm but light, the room darkened, but well-ventilated without draughts. Newly born babies can grasp objects, suck, and swallow, but movements of the arms and legs are not at first co-ordinated although by the end of the third month the child can usually lift up its head. By six months it begins to sit up, by the ninth month to crawl and by ten months to stand up. Walking begins about the twelfth or fourteenth month. Single words may be spoken by the end of the first year but anything that can be described as speech does not make its appearance until the end of the second.

In the general management of the infant one of the most neglected points is that the mother should be free from anxiety, relaxed, and not given to fussing. Many feeding difficulties arise from the infant's awareness of the mother's tension and in later life there is no surer way to make a child neurotic than to fuss over it thus giving it the impression that the world is a dangerous place. Neurosis is one of the most infectious diseases there is, even although it is not caused by germs. Feeding should be under the direction of the home nurse, health visitor or Welfare Centre but it is worth while pointing out that, no matter what advances have been made in our knowledge of breast-milk substitutes, the infant mortality in breast-fed infants is still much below that of the artificially-fed. This is partly because breast-milk contains antibodies (or is believed to do so) and the risk of infection is obviously much greater in artificial feeding. The idea that a fixed schedule of feeding should be ruthlessly adhered to regardless of the child's cries of hunger is no longer popular and it will be found that if the child is at first fed on demand it will gradually develop a regularity suited to its own needs.

Clothes: should be light and loose and preferably made of wool, silk and wool, or cellular material and it must be non-inflammable. The body should be able to get a reasonable amount of fresh air and sunshine and be free to move. After birth the baby is thoroughly washed in water a little above blood heat (100 degrees Fahrenheit) and this can best be tested by the mother's elbow. The stump of the umbilical cord is dried by swabbing, dusted with antiseptic powder, and covered with lint. Daily sponging is carried out thereafter whilst keeping the cord quite dry until it separates on or about the tenth day. In a month or so the temperature of the bath should be lowered to tepid and after the daily bath the child should be allowed to lie naked in front of the fire to kick and move freely.

Dentition: the lower central incisors appear from the 5th to the 8th month and the other incisors follow first in the upper jaw and then in the lower. The twenty milk teeth should all be present by the end of the second year and the permanent teeth begin to erupt from about the fourth.

Weaning should be a natural process and from the 4th month broth and egg yolk should be given, minced meat being used by the 9th month. The fruit juice and cod-liver oil supplements must always be given and the child should have something hard to exercise its teeth on. Weaning proper usually begins by the 9th month by omitting the midday feed and replacing it with cereal milk foods, broth, and hard crusts. A week later milk, hard crusts and butter, lightly boiled egg and bread-crumbs, porridge with milk, may replace the breakfast feed. In the third week, crisp toast with milk should replace the teatime feed and finally the other feeds should be stopped and replaced by milk or fruit-juice.

Amongst the symptoms and signs of ill-health are fever, restlessness and irritability, and persistent crying (crying in itself is not necessarily anything to worry about and the mother will soon learn to distinguish between the cry of pain or discomfort and the child who is merely exercising his lungs). Colds, which block the nose, are extremely distressing to babies and coughs should always be referred to the doctor or Welfare Clinic. Vomiting small amounts is not necessarily serious and the normal child brings up small amounts of food especially if it is overfed, but violent vomiting with or without diarrhoea should receive medical attention. Constipation is rarely a cause for worry and many babies who are perfectly healthy tend to be constipated; it is only worth considering when it is prolonged or accompanied by other signs of ill-

317

health. Here it should be pointed out that the habit of 'potting' regularly even at a time when the child is quite unable for anatomical reasons to control its bowels is a bad thing and to be avoided; most bowel troubles and neuroses in later life are caused by the parent's obsession with the child's bowel functions which should be allowed to develop control in their own good time.

Infantile Paralysis: (*see* Poliomyelitis).

Infarction: the process which takes place when an artery is suddenly blocked by a thrombus or an embolus leading to the formation (e.g. in the heart or lung) of a wedge-shaped mass of dead tissue in the area supplied, the apex of the wedge being at the point of entry of the vessel and the base on the surface of the organ.

Infection: infectious diseases are those caused by invasion of the body by organisms from outside and characterised by the fact that the disease can be passed on from one person to another or from an animal to a person either directly or through an intermediary such as an insect or even a water snail. Thus they gain entrance to the body and provoke a total reaction even although the area directly affected may be quite small, whereas *vermin* which live on the surface of the body, if in one sense infectious, are said to *infest* rather than infect the individual. A raised temperature is usually, but by no means always, present and some infectious diseases (often quite serious ones) produce very little fever whilst other conditions which are not infections may be accompanied by high fever, e.g. heatstroke. The bacteria causing disease are mentioned under that heading where they are classified according to shape as bacilli (rods), staphylococci (bunches), streptococci (chains), diplococci (pairs), vibrio (comma-shaped), etc., and the other pathenogens or disease-producing organisms can be classified as spirochaetes (these are corkscrew-shaped, move about by wriggling, and cause the two important diseases syphilis and spirochaetal jaundice), viruses, fungi, and amoebae. Viruses are usually too small to be seen under an ordinary microscope; they can, however, be photographed under an electron microscope which uses a magnetic field in place of a lens and a stream of electrons in place of a beam of light. Viruses cause such diseases as typhus, measles, mumps, poliomyelitis, smallpox, virus pneumonia and infective jaundice and chicken-pox and also such plant and animal infections as tobacco mosaic disease and foot and mouth disease which often have serious economic consequences. Other virus diseases are psittacosis (an infection of parrots and other birds which can be transmitted to man), swine fever in pigs, influenza, and myxomatosis in rabbits. They are responsible, so far as research has been able to show, for the common cold. The other main characteristics of these mysterious organisms may be briefly summarised. (1) They can only grow in living cells and must be cultured in the laboratory on portions of living tissue unlike the bacteria which readily grow on plates containing jelly made from meat broth, gelatin, milk, and other delicacies. (2) They are so small that they can usually pass through the pores of the finest bacteriological filter. (3) A first attack often produces immunity for life, second attacks of the diseases mentioned above being very rare save in the cases of influenza and the common cold. (4) Viruses reproduce themselves and show other traits of living things yet in other respects can act as non-living ones, e.g. they can be produced in crystalline form whilst remaining as dangerous as before. (5) Numerous viruses have shown themselves to be little affected by the new antibiotics and other drugs although vaccination and active and passive immunisation is possible in many cases.

Some infections are caused by fungi, i.e. organisms belonging to the same group as moulds, mushrooms, and toadstools. Penicillin and other antibiotics are also produced from moulds and these can kill fungi such as actinomycosis perhaps the most serious fungal infection. Most, however, are relatively trivial and restricted to the surface of the skin as in the case of ringworm and athlete's foot; the former shows markedly the tendency of fungi to grow in circles as do the 'fairy rings' of toadstools.

Amoebae are tiny, formless, jelly-like particles, the largest of which, the harmless amoeba of ponds and stagnant water, is just visible to the naked eye. Amoebae can move by flowing along and, like bacteria, reproduce by dividing into two halves each of which becomes a new amoeba. The main human diseases caused by amoebae are: amoebic dysentery (not to be confused with bacillary dysentery), sleeping sickness and trypanosomiasis which is caused by a special kind of amoeba known as a trypanosome, and malaria. These are three of the great scourges of mankind but now well on the way to be controlled; the measures to be taken to this end are well known and only human ignorance and lack of money prevents such diseases being wiped out altogether.

Other organisms which it would be more correct to describe as infesting the human body are animal parasites and worms. The former live on the skin and in Europe the main groups are fleas, lice, and the mite of scabies. These, if uncomfortable, are not in themselves dangerous but some together with the insect pests can carry the germs of dangerous diseases: the flea, plague; the louse, typhus; and the mosquito, malaria and yellow fever. Worms live in the human intestine and the only common types in Britain are the tiny threadworm, the round-worm somewhat resembling an ordinary garden earthworm, and tapeworms which are flat and segmented and may reach a length of 10 or even 20 feet. Many parasitic worms lead a kind of double life spending part of their life in the human intestine and the other in the muscles of some animal which is used for food. Eggs are laid in the intestine of the human host which pass out with the faeces and are then swallowed by pigs (especially in those parts of the world where human excreta are used as manure). In the pig the eggs form cysts in the muscles forming the flesh known as 'measly pork' which, being eaten by human beings, starts the cycle all over again. Less familiar are the Russian tapeworm which grows to nearly 30 feet and is spread by caviare or raw infected fish and the small leaf-shaped liver-fluke of Egypt and other tropical countries which lays eggs that are passed into canals and pools in the urine of infected people, hatch out and enter a water snail leaving it in the form of small parasites capable of piercing the skin of bathers, passing to the liver, and subsequently reaching the bladder or rectum. Bilharzia, as this disease is called, is a serious infestation described more fully elsewhere. Ankylostomiasis, filariasis (which causes elephantiasis), the disease known as dracontiasis spread by the Guinea-worm, and trichiniasis (which sometimes occurs in Britain from eating infected pork and ham), are all round-worm or nematode diseases.

The Spread of Infection, one of the commonest means of spread is by droplet infection when minute drops carrying the germs are coughed or sneezed into the air by someone already suffering from the disease. Such droplets can be projected at least 10–15 feet and when breathed in by another within range infection may result. Next commonest mode of spread is perhaps by way of infected food, water, and the infected hands of those who prepare or handle them; cholera, dysentery, food-poisoning, and typhoid fever are passed on in this way. Spread by direct contact is less common than might be supposed since the skin unless broken forms a formidable barrier, but parasites are generally spread in this way and when the mucous membranes of the mouth or genitals are involved protection is slight indeed. Hence sexual contact where this occurs is the common cause of venereal infection. Spread through an intermediary host has already been mentioned and the actual carrier from one to the other may be an insect or parasite as the rat-flea which carries plague from the rat to man. Lastly the infection may sometimes come from within one's own body from bacteria which are harmless in one part but not in another, e.g. the bacillus coli does no harm in the human intestine but can cause pyelitis or cystitis (inflammation of the pelvis of the kidney or bladder) when it gets into the urinary tract.

How the body deals with infection: the body has numerous methods of defence but the two main ones are, firstly, the substances known as antibodies and antitoxins produced in response to an infection the former rendering the invaders helpless by causing them to clump together (agglutinate) and the latter neutralising their poisons. Secondly, some of the white cells of the blood (phagocytes) act as amoebae engulfing and destroying the germs after they have been agglutinated by the antibodies. Antibodies and antitoxins can be transferred from one individual to another and are used in medicine both to prevent infection and to cure it. This is known as passive immunisation, the ready-made substances being taken from someone who has had the disease and given to another who either has just developed it or has been in contact with a case. Obviously it is much better if the body can be stimulated to produce its own antitoxins and antibodies and this is done by injecting a solution of killed bacteria (e.g. TAB for typhoid) or one of live but weakened organisms (vaccination). This type of immunity may last a long time but passive immunity is always short-lived. The manner in which the body deals with local infections is discussed under the heading of Inflammation.

Infectious Mononucleosis: (*see* Glandular Fever).

Infestation: the occurrence of animal parasites in the intestine or on the skin, hair or clothing (*see* Parasites).

Inflammation: the classical signs of inflammation noticed by the early physicians were described as: rubor, dolor, tumor, and calor, i.e. redness, pain, swelling, and heat. At the point of entry of the germs the blood-vessels initially dilate so that the blood circulates more quickly and the skin appears red and feels hot to the touch; but soon the circulation slows down, the white blood-cells begin to stick to the walls of the smallest vessels and finally push their way through them and move out into the surrounding spaces. The fluid part of the blood passes out also giving rise to swelling. The white blood-cells have several functions: they destroy and absorb germs as described under Infection, remove dead tissue, and when the attack has been overcome aid in the process of repair, although most of this is done by the surrounding tissues themselves. In addition the tissues proliferate to form a thick barrier which fences off the infected area and those germs which escape pass up the lymph vessels to be trapped at the nearest glands (q.v.). This is why in a bad infection of the hand or foot red streaks (lymphangitis) are seen spreading up the limb and the glands in the arm-pit or groin become swollen and painful. If the defence is less successful one of two things may happen depending on whether the infection has destroyed a good deal of tissue leaving many dead cells on the field to form an abscess filled with pus which ultimately bursts or is opened by the surgeon or, in the worst cases, the infection gets into the general blood-stream causing blood-poisoning or septicaemia, at one time usually fatal. Such cases are now treated at this, or preferably the earlier stages, by antibiotics and sulpha drugs locally and internally; the function of hot applications on the wound is to increase congestion and relieve pain.

Influenza: there are all types of influenza ranging from the minor epidemic happening almost every winter to the raging pandemics which swept the world in 1918–19 killing more people than the actual fighting. Many viruses cause diseases of the influenza type but there is no very close correlation between the actual symptoms during an epidemic and the strain of virus causing it. However, a sudden onset, aching in the muscles of the back and legs, and redness of the eyes with a moderately high fever would suggest influenza especially if followed by the general depression and weakness which is characteristic of this disease but not of the common cold which in other respects it often resembles. There is no specific treatment beyond rest in bed and (inevitably) aspirin although this has no *curative* value whatever even if it relieves the head and muscular pains. Post-influenzal depression, if severe, can be treated by concentrated vitamin injections in the form of Parentrovite. Influenza is known elsewhere as 'grippe' and during serious epidemics vaccination may be tried to prevent infection although this method is very much in the experimental stage, the practical difficulty being the great variability of the strain from one epidemic to another.

Infusions: are watery preparations of vegetable drugs made by steeping the appropriate part of the plant in water and straining. Following this they must be suitably standardised, one of the weaknesses of herbal preparations being the variability of the amount of drug in different samples. Senna, digitalis, quassia, gentian, cinchona, and other herbs are prepared in this way.

Inguinal Region: the groin (*see* Hernia).

Inhalation: a means of inhaling drugs in the form of gas, vapour, or finely divided particles. Anaesthetics are generally used in this way either as a gas or such volatile substances as chloroform or ether and volatile drugs are also used in the inhalers which clear the nose during a head cold. Apart from these purposes inhalants are generally used in diseases of the bronchi or lungs and here their usefulness is less highly regarded than formerly except in the case of asthma when it is certainly possible to dilate the bronchi by inhalants using a nebuliser, a mask, cigarettes containing stramonium, or aerosols under pressure in a tin container. However, eucalyptus, friar's balsam, pine oil, creosote, and all the other old favourites can at the most relieve but do not cure coughs, colds, bronchitis, and the rest; they are generally applied in steam or by burning over a spirit lamp. Antibiotics are sometimes inhaled but by and large the main function of inhalants is to ease breathing by dilating the bronchial tubes. Antiseptic sprays

323

to 'purify' the air or to destroy germs lurking in the dust on the floor are of very little use; to quote the *British Medical Journal*: 'There is no good scientific evidence that any of the chemical air-disinfectants can control the spread of infection in places such as schools, offices, or cinemas. Nor is there good evidence that any substantial effect on the spread of illness can be obtained by disinfection of dust.' Such substances may make the room smell cleaner (although with respect to manufacturers there are those which create an odour considerably less pleasant than that they strive to conceal) but they have no medical effect of any sort.

Inhibition: the process whereby one nervous process by its strength overwhelms another. At the physiological level this can refer, e.g. to the slowing-down of the heart's beat by the action of the vagus nerve, at a higher level one may speak of the inhibition of gastric secretion by worry, or at the highest psychological level of the inhibition of anti-social drives by the action of the self-regarding sentiment, superego, or conscience, i.e. by other dominant aspects of the mind which realise them to be inappropriate. In the popular (which is not the scientific) sense a person is said to be inhibited or to have 'inhibitions' when he is shy, unsociable, or afraid of expressing his emotions. Inhibition may be a conscious or unconscious process, repression is always automatic and unconscious, although both are used as equivalent to each other in everyday speech if not in psychology.

Injections: may be hypodermic (under the skin), intravenous (into a vein) or intramuscular (into a muscle). The intravenous route is the most rapid. Enemata are correctly, but not ordinarily, referred to as injections.

Innominate: (a) the large bone at each side of the pelvis; (b) the large artery from which the right subclavian and right carotid arteries separate out after it has left the aortic arch; (c) the corresponding vein, formed from the union of the internal jugular and subclavian veins at the base of the neck.

Inoculation: the accidental or intentional introduction of germs into the system through a small wound in the skin or mucous membranes. Vaccines may be live (as in the case of smallpox vaccination) or dead (as in most other types) (*see* Infection, Vaccine).

Insanity: (*see* Mental Illness).

Insects and Disease: (*see* Infection and the various specific insect-borne diseases mentioned under separate headings).

Insomnia: inability to sleep may take numerous forms: the inability to get to sleep on going to bed, waking up too early, disturbed sleep following which the individual does not feel sufficiently rested in the morning, or sleep accompanied by frightening dreams and nightmares. Its cause in the vast majority of cases is psychological being due to the sleeper's fear of relaxing control over his mind lest the fears or primitive desires from the unconscious should get out of hand or even enter consciousness in the form of dreams. In other cases the individual is unable to get to sleep because anxiety or worry makes him unable to relax, and a more normal form of this is the case of the brain-worker whose mind has been so active all day that he is unable to turn it off at bedtime, even although his thoughts are not necessarily unpleasant. His state of mind may well be (and in children often is) one of pleasurable expectation for the following day. Worry, however, is the chief killer of sleep and other factors are either obvious or uncommon. Thus it is hardly necessary to point out that pain can prevent sleep, that drugs which are mental stimulants such as amphetamine and numerous others can have the same effect, that there are some organic nervous conditions so rare as to be almost irrelevant which interfere with sleep, nor that there are some people who sleep so lightly that they are easily distressed by a full stomach, cold feet, noises, and so on – all of which are simply manifestations of an over-sensitive nervous system. The cure of insomnia depends first of all upon realising that no harm can come from it; the body is a self-regulating system and on the whole a very effective one and it ensures that everyone always in any ordinary circumstances gets enough sleep. Of course, as in the case of constipation, if one believes that a particular process is harmful then harmful it will be even if this is only manifestated in the way the person feels; for one is hardly likely to feel well when living in the belief that mysterious 'toxins' are slowly poisoning the system or that lack of sleep is about to lead to insanity. The latter belief is based on the assumption that because those who have subsequently become mentally ill previously could not sleep therefore the lack of sleep caused the mental breakdown. This is to put the cart before the horse since it was the inability to sleep that was caused by the approaching illness rather than the commonly-accepted reversed state of affairs. Insomnia is a sign of anxiety, not a cause of it, and many great men have slept very little whilst there have been claims from those who have never slept at all, e.g. a Dr Pavoni in northern Italy who died in his eighties did not sleep to any significant degree for over sixty years, but instead of complaining he made a virtue of necessity and amassed a comfortable fortune by doing other doctors' night calls. The treatment of insomnia is the treatment of its cause and, in mild cases, a hot soothing drink at night, warm but not too heavy bedclothes, the avoidance of intellectually stimulating activity late at night, and the avoidance of late tea or coffee, may be sufficient especially when combined with a state of mind which looks forward to sleep but allows a healthy indifference towards the possibility of failing to do so; nobody can sleep if his mind is filled with the thought that he will have a breakdown if he does not. Hence a good way of wooing somnolence is to read in bed choosing a book which is pleasing but not enthralling. Pain and other strictly medical conditions which interfere with sleep must be dealt with by the doctor as should the question of sleeping tablets. In general unless one is ill or old it is thoroughly bad to get into the habit of using sedatives (although it is unnecessary to be puritanical about this) and the natural ones such as a hot whisky can do no harm nor even the beverages advertised as suitable for 'night starvation' (although no such state exists) which are helpful in inducing sleep by withdrawing blood from the brain to the stomach. In severe insomnia such measures are unlikely to succeed and, if psychological problems seem to be at the root of this, it is best to ask the doctor's advice about a psychiatric opinion. It is unnecessary to discuss here the many types of sedatives regarding which the doctor's advice must be obtained in addition to his prescription since most of these are restricted drugs. The largest group is the barbiturates (q.v.) which are of course dangerous things to possess but the newer sedatives are fairly safe (*see* Sleep).

Insufflation: the blowing of suitable powder into a cavity in order to treat local disease, e.g. in the ears or vagina.

Insulin: the internal secretion of the islets of Langerhans in the pancreas is a hormone which acts to enable the tissues requiring sugar for their activity to absorb it from the bloodstream. When insulin is deficient the sugar accumulates in the blood in large amounts and overflows into the urine. This state is what is known as diabetes and severe cases of this disease (q.v.) were almost invariably fatal until insulin, the existence of which had been postulated by Schafer in 1909, was isolated in 1921 by the Canadians McLeod, Banting, and Best; for this piece of research McLeod and Banting received the Nobel Prize in 1923. All diabetics do not necessarily need insulin since mild cases can be treated by a carbohydrate-restricted diet alone but most do and today there are seven varieties which differ mainly in the length of time for which they act and the concentration reached in the blood. These are, insulin; protamine zinc insulin; globin insulin; isophane insulin; insulin zinc suspension; insulin zinc suspension (amorphous); insulin zinc suspension (crystalline) (*see* Diabetes).

Intercostal: connected with the bloodvessels, nerves, and muscles lying between the ribs.

Interferon: although many of the infectious diseases have been brought under control or in some cases almost eliminated, one large group stands out as resistant to most methods of treatment. This is the group of the virus diseases; for whilst smallpox has been reduced in the technically-advanced countries to a comparative rarity and an effective vaccine is now available against influenza, only the larger viruses are affected by modern antibiotics. Since the list of virus diseases for which there is no specific cure runs all the way from the common cold, chickenpox, measles, mumps, infectious hepatitis, poliomyelitis, and other infections found in the West to such very fatal conditions as typhus and yellow fever, it is obviously important to find some active agent which will cure these diseases once they have started. Of course, a number of them can be protected against *before* infection occurs (yellow fever, for example), but only good nursing is available after infection.

The substance now known as interferon was first described by Isaacs and Lindenmann in 1957 when they were studying the effect on live influenza virus in a chick embryo of killed virus introduced after the infection had taken. They noted that the fluid surrounding the cells that had been treated with

327

killed virus contained a substance which protected them against the live one and gave it the name of interferon. It is now known that many types of tissue exposed to live or dead viruses produce this substance which is apparently non-poisonous and effective against most viruses within the same species (i.e. rabbits would not be helped by chick interferon). Although nearly all the work so far has been carried out on animals, it has been shown that the great majority of virus diseases infecting chickens can be prevented or halted by this substance, and perhaps one of the most significant findings is its ability to halt the development of the form of cancer in chickens known as Rous sarcoma which is caused by a virus. Opinions vary about the use of interferon in controlling virus infections in man, and certainly a great deal of further research has to be done. Nevertheless, this discovery, like the initial discovery of penicillin, opens a new window on another approach to controlling infectious disease and possibly even cancer (*see* Cancer).

Intermittent Claudication: a condition found in middle-aged or old people in which cramps occur in the muscles of the legs on walking for a distance which varies with its severity. It is caused by arteriosclerosis of the arteries which leads to an inadequate blood-supply during exercise. The treatment is that of the cause, but the new vasodilator drugs (Dibenylene, Hydergine, Perdilatal, Priscol, Ronicol, and Vasculit) may be of considerable help.

Interstitial: the background tissue, usually fibrous in nature, supporting the active cells of an organ, e.g. interstitial nephritis is a disease of this tissue in the kidneys.

Intertrigo: chafing between two surfaces of skin that rub together, e.g. beneath the breasts, in the arm-pit, between the thighs, etc. (*see* Chafing).

Intestines: the whole of the alimentary canal after it leaves the stomach. The first part or duodenum into which the ducts of the liver and pancreas open is, as the name indicates, about twelve inches long; following this the jejunum (the word means 'empty' as this part of the intestine is nearly always found empty after death) occupies 8–9 feet and this is succeeded by the 11 feet of the ileum (meaning the twisted part) the coils of which fill much of the abdomen. The large intestine begins at the lower right-hand part of the abdomen where the caecum, a cul-de-sac to which the appendix is attached, lies just below its point of entry into the ascending colon which passes upwards to the right upper corner then turns across the top of the abdomen to form the transverse colon which going down the left side as the descending colon joins the pelvic colon on entering the pelvis. The functions of the intestines are described under Digestion and their diseases under separate headings (see Appendicitis, Cholera, Colitis, Constipation, Diarrhoea, Dysentery, Gastro-enteritis, Hernia, Ileitis, Intussusception, Obstruction, Perforation, Peritonitis, Piles, Rectum, Diseases of).

Intracranial: within the skull.

Intrathecal: within the meninges covering the brain and spinal cord, i.e. between the arachnoid or middle membrane and the intimate pia mater both enclosing a space within which lies the cerebro-spinal fluid. It is from this space that the fluid is drawn in lumbar puncture and into which drugs are sometimes injected.

Intussusception: is a condition in which the small intestine telescopes into the large intestine or in a few cases the upper segment of a part of small intestine telescopes into a lower one usually in the right lower part of the abdomen in the region of the caecum and appendix. Such a situation produces obstruction of the bowel, is seen almost exclusively in children under three years of age (in fact it is largely limited to males during the first eighteen months of life) and most hospital cases happen about the week-end when children are more likely to be given unsuitable food. The symptoms are attacks of severe colic, vomiting, the passage of blood and mucus by the rectum, and a lump usually can be felt on the abdomen at the affected site. Immediate operation is performed and by gentle pulling the small intestine can be taken out from its abnormal position. Recovery is the rule unless too much time has been wasted when strangulation or gangrene may have set in requiring a portion of bowel to be removed.

Inunction: a method of treating disease by rubbing in drugs mixed with oil or fat. This unpleasant and unsatisfactory procedure was once used for administering mercury in the treatment of syphilis.

In Vitro: means the testing of drugs in a test-tube (lit. in glass) as opposed to *in vivo*, in the living animal or human body.

Obviously the fact that a drug has a particular action in vitro need not necessarily imply that it can be used in vivo when it might be toxic or transformed into another product.

Involution: a return to the normal size as of the uterus after pregnancy. The failure to do so in a reasonable time is known as subinvolution. Also the shrinking with old age of other organs.

Iodides: the salts of iodine, e.g. potassium iodide. These are used in expectorant cough-mixtures, in chronic syphilis to absorb diseased tissues, and in some types of goitre since iodine has an affinity for the thyroid gland being the main constituent of its hormone thyroxin. Iodine is now used mainly in the radioactive form as an isotope (q.v.) but was formerly much used as the tincture to clean wounds or to apply to the skin before surgical operations; it has also been used as a means of applying counter-irritation to chronically inflamed joints or glands. Lugol's iodine (5% iodine and 10% potassium iodine in water) is sometimes given prior to operation for toxic goitre. Mandel's paint, a similar mixture dissolved in glycerine, is used to paint the throat in inflammatory conditions. In excess, iodine leads to 'iodism' with symptoms similar to those of a cold with an associated skin rash.

Iodoform: is obtained by the action of iodine on alcohol in the presence of potassum carbonate. Although much used on wounds, especially in the Latin countries, its antiseptic action is slight but it has a pleasant 'sea-weed' smell, diminishes pain, and forms a protective covering over the damaged tissues. 'Bipp' (bismuth and iodoform paste) was commonly used here but has largely been replaced by other dressings.

Iodophthalein: which is excreted quickly by the liver through the bile is used to outline the gall-bladder for the diagnosis of disease by X-rays. It is given by mouth or intravenously. *Iodoxyl* is similarly used in contrast radiography of the kidneys and their tubes by intravenous injection.

Ionization: the breaking-up of a substance by electricity into its constituent ions, e.g. sodium chloride into sodium and chlorine. In medicine the introduction by similar methods of suitable ions through the skin as treatment, e.g. sodium salicylate for rheumatic conditions.

Ipecacuanha: the dried root of Cephaelis ipecacuanha, a Brazilian shrub which contains alkaloids (q.v.) and tannic acid. The most important of the former is emetine. Ipecacuanha is a powerful emetic and in smaller doses, like all emetics, acts as an expectorant used in stimulating cough mixtures to liquefy sputum. It mildly depresses the heart and induces sweating (hence it is included in Dover's powders for use in fevers). Emetine is specific for amoebic dysentery when it is given orally in the form of the insoluble iodide of bismuth and emetine in cachets, or intramuscularly as emetine hydrochloride. The former is necessary if cysts are present in the motions.

Iproniazid: (*see* Isoniazid).

Iridectomy: a surgical operation performed either under local or general anaesthesia and usually for glaucoma (q.v.) in which a segment of the iris is removed to increase the size of the pupil of the eye and thus relieve tension.

Iris: from the Greek word for a halo, is the part of the eye behind the cornea which, by alteration of the size of the hole in its centre or pupil, controls the amount of light entering the eye.

Iritis: inflammation of the iris, the ciliary body, and the choroid which together make up the middle coat of the eye (q.v.) The disease is commonest in young adults and in 50% of such cases the cause is syphilis, iritis being the usual factor leading to serious eye-diseases in this condition. The other 50% of cases are children with ulcers of the cornea or adults with rheumatic conditions, diabetes, dental abcesses or infections of the nose. 'Sympathetic' iritis however usually develops as the result of an open wound or an unremoved foreign body in the other eye; probably infection from this area passes by way of the lymph vessels or through the blood to the new situation and serious penetrating wounds of an eye resulting in blindness and inflamed tissues are best treated by removal of the eye to prevent the other being affected. The symptoms of iritis are severe pain either in or just above the eye, watering, and photophobia (fear of light). The eye is red as in conjuctivitis for which iritis is often mistaken although in the former case severe pain is absent save for the typical 'gritty' feeling and the gumming together of the eyelids in the morning. The pupil itself is narrow and may be irregular in outline and its margins dull and lustreless. An acute attack may last several weeks and, if not quickly dealt with, vision may be greatly impaired or lost. The treatment is that of the original cause together with rest, dark glasses, cessation of reading, warm bathing, aspirin for the pain, and the use of atropine (belladonna) drops.

Iron: is used primarily in the treatment of iron-deficiency anaemias for which it is specific; in itself it is useless in the treatment of hyperchromic anaemias such as pernicious anaemia where liver-extract is necessary so supply the missing factor. There are three misapprehensions concerning the use of iron, which is a perfectly straightforward means of cure in the appropriate type of case, and these are worth mentioning here: (1) *It is untrue that iron need be given in some special form or that there is a substitute for iron.* The belief used to be common that 'organic iron' is more readily absorbed than inorganic and it is often contended that iron pills containing additional substances such as copper, vitamins of the B and C groups, stomach extract, etc., are better than the ordinary ones of the Pharmacopoeia. At one time it was even suggested that chlorophyll, which has the same structural formula as the haemoglobin of the blood (with the significant difference that it contains magnesium instead of iron), could be used in the treatment of anaemias. But iron is best given as the official preparations which are ferrous sulphate, ferrous carbonate (Blaud's pills), or iron and ammonium citrate mixture, or such proprietary preparations of these as Fergon or Fersolate. Complicated proprietary preparations with 'blunderbuss' formulae of the type mentioned above are not only no better than the official preparations – they are positively harmful since those containing stomach extract will conceal the existence of pernicious anaemia if it happens to be present so that it remains undiagnosed. There is no place for the use of liver or stomach extract in the treatment of simple anaemia. Injections of iron may impress the simple-minded rich but they too have no place in treatment save in those isolated cases where the oral route causes gastric upset. Iron-containing (chalybeate) natural waters are, by and large, useless since they do not contain iron in sufficient concentration to treat anaemia and those who are not anaemic do not require iron beyond that supplied in their diet. (2) *Iron is not a tonic and it is unscientific to give it in the absence of anaemia.* All talk of 'tired blood,' or 'bloodlessness' as a cause of fatigue which requires an 'iron tonic' is nonsense. Anaemia is either present in a measurable degree or it is not and it is easy to carry out tests to discover this, so iron should not be given unless tests have been done (unless one is living in the backwoods without even the simple apparatus necessary to do them). Neurosis and boredom are the common causes of undue fatigue and they will not of course be affected by iron; fatigue genuinely due to anaemia argues a quite profound degree of the condition. (3) *Iron, if given during meals need not upset the stomach and, if it does, it is usually possible to avoid this by the use of another preparation without additions.* It is extremely doubtful whether there are really many people who have a 'tendency to anaemia' requiring frequent courses of iron and certain that if they do there is something else wrong with them. Iron turns the motions black and in some may lead to constipation (*see* Anaemia).

Irrigation: the washing-out of a cavity or wound by large amounts of water, with or without other substances added.

Ischaemia: lack of blood to a part of the body caused by spasm of the blood-vessels, an embolism, or a clot which has formed on the spot.

Ischiorectal Abscess: an abscess between the rectum and the ischium bone of the pelvis often leading to fistula (q.v.).

Ischium: the lower and rear bone of the pelvis on which one sits.

Ishihara Test: a Japanese test for colour-blindness used in this country as the standard test for the fighting forces. It consists of several plates illustrated with a large number of spots in different colours; these are arranged in patterns which cannot be seen by the colour-blind and others which appear to the colour-blind but not to those with normal vision.

Iso-Immunisation: the immunisation of an individual by an antigen lacking in himself but present in other normal beings, e.g. the immunisation of an Rh-negative mother by an Rh-positive foetus which causes the mother to produce anti-Rh agglutinins which harm the foetus (*see* Icterus Neonatorum Gravis, Rh factor).

Isolation: is used for those suffering from infectious diseases and those who have been in contact with them (*see* Infection, Incubation Period).

Isoniazid: a drug used effectively in the treatment of tuberculosis; it is the official name for isonicotinic acid hydrazide, known for many years but only fairly recently found to be curative in tuberculosis. It is given by mouth and relatively non-toxic but, like streptomycin, tends to produce resistant strains of organism. This tendency is greatly reduced if it is given in conjunction with streptomycin or P.A.S. (para-aminosalicylic acid). Two interesting facts about isoniazid are firstly, that unlike most new drugs it is a simple chemical substance easily manufactured in the laboratory, and secondly, that its effect in improving the mood of tuberculous patients led to the discovery of the closely-related iproniazid (Marsalid) one of the new monoamine oxidase inhibitors which has a remarkable effect in psychiatric cases suffering from severe depression. However, the tendency of Marsalid to cause severe toxic jaundice in 1 in 250 cases has led to its partial replacement by Marplan (isocarboxazid) which is safer if slightly less effective.

Isotonic: solutions which have the same osmotic pressure, i.e. which will not bring about diffusion one into another. A 'normal' salt solution containing 80 grains of sodium chloride to the pint will not draw fluid from surrounding tissues nor be absorbed into them, being isotonic. On the other hand, *hypertonic* solutions will withdraw fluid from tissues and *hypotonic* solutions will be drawn into them until both become isotonic. Isotonic glucose is 5% in water.

Isotope: broadly speaking isotopes are elements with the same physical and chemical properties for most practical purposes but different atomic weights. Thus in the case of hydrogen (atomic weight 1) the isotopes are deuterium (atomic weight 2), and tritium (atomic weight 3) although all three are 'hydrogen' in the everyday sense. Radioactive isotopes are used in medicine both for investigation and in the treatment of disease.

Itch: a popular name for Scabies (*see* Parasites).

Itching: (see Pruritis).

Jaborandi: the leaves of a South American plant containing the alkaloid pilocarpine (q.v.).

Jacksonian Epilepsy: localised epileptic attacks usually without loss of consciousness named after the great British neurologist Hughlings Jackson (*see* Epilepsy).

Jalap: a powerful purgative obtained from the tuber of a Mexican plant but now rarely used.

Jaundice: or Icterus is the yellow to bronze coloration of the skin and mucous membranes (including the whites of the eyes) caused by the presence of abnormal amounts of bile pigment (bilirubin) in the blood (*see* Bile). Bilirubin is a product of the breakdown of haemoglobin from spent cells which is normally separated within the liver into iron to be stored and bilirubin which is excreted in the bile. Jaundice is therefore brought about: (1) by interference with the excretion of bile which is then reabsorbed into the blood; (2) by abnormal destruction of the red cells within the blood-vessels; or (3) by severe damage to the liver resulting in liberation of the bilirubin within the liver cells into the bloodstream. The first is known as *obstructive jaundice* and caused by anything blocking the bile passages (i.e. either the hepatic ducts from the liver or the common bile duct below the point of entry of the cystic duct from the gall-bladder). This may be a calculus or stone, a tumour, stenosis or narrowing, or inflammation, the latter being known as catarrhal jaundice and generally resulting from a virus infection occurring in epidemics. *Haemolytic jaundice* is the name given to the second type when the red blood cells have been destroyed in the circulation as in acholuric jaundice and icterus gravis neonatorum; in this type the motions and urine are unchanged in colour and in this respect it differs from the clay-coloured stools and dark yellow urine of obstructive jaundice where the bile cannot get into the intestines to give the motions their normal colour. *Toxic jaundice* as in acute yellow atrophy of the liver is caused by germs (yellow fever) or poisons such as phosphorus, chloroform, carbon tetrachloride, etc. Most cases of jaundice are of the obstructive type (*see* Bile, Gall-bladder, Liver, and the diseases mentioned). Jaundice is therefore a symptom rather than a disease and its cause must be dealt with first; gall-stones may have to be removed, but the treatment thereafter and for all types of jaundice is symptomatic. The diet should be low in fat but with adequate amounts of carbohydrate and protein and the itching of the skin which is a common problem may have to be dealt with by sedatives or anti-histamine drugs and calamine lotion with 2% phenol or a cortisone spray. Dyspepsia can be dealt with by the usual measures.

Jaundice, Epidemic: (*see* Hepatitis).

Joint Diseases: points are classified into movable and

335

immovable, the latter being those such as connect the bones of the skull or the teeth in their sockets whilst the former are further subdivided into perfect and imperfect. The best example of a movable perfect joint is the knee where the articular surfaces fit together closely but comfortably and, in this case, their cartilaginous surfaces are further separated by interarticular plates of cartilage (the semilunar cartilages). The joint is enclosed in a synovial membrane forming a closed sac containing a sticky lubricating material called synovial fluid. Outside this is a covering of fibrous tissue known as the capsular ligament and other sacs formed from synovial membrane develop at points where the joint is subjected to pressure, (e.g. the prepatellar bursa which becomes inflamed in 'housemaid's knee'). An imperfect joint is one in which the bones are connected by cartilages or ligaments the flexibility of which alone permits any movement, e.g. the vertebrae of the spinal column which are separated by thick plates of fibro-cartilage. Other types of movable joint defined in terms of the movement they permit are ball and socket, gliding, hinge, saddle, and privot. In general the joints most commonly affected by disease are the knee, the hip, ankle, and elbow since these are the most frequently exposed to injury. But even severe injuries of a joint are not as serious as they may appear provided the skin and the joint cavity are not penetrated or broken, but penetrating wounds of joints are amongst the most serious injuries (apart from abdominal injuries or those to vital organs) that can happen. *Synovitis* is the name given to any inflammation of the membrane lining the joint cavity; it may be caused by infection (especially tuberculous in chronic cases) or rheumatic diseases and gout. *Epiphysitis* is inflammation situated at the end of a long bone just outside the joint, the epiphysis being the end of spongy bone forming the terminal knob; since at the inner end of this knob there is a plate of cartilage which is the growing point of the bone, damage here during the early years may permanently affect growth. Gout, Rheumatism, and Arthritis, are dealt with separately. *Sprains* is a loose term implying any sort of twisting injury to a joint. If of moderately severe degree they probably result in a slight outpouring of the synovial fluid into the joint cavity with or without stretching or tearing of the ligaments supporting it outside. *Stiffness* may follow a sprain because of the additional fluid in and around the joint or may be a sign of arthritis in the early stages of spasm of the surrounding muscles. The treatment of such conditions is usually with pain-killing drugs such as aspirin, rest, and heat applied to the joint. Sprains are sometimes treated with injections of local anaesthetic which relieve the pain; strangely enough although the duration of anaesthesia is only about $\frac{1}{2}$–1 hour the pain does not usually return after the injection.

Jugular: the anterior, external and internal jugular veins which convey blood from the head and neck region to the chest.

Kahn Test: is used in the diagnosis of syphilis either in conjunction with, or instead of, the Wassermann reaction. In Britain the W.R. remains the preferred blood-test for syphilis.

Kala-Azar: a tropical disease also known as 'black' or 'dumdum' fever found throughout the tropics but most commonly in India, China, West Africa, and the Sudan; characterised by an enlarged spleen, wasting and irregular fever, and caused by infection with a protozoon carried by the sand-fly. The previous mortality of about 96% has been lowered by treatment with antimony to about 10%. The drug is given in the form of injections of sodium antimony tartrate (tartar emetic), Stibosan (von Heyden 471), or Neo-stibosan. Another type – or possibly the same – is found around the Mediterranean and, being found largely in children, is known as Infantile kala-azar. Kala-azar is an insidious disease which begins with diarrhoea, sweating, irregular fever, bleeding from the nose or gums, and loss of weight. In the later stages there is great emaciation and the skin is pigmented. The causative organism is the protozoon Leishmania donovani, a small oval-shaped body with two nuclei and the disease is one form of Leishmaniasis.

Kaolin: is aluminium silicate powdered and freed from grit. It is used as a dusting-powder (c.f. Fullers' earth), internally in the treatment of diarrhoea, and as kaolin poultice (cataplasma kaolin, Antiphlogistin) which is a mixture of kaolin, boric acid, methyl salicylate, and the oils of peppermint and thymol with glycerine in the treatment of any condition (septic sores, sprains, inflammation) where heat is helpful together with the hygroscopic or 'drawing' action of glycerine. This is by far the cleanest and most effective form of poltice and although it can be heated in the can and spread hot on lint the easiest method is to spread the kaolin on cold and toast the dressing under a grill. The mixture of kaolin and morphia is a favourite in the symptomatic treatment of diarrhoea.

Keloid: (see Cheloid).

Keratin: the substance of which horn, hair, and the surface layer of the skin is composed.

Keratitis: inflammation of the cornea in the front of the eye. This may accompany certain kinds of conjunctivitis or result from unremoved foreign bodies but *interstitial keratitis* in which the substance rather than the surface of the cornea is affected is caused by inherited syphilis. Other possible causes are infection with other organisms, general debility, and possibly local sepsis elsewhere. The dangers of keratitis are from ulceration of the cornea and the formation of opaque patches which seriously interfere with vision; syphilitic keratitis, however, does not lead to ulceration although first appearing from the 7th–20th years when it may be the earliest indication of congenital syphilis. The symptoms of keratitis in general are pain, light-sensitivity (photophobia), an overflow of tears, spasm of the eyelids, and deterioration of vision. Ulceration is readily demonstrated by the use of fluorescin drops and no time should be lost in getting treatment, preferably by an ophthalmologist, once the condition has been diagnosed. The eyes are ordinarily both affected, the corneas being dull and hazy, and the attack may last for several months. Hot compresses, atropine drops, and penicillin ointment are used in treatment as with iritis (q.v.) which usually accompanies the disease. Residual opacities of the cornea can be dealt with by the use of corneal grafts with recovery of full vision and minor scars are cleared up by the use of cortisone eyedrops. Corneal transplants are obtained from an Eye Bank and come from eyes with a healthy cornea removed at operation or from dead bodies; they are satisfactory in over 60% of cases but, of course, do not relieve blindness due to other causes (i.e. they can only help those whose defect is due to corneal scarring, or 1 in 25 of all cases of blindness). The graft is not visible. Cases due to syphilis require intensive treatment for this condition.

Kernicterus: the staining with bile of the basal nuclei of the brain occurring in icterus neonatorum gravis (q.v.) which may lead to toxic degeneration of the nerve cells with resultant disabilities. In 10% of cases the child becomes spastic and mentally defective with an accompanying cirrhosis of the liver. This is one of those interesting conditions many of which have but recently been discovered in which mental defect is due, not to heredity, but to influences operating within the womb during pregnancy, an excellent genetic plan being spoilt by often undetected maternal disease or metabolic defects.

Kernig Sign: is typical of meningitis where, when the thigh is bent at right-angles to the body, the knee cannot be straightened to complete the right-angle and there is great pain upon attempting to do so.

Ketogenic Diet: is a diet containing an excess of fats and a minimum of carbohydrate so that acetone and other ketone bodies appear in the urine. It was once used in the treatment of chronic pyelitis but has now been superseded by antibiotics and sulpha drugs; in epilepsy in children a ketogenic diet sometimes gives good results (attacks cease in about 30% of cases and remain absent even after return to ordinary diet) but in older and more severe cases no change is obtained although there is some hope of improvement in milder ones. Fat meat, butter, cream, and eggs are allowed in abundance whilst bread, sugar, and other carbohydrates are reduced to a minimum. Such a diet should only be carried out on specialist advice since it is not without its risks and drawbacks. Ketones are substances produced by the imperfect oxidation of fats and proteins and ketonuria is typical of severe cases of diabetes.

Khellin: (Benecardin, Viscardan) is obtained from the fruit of a Mediterranean plant which long had a local reputation for the relief of renal colic. It is an antispasmodic used in the treatment of distress due to this cause, e.g. angina pectoris, bronchial asthma, and similar conditions.

Kidneys: the Urinary System: it is essential to life that the waste products of metabolism should be excreted and this is done through the kidneys, the skin, the lungs, and the bowel. With the exception of the waste excreted by the bowel, the gaseous products excreted by the lungs, and the water with a small amount of salt excreted by the skin, the elimination of waste matter is almost entirely the work of the kidneys. These lie in the upper part of the abdomen, one on each side of the vertebral column and from each at the point known as the hilum there emerges a long tube, the ureter, which passes to the upper and rear part of the bladder in the pelvis. The tube leaving the bladder at its underpart is the urethra which carries the urine to the outside. Each kidney is bean-shaped and about 4 inches long and, when sliced longitudinally, thousands of lines can be seen radiating between the hilum and the outer portion or cortex; these are the uriniferous tubules which at the portion near the surface each take the form of a tiny cup or Malpighian corpuscle enclosing a bundle of capillaries (the glomerulus) and then move inwards towards the pelvis of the kidney where the urine collected passes finally into the ureters. Their course is not a straight one as appearance might suggest, for on microscopic examination the tubules are seen to make loops. It was formerly believed that the kidney acted merely as a filter which allowed certain constituents of the blood plasma in the glomeruli to pass through the walls into the tubules, but this is now known to be wrong since the latter actively excrete and urine is not simply a filtrate. In addition to their excretory function, the kidneys control the pH of the blood by excreting acid sodium phosphate in this way keeping the blood more or less alkaline. Any increase of the normal constituents of the blood or the appearance of abnormal ones is dealt with by getting rid of the excess or expelling the foreign substances, e.g. drugs such as bromides, iodides, and arsenic.

The activity of the kidneys depends upon three main factors: the blood-pressure in the capillaries, the rate of the circulation, and the activity of the cells lining the tubules. Thus should the renal arteries dilate bringing more blood to the cortex excretion becomes more active; this happens automatically when the blood-vessels in the skin contract, hence more urine is passed in cold weather. In heart failure on the other hand little urine is passed owing to a fall in general blood-pressure. The work of the tubules is often interfered with by bacterial toxins such as those of scarlet fever, diphtheria, tonsillitis, and typhoid and chronic alcoholism has a similar effect. But the tubules not only excrete; they also absorb. Indeed, of the total amount of 150–200 litres filtered through the glomeruli in 24 hours at least 99% is reabsorbed and when the constituents of the filtrate are classified according to the extent to which this happens, we find some which, being useful to the body, are actively returned (e.g. glucose, potassium, sodium, calcium, and amino-acids), others which simply diffuse out when their concentration in the filtrate exceeds that in the plasma of the blood, and unwanted products which are not returned at all.

When the urine passes down the ureters it is passed in short spurts aided by the contractions of the ureters into the bladder. By the use of a cystoscope (q.v.) passed into the bladder this can be observed and the function of each kidney assessed, especially if the blood has previously been coloured by intravenous injection of such dyes as indigo carmine. The time taken for this to appear at each opening enables the relative efficiency of each kidney to be observed. On the other hand, drugs such as uroselectan similarly injected can outline the kidney to X-ray examination as well as their pelves and ureters. When the bladder is full, or nearly so, the sensory nerves in its walls send a message to the micturition centre in the lower part of the spinal cord initiating the reflex of micturition whereby the bladder muscle contracts and the circular muscle or sphincter at its exit relaxes to allow the urine out. But training enables the higher centres of the brain to inhibit this, at first in the daytime and only later at night, hence control over the latter action takes much longer to develop than the other and some children and young men, especially neurotic ones, wet the bed to quite a late age. Anxiety in general tends to cause frequency which is often mistaken by those who believe in the 'ghost in the machine' theory of the relationship between body and mind for organic disease.

The commonest disease of the kidney is called Bright's disease or nephritis (q.v.) after the physician from Guy's Hospital who in the last century showed the connection between degenerative changes in the kidneys and albumen in the urine. In some cases albuminuria (q.v.) indicates degenerative kidney disease and the same sort of changes interfere with the kidney's ability to excrete water which results in oedema with swelling and puffiness which begins first in the soft or dependent tissues such as the ankles or beneath the eyes. Disease of this nature may lead to uraemia (q.v.) with the accumulation of waste products in the body and ultimately death. Stone in the kidney or renal calculus ('renal' meaning relating to the kidney) is discussed under the heading Renal Calculus. Infections may be tuberculous when the treatment is similar to that of tuberculosis in general, with streptomycin and other drugs, but more commonly infections of the urinary tract are caused by the bacillus coli from the bowels or sometimes they are carried to the kidneys from infections elsewhere – that is to say, the infection may come upwards from the lower urinary passages or from some other part through the blood-stream. Injuries to a kidney are always very serious although less so than formerly and tumours, which are not common, are likely to be congenital cystic disease or a hypernephroma (q.v.); the former may exist without symptoms for many years, the latter is rapidly-growing and malignant. Undue mobility of a kidney is usually part of a general visceroptosis (q.v.) and sometimes leads by kinking of the ureter to hydronephrosis (q.v.).

Amongst the characteristic symptoms of diseases of the urinary system are pain usually in the loins (although this is absent in many kidney diseases and aften present in diseases which have nothing to do with them); much more typical is renal colic with spasms of agonising pain which is intermittent and shoots down from the loins to the groin at the front. Oedema or dropsy, like that found in heart failure, occurs too in nephritis but that of kidney disease is usually worse in the mornings when the circulation is sluggish and more generalised whereas that connected with heart failure is least obvious in the earlier part of the day when the legs have been raised in bed and is always most obvious in the lower parts of the body. One would have to have a very severe degree of heart-failure to produce the swelling of the face and under the eyes which is common in nephritis. Disorders of micturition are shown in frequency of the desire, difficulty in passing urine or inability to control it, pain on urinating, or the passing of larger or smaller amounts of urine than normal with or without abnormal constituents such as blood or pus (*see* Urine). These may be due to bladder, urethral, or ureteric disease, to kidney disease, or to disease of structures outside the system (e.g. enlargement of the prostate gland in men).

Kinaesthetic Sensations: the sensory impulses underlying muscle tension and posture which, sent to the brain, enable it to send out motor impulses controlling and correlating the positions in relation to each other of muscles, groups of muscles, and joints. They are, for example, those impulses by virtue of which one may remain standing or touch the tip of the nose with the eyes shut. Very often the first sign that they are diseased comes from the individual's discovery that he totters when bending over a wash-basin with the eyes closed in order to wash his face.

King's Evil: or scrofula is tuberculosis with swelling of the glands of the neck which in former times was believed to be curable by the touch of the royal hand. The power was claimed by (or imposed upon) the royal houses of England and France and maintained here until the time of the Stuarts but died out under the Hanoverians, although the Stuart claimants practised it during their exile and even during their invasions of the country. This does not necessarily imply that they believed in the power and Charles II, for one, certainly did not.

Kino: is obtained from the dried trunk of the Indian tree Pterocarpus Marsupium and is an astringent owing to its content of tannic acid. It is (or was) used internally for diarrhoea and also as a gargle for a so-called 'relaxed' throat, assuming we believe that such a condition exists.

Kleptomania: the pathological urge to steal objects which are not necessarily, or even usually, wanted. Those who steal compulsively in this way are commonly elderly or middle-aged women of impeccable character who have a compulsion to steal objects which are trivial, useless, and which they would be well able to buy. The unconscious motive is usually a symbolic stealing of love or an attack against the virtuous, dull, or disinterested husband who will be most injured by the publicity given to his wife's shocking behaviour. Kleptomania has, of course, no connection whatever with ordinary shoplifting for which excuses are sometimes made along these lines, nor is it a specific disease entity but rather a symptom of general neurosis or unhappiness.

Knee: the knee-joint is one of the strongest joints in the body and as a hinge-joint is described elsewhere (*see* Joints). The ligaments holding it together are the strong internal and external lateral ligaments, a weaker posterior one, and the very strong patellar one attaching the knee-cap to the front of the tibia. Within the joint are the two crucial ligaments and the two fibrocartilages between the joint surfaces of the tibia and femur at both edges (the semilunar cartilages). The knee is therefore very rarely dislocated, but it is exposed to the risk of wounding and when the inner cavity is affected this can be serious. Tuberculosis also occurs. One of the commonest of the ailments to which the knee is subject is loosening of one or other of the semilunar cartilages, especially the inner one. When this happens the knee is likely to become locked so that the joint can only be moved by forcible straightening and this is liable to be followed by an attack of synovitis with swelling and pain on movement which lasts for some time. The knee may be supported by a suitable bandage or, if necessary, the cartilage may be partially removed by a surgical operation.

Knee-Jerk: (*see* Nervous System).

Knock Knee: (genu valgum) a condition in which the knees are close together and the feet widely separated. In infants it is usually the result of rickets which is now a rare disease. Knock-knee sometimes results from injury to the femur or thigh-bone such as a fracture and in this case an operation may be necessary to correct the deformity. In this the prominent part of the lower end of the femur on the inner side is cut away. Knock-knee is the opposite of bow-legs.

Koilonychia: spoon-shaped finger-nails, sometimes resulting from prolonged anaemia. The nails are usually abnormally brittle.

Kola: the nut of the African tree *kola acuminata* which contains caffeine in about double the amount of that in coffee but approximately the same amount as in tea. Figures are: tea 3–5%, kola 3%, coffee 1·3%, and maté (Paraguay tea) 0·5%. Kola is used as a beverage in Africa and in minerals elsewhere but has no medical applications (*see* Caffeine).

Koplik's Spots: these are bluish-white spots appearing in the mouth on the inner surface of the cheeks in cases of measles. They appear about the third day and prior to the generalised rash on the body.

Korsakof's (Korsakow's) Syndrome: a mental disorder occurring in toxic states resulting from both organic and inorganic poisons and frequently associated with polyneuritis. Its typical features are: poor memory for recent events, a tendency to fabricate (i.e. to invent tales of non-existent happenings in order to make up for memory blanks), and disorientation for time, place, and person, e.g. the patient does not recognise the doctor nor does he know where he is or the date or what he was doing the day before, but may make up for this loss by addressing the doctor by another name and giving a long and circumstantial account of a fictitious visit to London that very morning although he may have been in the hospital for many weeks. The commonest toxin is alcohol and this is one of the many forms that may be taken by chronic alcoholism, but other poisons such as lead and bacterial toxins in typhoid and malaria may be responsible. The outlook depends on the initial cause but, by and large, a considerable measure of recovery is likely in a few weeks with concentrated vitamin therapy (particularly those of the B group since this is partly a vitamin deficiency disease brought about by defective absorption or intake resulting from the poison). However, complete recovery is likely to take a long time and in many cases there remains a varying degree of memory defect and emotional deterioration evidenced by an easy suggestibility, emotional facility, and lack of efficiency.

Krameria: or Rhatany is the root of a South American plant which has much the same astringent action as kino due to its tannic acid content.

Kummell's Disease: results from an undiagnosed crush fracture of a vertebra, the patient complaining of backache, stiffness, and varying degrees of deformity.

Kupffer Cells: the star-shaped cells in the liver which are responsible for the breakdown of haemoglobin into the bile pigments. They form part of the reticulo-endothelial system (q.v.).

Kyphosis: a pathological curvature of the spine in which the concavity of the curve is directed forward, i.e. hunchback.

Labium: part of the vulva or female genitals (*see* Vulva).

Labour: in animals and most primitive races labour or parturition is not a great problem. In the animals this is due to anatomical differences but there can be little doubt that, whatever anatomical differences may be present, the relative ease with which primitive peoples bring forth children is in the main due to (*a*) better muscular development which is associated with a more active life, and (*b*) a different psychological attitude to pregnancy and childbirth. Many modern women secretly resent their role or have been adversely affected by tales of the terrors of labour and the resulting tension may lead to difficulties. That this is so is shown by the good results obtained by hypnosis or relaxation therapy of the Grantly Dick Read type which would hardly result if the problem was purely one of structure. When pregnancy has lasted, more or less, for 280 days the contractions of the uterus known as labour pains begin. Why this should occur at a specific time is unknown although many factors, taken singly or collectively, have been mentioned including distension of the uterus or womb, the accumulation of carbon dioxide in the blood, degenerative changes in the placenta (the large plate of tissue by which the child is attached through the umbilical cord to the wall of the womb), and the actions of hormones produced in the foetus, placenta, or pituitary gland at the base of the skull. However, the pains initiate the act of expelling the child from the womb. Labour is divided into three stages: (1) the child is lying head downwards in the womb surrounded by the amniotic fluid and enclosed within the cellophane-like membranes and as the contractions proceed the opening of the womb or cervix which projects into the upper part of the vagina begins to dilate, the process being aided by the thrusting forward of a part of the membranes like a finger of a rubber glove into the space. Soon the pressure and the stretching causes the membranes to burst and with a rush of clear fluid mingled with blood to the outside the first stage ends. (2) The head of the baby now takes the place of the membranous projection and is thrust downwards first through the cervix which stretches even more widely and then through the vagina itself. The contractions become stronger, more frequent and prolonged, and the abdominal muscles begin to play a part until the child is finally expelled. Sometimes in a so-called breech presentation the buttocks present first and this, if not diagnosed earlier, will lead to difficulties unless the child is turned round. The third stage of labour consists in the expulsion of the placenta and the membranes when, after a resting-period of 20–30 minutes, the contractions begin again until they, too, have been expelled and the mother is able to rest whilst the nurse attends to the cleaning-up of the baby and its comfort. Most pregnancies would terminate normally even in the absence of skilled help, but obviously it is desirable for a trained midwife to assist what is, after all, a normal process. As soon as the child is born and before the third stage begins the umbilical cord binding it to the placenta in the mother will have to be tied and cut and the usual lusty yells which begin immediately after birth help to establish the unfamiliar process of breathing. Apart from breech presentations ($3\frac{1}{2}\%$ of all cases), there may be face presentations (0·4% of cases) or the rather rare cross presentation in which the child is lying transversely across the womb and the pelvis. These, like the breech presentation, require skilled attention. The great dangers of the peurperium (the period after childbirth in the mother) are haemorrhage and sepsis. Post-partum haemorrhage can be dangerous and occasionally fatal but now it is nearly always controllable. Immediate measures to deal with it are compression of the womb which has not contracted down sufficiently through the abdominal wall and the administration of very hot vaginal douches with injections of ergometrine or pituitrin. A very common source of bleeding in the weeks just before labour which creates difficulties during it is placenta praevia in which the placenta is situated too low down in the womb sometimes completely blocking the exit of the cervix. Sepsis was formerly a very grave condition and many mothers died of 'child-bed fever' before the Viennese physician Semmelweiss was able to show its connection with faulty hygiene in the early 19th century and with the advent of the sulpha drugs and the antibiotics it is almost a thing of the past in civilised communities.

Lachesine: is a mydriatic to dilate the pupils and sometimes used in place of atropine when a shorter-acting drug is required as for examination of the retina.

Lachrymal Apparatus: the system concerned with the secretion, storing and absorption of tears (*see* Eye).

Lactation: the period during which the infant is suckled at the breast. The secretion of milk is initiated by the pituitary gland but affected both by the infant's sucking and the mother's emotions. Hence emotional upset or inadequate stimulus from the child causes the flow to dry up. If the child is not to be breast-fed the flow must be stopped by the administration of ovarian hormones otherwise painful engorgement or even abscess-formation will result.

Lactic Acid: is made by the fermentation of milk-sugar or lactose by a bacterium as in the souring of milk. Muscular fatigue results from the accumulation of lactic acid in the muscle cells. Sour milk in the form of koumiss (originally produced from mare's milk) or yogourt is a healthy form of food as also is cream cheese which contains lactic acid too but the exaggerated claims made earlier in this century by the Russian Metchnikoff concerning its alleged effects in prolonging life are nonsensical.

Lactose: milk-sugar.

Laevulose: one of the constituents of grape-sugar or dextrose.

Lambliasis: lamblia intestinalis are single-celled organisms with flagellae (i.e. whip-like appendages for propelling themselves along). The organism was introduced to this country from the Middle East during both wars and sometimes, although by no means always, gives rise to diarrhoea with loss of appetite. In children the motions may be large and pale from undigested fats and wasting or dwarfism may occur in the very young as in coeliac disease (q.v.). Lambliasis is readily cured by a brief course of mepacrin.

Lamellae: are tiny confetti-like discs of glycerine impregnated with a drug for applying to the eye where they dissolve when placed behind the lower lid. The official lamellae contain atropine, homatropine, physostigmine, cocaine, and penicillin.

Lameness: (*see* Gait, Joints).

Laminectomy: when operating upon the spinal cord it is first necessary to remove parts of the arches of the overlying vertebrae and this operation is known as laminectomy. Thus pressure from a fracture may be removed or a tumour dissected out.

Lanolin: is obtained from sheep's wool and used as a base for ointments because it does not go rancid and can penetrate the skin as mineral substances cannot. Lanolin is capable of absorbing and mixing with water.

Laparotomy: the opening of the abdominal cavity either as an exploratory operation or as the initial stage of further surgery.

Laryngismus Stridulus: a term applied to a condition of spasm of the glottis or larynx each attack lasting some seconds and ending in a long crowing inspiration. It is a manifestation of rickets and therefore rare being part of the nervous complications of that disease to which the name spasmophilia has been applied. Treatment is as for rickets.

Laryngitis: acute simple laryngitis may occur as a symptom of the common cold, as an early sign of measles, from irritation of the throat by harmful dusts or vapours, or by misuse of the voice. It is characterised by redness of the vocal cords with production of mucus, a harsh or hoarse voice, a feeling of 'rawness,' slight fever, and an irritating cough which is, and remains, dry. A danger in children is descending infection. The condition is usually quickly relieved by resting the voice, a suitable linctus, inhalations, and hot applications to the neck. Chronic laryngitis results from irritants, over-smoking, prolonged coughing as in bronchitis, or faulty voice production (it should be noted that mere unwillingness to use the voice even when unconscious may produce similar results by causing the patient to use his voice in an unnatural way). The 'diplomatic sore throat' of public figures may sometimes be a diplomatic lie, but it is often one told by the sufferer to himself. In a few cases laryngitis is a manifestation of syphilis or tuberculosis.

Laryngoscope: the laryngoscope is a long stem with a small round mirror placed at one end at an angle of about 120 degrees. The beam from a light at the patient's side reflected from a mirror on the doctor's forehead into the throat, or a direct light from the doctor, enables him to see the vocal cords in the mirror when placed at the back of the throat.

Larynx: the larynx is a fairly rigid framework of cartilages held together by ligaments and moved by attached muscles. It is lined with mucous membrane which is continuous above with that of the throat and below with that of the trachea or windpipe. It is the organ which, on the outside of the neck, forms the lump known as the Adam's apple and its chief functions are speech (brought about by the movement of air through its passage while the vocal cords narrow or widen its aperature), breathing (since when the vocal cords are opened air passes up and down on its way to and from the lungs), and the protective function which by the lid-like action of the epiglottis prevents food going down the wrong way. Apart from the conditions mentioned elsewhere, the three main categories of disease in the larynx are obstruction, paralysis, and tumour.

The commonest causes of obstruction are abscess formation of the lining of the laryngeal cartilage (perichondritis),

349

croup, acute infections of the throat or floor of the mouth, injuries or wounds, foreign bodies, burns from scalding liquids or steam, and irritation from harmful vapours. *Obstruction* begins suddenly and progresses quickly; there is difficulty in breathing, pallor, restlessness, and later cyanosis (blueness). Treatment must be immediate and if the cause can be removed this must be done at once. But when life is threatened and the cause cannot be removed, tracheotomy must be performed as quickly as possible. In this operation an incision is made low in the front of the neck cutting three rings of the trachea, a tube is inserted and the bleeding points tied. The tube must be anchored to the neck by tapes and relief is almost immediate. Later, when the cause has been dealt with the opening can be closed and breathing once more takes place in the ordinary way. *Paralysis* of one vocal cord causes hoarseness and change in the voice, but when both are paralysed and relax towards the midline breathing in, although not breathing out, is severely affected. This may be caused by bulbar poliomyelitis (poliomyelitis of the base of the brain), injury to the nerves supplying the larynx (occasionally during surgical removal of the thyroid gland), and cancer of the thyroid, oesophagus, or neck glands involving the laryngeal nerves. When both cords are paralysed an operation can sometimes be done to fix one in an open position thus relieving the situation. *Tumours of the larynx* are relatively common and it is a general rule that *anyone who is hoarse for more than two weeks should forthwith see a doctor*. Most laryngeal tumours are benign but nevertheless these must be removed and cancerous growths, commonest in men over the age of fifty, will require both operation and X-ray therapy. The latter seem to be associated with the excessive use of tobacco, overuse of the voice, and the habit of drinking too hot liquids. Both partial and complete laryngectomy are performed in this type of case and although the complete operation necessitates breathing through a hole in the neck for the rest of the patient's life, quite a good voice may be achieved without a larynx.

Lassar's Paste: a paste used in the treatment of dermatitis and composed of zinc oxide and starch in 'Vaseline' Brand Petroleum Jelly with a small amount of salicylic acid added. It is soothing, softening, and antiseptic.

Lathyrism: a disease caused by eating vetch seeds or varieties of chick-pea. There is pain in the loins and spastic paralysis of the legs.

Laudanum: tincture of opium.

Laughing-Gas: nitrous oxide gas, used in dental and other short operations.

Lavage: washing-out of the stomach for severe alcoholic intoxication or in chronic gastritis (for Colonic lavage *see* Enema).

Laxatives: (*see* Constipation).

Lead: like most metals lead is only poisonous in the form of its soluble salts and used to be important because of the relative frequency of poisoning both in industry and from lead water-pipes. But now that few paints contain lead and water-pipes are carefully supervised poisoning is uncommon. Its earliest symptoms are abdominal colic and constipation and subsequently there is anaemia, a blue line on the gums, neuritis with wrist-drop or foot-drop, optic neuritis with blindness, and insanity of a specific type (*see* Korsakof's Psychosis). Acute poisoning is rarer still and usually due to lead acetate solution which causes burning in the mouth, colic, thirst, and vomiting leading to cramps in the legs and convulsions. The treatment is administration of ammonium chloride and parathormone. In medicine lead is little used, although lead lotion (Goulard's water q.v.) is still popular for sprains and itching of the skin. Lead also causes abortion.

Leaders: a popular name for tendons or sinews.

Leber's Disease: or hereditary optic atrophy is inherited and comes on about the age of 20 leading to total blindness.

Lecithin: a complex fat found in large amounts in the brain and nerves as well as in the yolk of eggs.

Leeches: the medical leech was formerly used to reduced congestion in headaches, congestion of the lungs, etc. It is worm-shaped and has a sucker for a mouth at one end armed with three teeth with which it breaks the skin and sucks blood.

Left-Handedness: or mancinism is a much more deep-rooted and all-pervading problem than is usually thought. Being due to dominance of the right side of the brain rather than the left as is usual in right-handed people, it is not merely a matter of a preference for the left over the right hand; for such people are often 'left-eyed' too and their natural tendency to read from right to left and even to produce mirror-writing

351

(i.e. writing which is wholly reversed and can only be read by its reflection in a mirror) may result in considerable retardation in learning to read and often unhappiness and frustration. In a world of right-handed people the left-handed person is at a disadvantage when it comes to opening bottles, playing cricket or golf, and in numerous everyday situations. It is difficult to believe that there can be any harm in causing such a child to use its right hand from the earliest days, but it is equally difficult to believe that it does much good and, of course, although the *fact* of so training him is harmless it is likely to be carried out in a spirit of annoyance on the part of the parent and resentment on the part of the child which is bad for both. Nor is the tendency 'cured' and such a child, no matter how competent he has become with his right hand will in moments of tiredness be found reading MAT as TAM. Probably the best solution is to allow the child his left-handedness (making it clear that it is not regarded as an abnormality) and in later years encouraging him to become equally proficient with his right hand as a right-handed person would with his left when suffering from an injury to his normally-used hand or wrist. Left-handedness is occasionally associated with stammering and squint but it is probably true to say that it is equally often associated with exceptional achievement.

Leg: the lower limb is attached to the pelvis by the strong muscles of the gluteal region (i.e. the seat), the hamstring muscles behind the thigh, and the abductor muscles on its inner side. The femur or thigh-bone is the longest and largest bone in the body which articulates with the pelvis at the hip-joint where its ball-shaped end fits into the cup known as the acetabulum; at the lower end it articulates with the upper surface of the tibia of the leg proper. Along the outer side of the tibia lies the long, thin, fibula (the name means a pin) which does not articulate with the femur at the top but together with the lower end of the tibia helps to form the ankle joint below (the two bumps on either side of the ankle are formed by the fibula on the outer side and the tibia on the inner). The tarsal bones are seven in number and form the rear part of the foot with calcaneus as the heel and the astragalus taking the main weight from the tibia and fibula. As in the hand the metatarsal bones are five and each toe has three phalanges except the big toe which has two. The body is kept erect and the leg straightened by the quadriceps extensor muscle in front of the thigh which is attached to the knee-cap or patella. The muscles of the calf (gastrocnemius) which are attached to the heel by the tendon Achilles raise the heel from the ground in walking and in front of and to the outer side of the leg the tibial and peroneal muscles bend the ankle upwards and raise the toes. The toes are bent downwards by the small muscles of the foot (see Foot). The main blood-supply to the leg is through the femoral artery which, entering the limb at the middle of the groin, passes down the inside of the thigh to the back of the knee where it becomes the popliteal artery. Just below the knee this divides into the anterior and posterior tibial vessels, the first of which passes down the front of the leg to the top of the foot, the other down the back of the leg beneath the external projection of the ankle (malleolus) where it can be felt as a pulse. The veins are mostly deep within the tissues and lie alongside the corresponding arteries, but the superficial ones pass into the saphenous vein which can be felt and seen passing up the inner side of the leg and thigh to enter the femoral vein at the groin. The chief nerve is the sciatic nerve in the middle of the back of the thigh which divides into internal and external popliteal nerves, the former running down the back of the leg to the foot, the latter passing round the top of the fibula to the side of the leg.

Leiomyoma: a tumour of unstriped muscle fibres, i.e. the muscles of the internal organs.

Leishmaniasis: a group of diseases, notably kala-azar (q.v.), infantile kala-azar, and tropical sore, caused by protozoa of the Leishmandonovan type.

Lemon: is used as a source of vitamin C, its juice containing 60 mgm of ascorbic acid per 100 grams. The vitamin can be obtained of course from many other sources or from tablets ('redoxon') and is the main reason for using lemon medically, although hot lemon drinks promote sweating during a cold (why this is supposed to be a benefit is another matter!) Lemon juice is *not* slimming whatever the bottlers say.

Lempert Operation: the fenestration (q.v.) procedure for deafness.

Lens: the lens of the eye (q.v.) by its bulging or flattening brought about by the ciliary muscle causes the image to be correctly focused on the retina whatever the distance of the object. The lens loses some of its elasticity from the forties onwards and glasses are often needed for reading. Cataract (q.v.) is a disease of the lens.

Lenticular Degeneration, Progressive: a familial disease starting in youth and associated with degeneration of the basal nuclei at the base of the brain and cirrhosis of the liver. There are tremors, muscular weakness, spastic paralysis and contractures together with difficulty in swallowing or speaking and mental deterioration. It is progressive and fatal in a few years.

Leprosy: occurs especially in India and China, the West Indies, and South Africa. Its highest incidence in Europe is in Iceland and the disease was once common in other countries. The bacillus leprae in many ways resembles that of tuberculosis being 'acid fast' and forming typical nodules of granulomatous tissue containing the organism. The two main types of leprosy are the nodular or lepromatous and the neural or anaesthetic. In the former there are repeated attacks of fever and reddish swellings on the face which gradually harden and become painful spreading until they coalesce in areas which are insensitive to touch. The ears, face, inside the nose, forearms and thighs become involved and in the late stage the face is 'leonine' in appearance (i.e. round, puffy, the eyes sunken in the swollen tissues, the nose flattened). There is also ulceration of the tongue, larynx and pharynx, and severe scarring occurs on healing. In the neural type the nerve trunks are first affected and large atrophic patches appear on the buttocks and body which gradually become pale and without feeling. Because of this loss of sensibility ulcers, sores, and finally gangrene of the fingers and toes appear. In treatment isolation is usually necessary although the disease is not very infectious and much of the horror it aroused in former times must have been due to the fact that leprosy persists for a long time, is readily distinguishable, and very disfiguring. The specific has been chaulmoogra oil in the form of injections of sodium or ethyl chaulmoograte, or hydnocarpus oil in the form of sodium hydnocarpate, but more recently the sulphone preparations, allied to the sulpha drugs, e.g. sulphetrone, diasone, promin, etc., have given good results as also has thiacetazone. There is little danger of contracting leprosy, even in a leper colony, provided that intimate personal contact be avoided.

Leptazol: also cardiazol and phrenazol is a respiratory stimulant which later came to be used in the chemical induction of convulsions for the treament of mental illness (*see* Electroconvulsant treatment, Mental Illness). It has been largely replaced by the use of electricity.

Lesion: a non-specific term meaning any disease change whatever in any part of the body.

Lethane: is used in the treatment of head lice (*see* Parasites).

Leucocyte: the white cells of the blood. They are classified as granulocytes or *polymorphonuclear leucocytes* which normally form 70% of the total, and according to their staining reactions are subdivided into neutrophils (65–70%), eosinophils which stain with acid dyes (3%) and basophils which stain with basic dyes (0·5%); *Lymphocytes* (25–30%) are subdivided into small and large; and *monocytes* (5%).

Leucocythaemia: (*see* Leukaemia).

Leucocytosis: an increase in the number of white cells in the blood usually in response to an acute infection.

Leucoderma: a condition of the skin in which patches of white appear often in negroes. The sole harm done is the social embarrassment it causes.

Leucopenia: reduction in the normal number of white cells in the blood.

Leucoplakia: a condition in which the patient, usually a man over 40, develops thickened white patches of the tongue due to hardening and overgrowth of the tissues. The usual causes are sepsis in the mouth, excessive smoking of strong tobacco, alcohol, and syphilis (or, as commonly happens, all four).

Leucorrhoea: abnormal white vaginal discharge (*see* Vagina).

Leucotomy: a brain operation severing in varying degree the connections between the cerebral cortex and the lower centres of the thalamus and hypothalamus. Devised in the 1930's by Moniz of Portugal for the treatment of otherwise incurable mental disease, the operation has taken different forms and varies in the extent of the incision or its locality but there are still those who strongly disapprove of it in spite of an equal or greater number who have made exaggerated claims on its behalf. On the whole the possibility of serious and permanent damage to the mental functions makes it advisable to reserve leucotomy for cases where all other methods have been tried and failed and there is no reasonable hope of spontaneous recovery. A leucotomised patient whose emotions are shallow and behaviour unreliable may be better than a demented one but he has certainly lost something which cannot be recovered. The recent tremendous progress in the drug therapy of such conditions should make one even more cautious about taking irrevocable measures.

Leukaemia: a disease in which the white cells of the blood are greatly increased in number with a corresponding decrease in the number of the red cells; the spleen is enlarged as usually are the lymph glands throughout the body and there are changes in the bone-marrow. According to the type of white cell mainly present the disease is described as (1) lymphatic leukaemia, (2) myeloid or spleno-medullary leukaemia. There also exists an acute form in children and young adults which, however, is rather rare. The granular or polymorphonuclear leucocytes are normally formed by the bone marrow, the lymphocytes by the lymphoid tissue in the lymph glands and spleen and these facts influence the symptoms in each type. *Lymphatic leukaemia* is primarily a disease of later life to old age (40–70) and in this case the disease may go on for 10 years or more with some enlargement of the spleen and considerable enlargement of the lymph glands. There is moderate anaemia and the white cells may be increased to 50,000 or 100,000 per cu. m.m. from the usual 5–6,000. Somewhat different is *myelogenous leukaemia*, occurring between the ages of 25–40 with as its main symptoms enormous enlargement of the spleen, swelling of the abdomen, and shortness of breath. There is usually pallor, occasionally a rash, and a slight intermittent fever often with swelling of the feet, attacks of bleeding from the gums, nose, or bowels, and diarrhoea. In this type the bone-marrow is entirely replaced by greyish-red tissue engaged in the enormous overproduction of polymorphonuclear leucocytes which may number as many as 1,000,000 per cu. m.m., so much so that the blood sometimes becomes greenish-yellow and clotted like pus. No cure has yet been found for leukaemia, nor has its cause been discovered, but acute leukaemia often resembles (although it probably is not) an infection, chronic leukaemia has many of the characteristics of a cancerous condition. The chronic types both respond to X-rays and, even untreated, may be consistent with some years of fair health. Various useful drugs have been discovered: mercaptopurine and cortisone in the acute type and in the chronic types when radiotherapy fails, urethane, busulphan and demecolcine are used for the myeloid form and mustine or tetramine for the lymphoid. Blood transfusion, too, plays an important part in prolonging life. Atomic radiation has been alleged to cause leukaemia, but the real state of affairs is uncertain (*see* Cancer).

Lice: (*see* Parasites).

Lichen Planus: a skin disease consisting of an eruption of small papules, lilac in colour, smooth on the surface and each with a dent at the top. These increase in number and often form a lace-like pattern on the skin which leaves staining behind as it fades. Any part of the body may be affected but most commonly the flexor surfaces of the arms and legs (i.e. the upper surface of the forearm and the front of the legs). There is severe itching. The condition should be treated by a specialist as it can become quite severe but there is no specific treatment and the disease has been attributed to mental stress. Cortisone preparations help as in other itchy skin rashes.

Ligaments: strong flattened bands (occasionally cord-like) which hold the bones together and support them at a joint.

Light Treatment: the ordinary medical lamps sold for use at home ordinarily produce both ultra-violet and infra-red rays. The former give the effect of sunlight, the latter of deep heat. Ultra-violet treatment was regarded by some about thirty years ago as almost a cure-all and the poor man's substitute for treatment in the sunlight of the Alpine sanatoria, but, alas, those days are gone and anybody who believes that ultra-violet rays do anything more than stimulate the skin and produce unnecessary vitamin D by irradiating the ergosterol of the body must be exceptionally credulous. Sunlight, of course, is good and it makes most people look good (often a great deal better than they actually are) but its effects as a *general* stimulant and tonic are largely psychological. Indeed, in an experiment carried out during the war when sun-bathing under ultra-violet lamps was provided for the benefit of industrial workers it was found that everybody who had this treatment felt better than those who had not been given it – but the workers who had been unknowingly exposed to lamps with an invisible screen cutting out all the 'health-giving' rays felt just as well as those who had been given the real thing.

Infra-red rays are those emitted by an ordinary hot body of any sort, e.g. a coal or electric fire; they penetrate sometimes to a depth of 1 inch and increase the blood-flow to the part. Hence they are used in muscular and rheumatic pains and are quite as effective as heat from an ordinary fire or a hot-water bottle, but not markedly more so. Really deep penetration requires a diathermy apparatus. Ultra-violet rays by their action in irritating the skin are also sometimes used in rheumatic conditions where they work by a process of counter-irritation but it must be remembered that such rays can be very dangerous and cause severe burning from overexposure. Most 'sunlight lamps' do not produce bronzing of the skin and sunburn as many advertisements claim.

Lignocaine: or xyclocaine is a local anaesthetic.

Linctus: any syrupy medicine, usually a cough-mixture.

Liniments: or embrocations are oily or spirit applications ordinarily rubbed into the surface of the body for muscular or joint pains. Older applications contained such substances as aconite (which is a local anaesthetic and very poisonous), belladonna, camphor (camphorated oil), and methyl salicylate, but with the exception of the last these are little used today, being both messy and poisonous. Most proprietary applications contain salicylates, presumably because of their association with rheumatism when taken internally, but the real function of a liniment is to increase the blood-supply to the part and soothe by warmth and counter-irritation. Demands are frequently made of the doctor for a 'strong' liniment but there is no evidence that these are much more effective than the milder ones and they may cause quite a severe rash on the skin. Some proprietary preparations claim to penetrate the skin bringing derivatives of nicotinic acid and salicylates into contact with the affected area, but there is little proof that they do so and even less that, if they did, the effect would be beneficial. For practical purposes lin. methyl. sal. is probably the best and safest and some of the proprietary preparations equally good and certainly cleaner, most of them being in the form of creams which have the further advantage of not being liable to be swallowed by mistake. The so-called 'horse oils' are best left to horses.

Lipoma: a fatty non-malignant tumour.

Lips: there are not many disorders to which lips are subject, but amongst the commonest are *fissures* and *cracks* which, although they often appear in cold weather are frequently associated with septic conditions of the mouth (this is particularly the case when the corners of the mouth are affected). Ordinary remedies can be tried, but if they prove inadequate it may be necessary to cauterise the fissures with silver nitrate. *Herpes simplex*, not to be confused with herpes zoster, is commonly called a cold sore and may be painted with 'new skin' or collodion which protects it but does not cure the condition which departs spontaneously. *Ulcers* on the inner surface of the lips are another sign of a mouth infection and should be treated accordingly, but any form of *septic sore or boil* must be regarded seriously since the infection can be carried into the skull and therefore the doctor should be seen. Of more serious conditions *hare-lip* is dealt with under Palate, and *cancer*, usually of the lower lip in elderly men (since women stopped smoking dirty pipes) is dealt with under Cancer.

Liquorice: the peeled or unpeeled root and underground stem of glycyrrhiza glabra common in S. Europe and Asia. Used in sweets and, in medicine, to cover the bad taste of other drugs, e.g. cascara sagrada. Recently it has become prominent in the treatment of peptic ulcer.

Lithotrity: the operation of crushing a stone in the bladder by an instrument passed along the urethra so that the fragments can be passed in the urine (also known as litholapaxy). A *lithagogue* is a drug which supposedly helps stones to pass out and *lithontriptics* are drugs which allegedly dissolve stones. No such substances exist although fortunes have been made in selling those which purport to do so. The *lithotomy* position in an operation is one in which the patient lies on his back with the legs held up in the air and bent at the knee in order that the surgeon may reach the perineum to remove the stone. These numerous names derive from the 18th century when 'cutting for the stone' was one of the few operations, apart from amputations, that doctors could do successfully. In fact, there was even a special class of surgeon expert in the operation and described as a *lithotomist*; from which we may deduce either that stone was much more common then than it is now or that many non-existent ones must have been removed.

Little's Disease: or congenital cerebral diplegia was formerly

359

thought to be a birth injury but is best regarded as a generic title for a group of diseases of various origins due in most cases to defective formation of the brain. Nothing is noticed at first but the child is backward, sitting up late and walking with difficulty if at all. The legs are stiff and rigid and cross-legged or 'scissors gait' as it is called is common. Fits and increasingly obvious mental deficiency make their appearance. Some cases improve greatly but in most there is progressive deterioration and generally death from some otherwise minor infection.

Liver: the liver is the largest gland in the body lying mainly on the right-hand side of the body beneath the ribs but extending slightly over the midline to the left side. It is lobulated, being made up of an immense number of units of glandular substance each about 1/16th of an inch in diameter and consisting of a number of cells clustered around a group of blood-vessels and bile capillaries. The blood-vessels are those coming from the portal vein which brings substances absorbed in the process of digestion from the intestines and their plasma bathes the cells of the organ. Eventually this plasma and blood passes into another system which finally becomes the hepatic veins flowing into the inferior vena cava, the main vein of the body. Bile formed in the liver cells similarly is gradually collected by ever larger capillaries until it passes into the bile ducts (*see* Gall-bladder). Bile is both an excretion and a secretion, i.e. it not only is a means of getting rid of waste in the form of the pigments bilirubin and biliverdin which result from the breakdown of the haemoglobin of spent red blood cells but is also an aid to the digestion, particularly of fats. Hence any interference with its flow tends to produce indigestion and flatulence in the bowels. Amongst the more important functions of the liver are: (1) the production of bile. (2) The neutralisation of poisons absorbed from the alimentary canal, e.g. bacterial toxins, drugs, and alcohol. The liver is therefore always of great interest to the pathologist in cases of alleged poisoning, and when it is damaged (as in chronic alcoholism) the body may lose its power to detoxicate drugs so that barbiturates and other substances are less well toxicated. Cirrhosis of the liver is an example of this and acute yellow atrophy occurs when the defences are completely overwhelmed as with severe degrees of phosphorus or chloroform poisoning. (3) The liver keeps the level of sugar and other substances at a constant level in the blood, storing excess glucose from the alimentary canal as glycogen or animal starch which is broken down equally rapidly when sugar is required; it is a sugar store. (4) The major part of the urea and uric acid excreted by the kidneys is formed in the liver as by-products of protein breakdown both from the food and the breaking-down of body tissues. (5) The liver is like a great sponge and can therefore store a large amount of blood; this it pours out when there has been loss of blood or retains when there is risk of over-distension of the heart by too much blood (in cases of heart-failure the liver is enlarged). (6) It has the function of breaking-down the old blood-cells, retaining their iron for further use, and expelling the rest in the bile.

Liver Diseases: since the liver plays such an important part in the economy of the body it is obvious that many troubles may theoretically befall it but fortunately these are minimised by the fact that unlike other tissues it is capable of regeneration and the amount of liver tissue is always in vast excess of what is needed. In fact extraordinarily few diseases are primarily liver conditions although there are many in which the liver is secondarily affected if not commonly to an extent which makes itself felt. Thus there is no reason to think that there is really such a state as being 'liverish' as one class of Englishmen and all Frenchmen seem to suppose when an evening of ill-chosen food or too much drink leads to gastritis where, of course, the stomach and not the liver is affected. Some people are unduly impressed when vomit contains bile and believe this to be an infallible sign that the liver is affected; but anyone who has vomited the contents of his stomach must inevitably if he vomits again produce the contents of his duodenum which are likely to contain bile – that is, if the liver is working properly. Bile in the vomit is a sign that the liver is doing its usual work. So we must consign 'liverishness' and 'biliousness' if not to limbo, at any rate to another category altogether; they are caused by irritation of the stomach. Similarly, in spite of the vast number of potions and pills sold for liver disorders and in spite of the fact that all drugs pass through it, there are very few which significantly influence liver function or disease. There is nothing that in the liver corresponds to the alkalies so freely and satisfactorily

361

given for stomach affections and most medicines designed to influence it are, in fact, cholagogues which increase the flow of bile on the assumption that its retention has some connection with 'biliousness.' But the only effective cholagogues are bile itself, its salts, and magnesium sulphate (Epsom salts) which draws the bile into the intestine as it draws fluids in general by osmosis. These are sometimes given in chronic infections of the gall-bladder or in cirrhosis of the liver but, even so, the value of stimulating the flow of bile is doubtful. *Hepatitis* may be local when the inflammation is caused by a blocked bile-duct or part of a general disease such as malaria, yellow fever, or amoebic dysentery. The commonest type is Epidemic Infective Hepatitis (q.v.) a virus infection. Amoebic dysentery frequently gives rise to *liver abscess* which is treated by drawing out the pus through a needle and the administration of emetine (*see* Dysentery). *Congestion of the liver* occurs obviously in cases of hepatitis and is also a meaningless word synonymous with 'biliousness' but its main form is the passive and often gross congestion of chronic heart-failure and lung diseases in which the flow of blood is impeded. *Fatty degeneration of the liver* is a side effect of some other disease; the fat does not, as used to be thought, come from the diet but is the result of degeneration of the liver cells. The only good reason for avoiding fats in liver disease is that, if the flow of bile is impeded, it will be difficult to digest them – they do not as such do the liver any harm. *Acute yellow atrophy* is very rare and results from the absorption of some poison which may be from without but can also arise within the body as in abnormal pregnancies. It is most common in women and always fatal. *Cirrhosis* of the liver is dealt with in the appropriate section, and *cancer* is nearly always secondary to cancer in other parts. Primary cancer is rare outside Asia.

Liver Extract: known under such proprietary names as Anahaemin, Hepatex, Perihemin, etc., is used in the treatment of pernicious and other macrocytic anaemias (*see* Anaemia). It is useless in ordinary anaemia and is given by intramuscular injection.

Liver-Fluke: (*see* Worms).

Liver Pills: (*see* Cholagogues, Liver Diseases).

Lobectomy: the operation of cutting out a lobe of the lung in such conditions as lung abscess, tuberculosis, and bronchiectasis, or for cysts or tumours. In the more extensive or potentially extensive conditions the whole lung may be removed (pneumonectomy). These are serious operations but operative recovery takes place in 95% of cases of lobectomy and 90% of cases of pneumonectomy.

Lobelia: the dry flowering herb of lobelia inflata, the Indian tobacco which amongst its alkaloids contains lobeline which has the same action as nicotine in increasing the force of ventilation of the lungs and dilating the bronchi. It is used in asthmatic powders for burning in cigarettes, and as an expectorant in asthmatic cough mixtures. Injections of lobeline are sometimes given to stimulate respiration in poisoning or asphyxia from coal gas. Recently it has been used in tablet form by those who wish to stop smoking (*see* Smoking).

Lobotomy: the operation performed in leucotomy (q.v.) which is carried out by cutting the fibres connecting certain areas of the brain for mental disorders or the relief of intractable pain.

Lochia: the discharge from the womb in the one or two weeks following childbirth.

Lockjaw: (*see* Tetanus).

Locomotor Ataxia: or tabes dorsalis is a form of syphilis of the nervous system occurring usually in men after middle-age. Basically the parts affected are the posterior nerve roots (i.e. the points at which the sensory nerves enter the spinal cord), the columns inside the cord in which they ascend to the brain, and to some extent the peripheral sensory nerves. That is to say, there is first inflammation and then degeneration of all the sensory paths. The patient has a history of syphilitic infection and the first sign that the disease has only been lying dormant is likely to be difficulty in passing water, impotence, or 'lightning' pains often in the outer side of the knee or in the calf, heel, or foot. There may be passing attacks of double vision and unsteadiness in the dark or when shutting the eyes to wash the face since the messages that usually give indication of the position of the limbs are unable to pass. The inability to stand with the eyes closed is known as Romberg's sign, and in addition the ankle-jerks and knee-jerks are likely to be absent and there are patches of anaesthesia to pin-prick throughout the body. The patient becomes very clumsy (ataxic) in his gait and later paralysed and bed-ridden, but the disease may either be arrested for quite long periods or kill very quickly. Treatment has been revolutionised by the use of penicillin sometimes supplemented by pyrexial therapy with malaria as in G.P.I. which is the same condition confined largely to the brain.

Lorrain Infantalism: one type of defect arising from under-function of the pituitary anterior lobe. The child does not grow and the secondary sex characters do not appear but the mentality may be normal. The famous Tom Thumb was of this 'miniature adult' type.

Lordosis: a forwards curvature of the spine usually in the lumbar region where the natural curve is in this direction.

Lues: syphilis. (Luetic).

Lugol's Iodine: (*see* Iodides).

Lumbago: pain of rheumatic origin in the lower part of the back. The condition is supposed to be a form of fibrositis in which the connective tissues become inflamed and the blood-vessels dilated with consequent pressure on the nerve-endings and pain, but similar results follow numerous other circumstances, e.g. a pulled muscle, a slipped disc, or even the strain of carrying out some movement to which one is not used and possibly the muscle spasm which results from nervous tension in some parts of the body. The pain may be so severe as to suggest disease of internal organs such as the kidneys which leads to similar sensations but this is easily excluded by the fact that in lumbago no other signs of disease are present. Cold, damp, and the other causes which are usually given for rheumatic diseases are often used to explain the onset of lumbago but it is extremely difficult to see how these could influence the body in any way and we are becoming critical of facile explanations which contradict experience, e.g. we now know for certain and in spite of tradition that colds are not caused in this way and that volunteers can run inadequately clothed in the rain, sleep in wet clothes, do, in fact, all the 'wrong' things and be not a whit the worse. It seems that lumbago is best regarded as a blanket term meaning a pain in the back which can be due to specific causes such as strain or spasm when it is best described as such or to certain unknown causes when the word lumbago may legitimately be used. The treatment, provided no other lesion is found, is aspirin, rest, and heat. Sometimes injections of novocaine are given into tender points.

Lumbar Puncture: the procedure for removing cerebrospinal fluid from the spinal canal in the lumbar region. This is done in order to diagnose disease of the nervous system, to relieve pressure as in meningitis, or to introduce drugs, dyes for X-ray examination, sera, or spinal anaesthetics.

Lumbricus: the roundworm (*see* Worms).

Luminal: the proprietary name devised by Bayer for phenobarbitone.

Lunar Caustic: silver nitrate.

Lungs: the Respiratory System: the respiratory tract includes the nose and naso-pharynx (i.e. the area at the back of the nose and throat), the trachea or windpipe, the bronchi, and the lungs. The whole tract is lined with mucous membrane and some of the cells secrete mucus to keep its surface moist whilst others are ciliated carrying hair-like processes which keep moving foreign particles in the direction of the mouth. The function of the hairs in the nose is to keep out larger particles and its lining is well supplied with blood-vessels which ensure that the air is kept warm as it passes through. If nevertheless particles or irritants enter the lower parts of the tract they are expelled by the reflex of coughing. Thus coughing may be a nuisance but provided it is not merely due to a false alarm as a 'tickle in the throat' the very last thing the doctor wants to do is to stop it – on the contrary, the general purpose of cough-mixtures is to enable the patient to cough to better effect although if it is unnecessary or too exhausting a sedative medicine may be necessary. The trachea is about 4–5 inches long, beginning with the glottis or larynx and ending in the upper part of the chest by dividing into the two bronchi, one to each lung. Each divides and subdivides into smaller branches known as bronchioles and these finally enter the air cells of the lungs which may be likened to the leaves of a tree of which the bronchioles are the small branches, the bronchi the large ones, and the trachea the trunk. The air cells or alveoli have epithelial walls of extreme thinness and are lined with a capillary network where the exchange of gases takes place, carbon dioxide being given out and oxygen taken in. It is the pulmonary artery, the only artery in the body containing venous blood, which brings the used blood to the lungs from the right ventricle and the pulmonary vein, carrying oxygenated blood, which returns it to the left auricle thence to be

365

distributed to the whole body by the left ventricle. Artery and vein together with the bronchus are attached to the hilum of the lung at the upper and inner side. Each lung, divided into several lobes, is surrounded by a double layer of a cellophane-like membrane known as the pleura and ordinarily the two layers slip over each other easily as the lung expands and contracts, but in pleurisy there is inflammation and therefore friction between the two which causes pain and brings about the rubbing sound which the doctor can hear through his stethoscope. The chest is airtight and therefore when it expands, which happens with the raising of the ribs and the lowering of the diaphragm, air is drawn in to the air passages. Expiration is brought about by a dimunition of the capacity of the chest by depressing the ribs and raising the diaphragm which normally takes place as a result of the natural elasticity of the tissues. This being the mechanism of breathing, any breech in the airtight box of the chest will result in the lungs collapsing, a fact which is made use of in creating an artificial pneumothorax for collapsing a lung to allow it to rest in certain chest diseases, but which causes trouble when wounds of the chest result in an unintentional collapse. Although most of the work of the lungs is done passively, the bronchi and bronchioles are surrounded by a thin layer of muscle and so are able to expand and contract and many cough-mixtures contain drugs to cause dilation to ease the breathing; this is especially necessary in the case of asthma which results in muscular spasm of the bronchioles. The act of breathing can, of course, be voluntarily speeded up or slowed down to a certain extent, but primarily it is automatically controlled by the breathing centre in the medulla at the point where the brain meets the spinal cord. Here, when the carbon dioxide content of the blood increases, breathing is speeded up to get rid of it, and slowed down again as the content decreases.

Lung Diseases: these are mostly dealt with under their ordinary names, e.g. Bronchitis, Colds, Emphysema, Pleurisy, Pneumonia, Tuberculosis, but those not so discussed are included here. *Abscesses* are not common but usually result from one of three causes: pneumonia which has failed to clear up, wounds, or the inhaling of foreign bodies down the air passages. Sometimes they burst into a bronchus and pus is spat up with resultant healing of the condition but most often, after diagnosis, the abscess has to be opened and antibiotics given. *Congestion of the lungs* is a popular term for pneumonia but it is more appropriately applied to hypostatic congestion of the base of the lungs (*see* Hypostasis) in old or weak people. *Collapse of the lung* happens (when not carried out intentionally in pneumothorax) following a wound, or when fluid is formed within the pleural cavity, or if a bronchus is blocked by secretion or a foreign body. The treatment depends on the cause, but with its removal the lung soon fills up once more. *Lung cancer* has become increasingly frequent and was responsible for 18,186 deaths in England and Wales in the year 1956 contrasted with 13,953 deaths from cancer of the stomach and 8,580 from cancer of the breast. Its connection with cigarette smoking is well known and some of the relevant facts are these:

(1) between the ages of 50–64 those who smoke more than twenty cigarettes a day have a death-rate more than twice as high as non-smokers although not necessarily from lung cancer.

(2) Five moderate smokers die of lung cancer for every one non-smoker and fifteen or sixteen heavy smokers.

(3) Other factors seem to be important, e.g. the death-rate from lung cancer is very much higher in cities than in the country, in cigarette smokers than amongst those who smoke pipes or cigars, amongst men than amongst women. This would suggest that the atmosphere of cities has something to do with lung cancer.

(4) The above figures do not *prove* that lung cancer is *caused* by excessive cigarette smoking; they prove that the two are *correlated* together which is quite another matter. One could, for example, correlate the incidence of coronary thrombosis with the number of cars in a man's garage, but this would not prove that the latter state of affairs caused the former. On the assumption that coronary thrombosis is caused by a high level of cholesterol in the blood, the connection would be: rich foods tend to contain a good deal of cholesterol; rich people often eat rich foods; they also are likely to have more cars than the less wealthy. Thus it is perfectly possible to hold, as did one of the leading experts in Britain, that there is something within the individual which predisposes him to cancer (possibly a genetic factor) and cigarette smoking merely de-

367

termines *where* in the body he will get it. Another possible theory (although perhaps a less feasible one) is that a tendency to lung cancer predisposes a man to smoke too much or that lung cancer and excessive smoking are associated with the same physical and psychological type of individual. But few would deny the risk involved in heavy smoking.

Unfortunately, lung cancer comes on insidiously with few early symptoms and many cases are found by accident when examinations are being carried out for another reason. Loss of appetite, weight loss, chest pain, and the coughing of blood are late symptoms when operation is likely to be too late and the only treatment possible is X-ray therapy (*see* Smoking).

Lupus: the term lupus includes two diseases which appear to have different origins: *lupus vulgaris*, a tuberculous infection of the skin, is the condition ordinarily described as lupus, *lupus erythematosus* is an inflammatory condition of the skin of so far unknown origin although some have believed it, too, to be tuberculous.

Lupus vulgaris is commonest in young people and more frequent in females than males; it is also perhaps commoner amongst poor and badly-housed people than among the well-to-do. The disease usually attacks the face and especially the nose and cheeks. It appears as small 'apple-jelly' nodules which increase in number and the skin in the surrounding areas becomes inflamed and thickened producing an irregular raised patch. As the condition heals scarring is produced and the contraction of the fibrous tissue formed may produce terrible deformities of the face and quite commonly the cartilages of the nose itself are destroyed. Lupus is very chronic and may last for many years. In treatment the general way of life should be improved in respect of food and hygiene and the ultra-violet lamp (Finsen lamp) has been in use for a long time. Sometimes it is possible to remove and cauterise individual nodules with surgery followed by trichloracetic acid, but the main standby today is that for general tuberculosis, i.e. isoniazid and streptomycin which give excellent results.

Lupus erythematosus is an inflammatory eruption of the skin of unknown origin although the relatively uncommon generalised form which runs an acute course is an extremely serious disease involving the heart, spleen, and kidneys. The ordinary type is chronic with a very characteristic rash which consists of symmetrical patches of red skin which are smooth and covered with small scales composed of sebaceous matter from the grease glands; these are arranged on both cheeks with a narrow bridge across the root of the nose giving the appearance of a butterfly with wings extended. The disease tends to extend at the edge and heal at the centre, the healed portions becoming scar tissue with a thin, white, shiny, appearance. It is more common in middle-aged women than men, superficially similar in appearance to rosacea, and may last for many years. The generalised form is also more common in women. The most satisfactory treatment for this very chronic disease is mepacrine or chloroquine, the anti-malarial drugs, and for the generalised form cortisone or A.C.T.H.

Luxation: dislocation.

Lymph: (*see* Glands).

Lymphadenitis: inflammation of the lymph glands (*see* Inflammation, Adenitis).

Lymphadenoma: another name for Hodgkin's disease (q.v.).

Lymphangitis: inflammation of the lymph vessels seen in the red lines which pass up the limb from a source of infection (*see* Inflammation).

Lymphocyte: (*see* Leucocyte).

Lymphogranuloma Inguinale: *lymphogranuloma* is another name for Hodgkin's disease (q.v.). *Lymphogranuloma inguinale* is a venereal disease caused by a virus, the main symptom of which is enlargement of the glands in the groin.

Lymphosarcoma: a cancerous condition of the lymphoid elements in the body with enlargement of the glands, spleen, and liver. Usually occurring in later life, it is treated by X-ray therapy but the outlook is poor.

Lysol: is a soapy solution of cresol once almost as popular in suicidal attempts as it was as a general disinfectant for cleaning. These are now much less common as lysol has come to be less frequently used in the home. As a caustic it is a very unpleasant method of suicide, producing burning wherever it touches. The treatment is to give large amounts of salt and water as an emetic followed by Epsom salts which act as an antidote. Subsequently milk may be given. The antiseptic qualities of lysol are discussed under the heading of Antiseptics but in general, although both cheap and effective, it has

369

been given up in favour of more elegant substitutes which are equally or more so.

Lysozyme: a bactericidal substance of an enzyme nature found in tears.

McBurney's Point: the point over which maximum tenderness is felt in the abdomen in appendicitis. It is on a line drawn from the umbilicus to the anterior superior spine of the right iliac bone (in ordinary language, the most prominent part of the front of the pelvis) about two inches away from the latter point.

Maceration: the softening of a solid by a fluid; in medicine the softening and damaging of tissues by water as in immersion foot or drowning.

Macules: whilst papules are raised spots, macules are flat brownish or purplish areas of a rash whatever type it may be, e.g. freckles are theoretically macules.

Madura Foot: a tropical disease found largely in India in which the foot swells and its tissues and bones become riddled with sinuses caused by a specific fungus.

Magnesium: is used in medicine in the form of its salts; magnesium oxide and carbonate are both used as antacids in indigestion and liquid magnesia or 'milk of magnesia' also has a slight aperient action used especially in children. Magnesium sulphate is Epsom salts (q.v.)

Malaise: a general feeling of feverishness and unwellness often preceding an acute fever.

Malaria: malaria is still one of the world's deadly plagues killing a man or woman every ten seconds in spite of the fact that a cure has long been known and preventive measures are only hampered by ignorance and lack of skilled personnel or money. It is prevalent in India, parts of America, and Africa (especially the Gold Coast which used to be called 'the white man's grave'). Low-lying marshy land where the climate is hot and humid favours its distribution. The parasite is injected by the mosquito anopheles maculipennis in the form of spores which give rise to the small amoebic-like organisms in the blood corpuscles known as trophozoites which divide into schizonts (about 2–4) and these in turn into 8–16 merozoites which escape into the plasma and invade other blood cells.

The spells of fever correspond with the setting-free of the merozoites into the blood-stream. This form of division is known as asexual reproduction since there is division but no separate sexes to unite with each other. But soon gametocytes begin to appear in the blood, and when a mosquito bites and sucks it up it, too, is infected; for the gametocytes turn into male microgametes which move about with the aid of a flagella to seek and penetrate the female macrogametes and produce a zygote. This penetrates the mosquito's stomach wall and there forms a cyst which breaks up into sickle-shaped spores (sporozoites) that make their way to the salivary glands ready to be transferred to the first human being who is bitten and complete the cycle. If the parasite be that of tertian fever (Plasmodium vivax) attacks occur on alternate days, in quartan fever (P. malariae) they occur every seventy-two hours, and in malignant malaria (P. falciparum) also known as aestivo-autumnal or subtertian fever the patient is continuously with a raised temperature. In quotidian fever there is a daily temperature rise from infection with both tertian and quartan malaria. The fever has three stages: the *cold*, when the patient shivers and feels cold and his temperature begins to rise; this lasts about one hour and is followed by the *hot* stage when he becomes flushed and heated with a dry and burning skin and great pain in the back and limbs; this lasts 4–8 hours and is succeeded by the *sweating* stage with profuse perspiration and a return of the fever to normal. In most cases malaria is unmistakable but in the chronic condition where there is a great deal of wasting, almost continuous fever, severe anaemia, and enlargement of the spleen and liver, malaria may easily be mistaken for typhoid fever until bacteriological tests and blood examinations have been carried out. *Blackwater fever* (q.v.) in which the urine is blackish in colour from breakdown of the blood cells may occur in such cases mainly due to damage done by large doses of quinine. The treatment of malaria begins with the first specific drug known to man, i.e. the first drug which could single out the cause of the disease and kill it without also killing its host, and this, of course, is quinine. Quinine was first discovered as the bark of a tree by the South American Indians who communicated their knowledge to the Jesuit priests from whom the Countess of Chichon, wife of the Viceroy of Peru, obtained specimens of the bark to bring to Europe. This was called 'Cinchona bark' or 'Jesuit's bark' and subsequently quinine was isolated from it. The curative treatment of malaria depends upon quinine, mepacrine, proguanil hydrochloride (paludrine), and chloroquine. Quinine is given in the form of the sulphate or bi-hydrochloride; plasmoquine or pamaquin is a synthetic drug which is of no value in the acute attack but useful in killing the sexual forms of the parasite. Mepacrine is also known as atebrin.

The essential measures in the prevention of malaria are: (1) the protection of houses and beds by mosquito netting and the use of repellent creams on the skin and caution on the part of those who go out at night; (2) warfare against the mosquito in the pools where its larvae and pupae swim in stagnant water breathing through a tube which projects just above the surface and can be destroyed by crude petrol or the special oil known as malariol spread over the surface; (3) destruction of mosquitoes by D.D.T. sprays or the use of gammexane which have become the main weapons in the fight; (4) the use of quinine, mepacrine, proguanil, and chloroquine taken regularly as prophylactics by all those living in malarial districts (mepacrine and proguanil may not be so universally efficacious as the others).

Male Fern: (*see* Fern-Root).

Malignant: of a tumour means cancerous, but the word is also used of particularly severe forms of a fever, e.g. m. smallpox, m. malaria, m. scarlatina.

Malingering: is the feigning of illness of which there are many different degrees ranging from the cold-blooded pretence to a non-existent disease purely for reasons of financial gain as is common in the East on the part of beggars, or indeed in any country where people live below a reasonable level of subsistence, to the kind of malingering which is virtually a sign of mental disorder, e.g. the 'Münchausen syndrome' where patients will go from one hospital to another seeking operations for pretended illnesses the symptoms of which have been carefully studied beforehand. In between are those who malinger in order to obtain, not money, but love and attention or the chance to evade unwelcome duties, and this may be almost entirely conscious or quite unconscious, e.g. hysteria in one sense is a form of unconscious malingering in many cases as, indeed, is writer's cramp since the person who is unable to write will brazenly use the 'paralysed' muscles to handle his knife and fork whilst remaining quite unaware of his unconscious rebellion against writing.

Malleolus: the bony projections at either side of the ankle.

Malta Fever: undulant fever or abortus fever is caused by the Brucella melitensis or abortus group of organisms, the former infecting goats and the latter cows and pigs. The disease is transmitted by drinking infected goat's or cow's milk and was first noticed in the Mediterranean coast towns and especially among British troops and their families in Malta. It was recognised to be caused by goat's milk and, after the organism had been discovered, a similar one was noted as causing abortion in cattle and sows. More recently the fever has been found in Britain, France, North America, and elsewhere. The incubation period 1–2 weeks and the disease begins with weakness, aching throughout the body, headache, sweating, constipation, and bronchitis. The spleen is enlarged and the temperature rises in a step-ladder fashion persisting irregularly between 100–103 degrees for 2–3 weeks, settling for a week or two more, and then rising for perhaps four weeks or many months. The high fever in the later stages is often associated with an appearance of general well-being which is quite striking and blood tests are positive after the first week, the organisms being found in the blood and urine. In preventive treatment goat's milk should be avoided or boiled and, in suspicious areas, cow's milk also. In Malta the disease is rare since goat's milk was given up. Malta fever responds well to antibiotics such as chloramphenicol and the tetracyclines but in chronic cases the tetracyclines along with streptomycin are more effective.

Mandelic Acid: a drug used in the treatment of urinary infections, especially those due to the bacillus coli and certain streptococci. It is only effective in an acid urine and therefore given along with ammonium chloride or, more commonly nowadays, in the forms of methenamine mandelate (Mandelamine) or calcium mandelate (Mandecal). To some extent mandelic acid has been replaced by the antibiotics and sulpha drugs.

Mandel's Paint: (*see* Iodides).

Manganese: is used in medicine only in the form of potassium

373

permanganate, the antiseptic, although it was formerly used to increase resistance in cases of multiple boils. Manganese is one of the trace elements in the body and minute quantities seem to be necessary to life. In industry, the inhalation of manganese dust or fumes over a period of time may lead to symptoms similar to those of paralysis agitans caused by damage to the basal ganglia of the brain.

Mania, Manic-Depressive Psychosis: (*see* Mental Illness).

Mantoux Test: for tuberculosis consists in injecting into the superficial layers of the skin a small amount of old tuberculin. A red and swollen area indicates the presence of tuberculosis.

Marasmus: progressive wasting, especially in young children.

Marie's Hereditary Ataxia: or spino-cerebellar ataxia is an hereditary and familial disease of the nervous system in which the spino-cerebellar tracts between the cord and cerebellum degenerate at some time after the age of twenty years. The gait is reeling like that of a drunken man, speech is slurred, and there is frequently optic atrophy leading to blindness. There is no treatment and the cause is unknown.

Marihuana: cannabis indica, Indian hemp, or hashish (*see* Drug Addiction).

Marrow: the marrow of the bones is red or yellow, although there is no essential difference between the two. The former is found in the spaces inside the ribs, sternum, and the bodies of the vertebrae, the latter (which contains more fat) in the shafts of the long bones the ends of which are also filled with red marrow. It is in these sites that the red blood cells, blood platelets, and granular white corpuscles are formed.

Marplan: a drug of the monoamine-oxidase inhibitor group used in psychiatry; it is isocarboxazid and considered to be effective in certain types of depression whilst safer in use than iproniazid (Marsalid) which is used effectively in the treatment of certain types of depression but liable (in 1 in 250 cases) to lead to severe toxic jaundice. Like Marplan it is a monoamine-oxidase inhibitor.

Massage: is a manipulative treatment applied to the soft tissues in certain diseases mainly of the rheumatic type or in convalescence when the normal movements of the body which stimulate metabolism and the flow of lymph are difficult or impossible. The masseur or masseuse aids passive movements of the muscles, limbs, and joints and by such movements as stroking, pinching, pressing, kneading, stimulates the tissues. Such movements are undoubtedly useful when limbs are paralysed or immobolised by fractures, having the effect of exercises; they are refreshing and have a considerable psychological effect, but, although often hastening cure, they are not themselves a cure and the sometimes exaggerated claims cannot be substantiated. Massage is essentially ameliorative rather than curative. The various movements are described as *effleurage* or stroking towards the heart, *stroking* which is the same movement away from the heart, *petrissage* or kneading, *frictions* or circular movements, *tapotement* or percussion which is beating or hacking the tissues with the edge of the hand. The efficacy of a treatment is often to be measured by the vagueness or otherwise of the conditions it is supposed to benefit and one which is concerned with 'rheumatism,' 'nervous affections' (meaning neuroses), 'insomnia,' etc., is likely to produce a good deal of its results psychologically rather than physically. There is a certain amount of hocus-pocus about massage although nobody can doubt its value in the instances mentioned. Certified masseurs have to undergo a period of training and a diploma is granted by the Chartered Society of Physiotherapy which holds a register.

Mastoiditis: when an acute middle ear infection has spread to the mastoid cells behind the ear the signs are as follows: abrupt rise in temperature with swelling of the glands in the neck, pain behind the ear over the protuberance known as the mastoid bone (this is usually worse at night), varying degrees of deafness and puffiness behind the ear which may give it the impression of being bent forward. Formerly these signs were an indication for immediate surgery but with the advent of the antibiotics the situation has completely changed and the administration of a suitable drug usually causes the inflammation to subside in under a week. In the rare case that does not respond mastoidectomy is carried out. In chronic mastoiditis where deafness and discharge have been present for many years the results from antibiotics are less satisfactory and in these patients a radical mastoidectomy with removal of the contents of the middle ear and all the mastoid cells may have to be performed. The two operations are the simple and the radical. In the former the mastoid cells are approached either from within the canal of the external ear (endaural approach) or from an incision about 2 inches long behind the ear and the bone chipped away until all diseased cells are removed and healthy bone exposed. In the latter, the operation is the same save that all the contents of the middle ear are removed leaving nothing but a bony cavity opening into the inner ear. The simple operation does not impair hearing but the radical one means loss of hearing in the ear affected; untreated the condition may lead to such serious complications as paralysis of the facial nerve, general blood-poisoning, bone infection, and meningitis or brain abscess leading to death. Acute mastoiditis is commonest in children between the ages of 2–12 and rare in adults.

Masturbation: or self-stimulation of the sexual organs is almost universal and, in fact, a normal stage in sexual development. It is found in nearly all boys and most girls (although the sexual impulse in women tends to be less conscious than in men until awakened). Masturbation produces no harmful effects physically and the only harm that can happen mentally is when a feeling of guilt is attached to the act which is abnormal (a) if carried out to excess, which indicates severe anxiety rather than excessive sexuality, and (b) if carried out in preference to normal sexual relations when it indicates something seriously amiss with the individual's personal relationships.

Maternity and Child Welfare: public interest in maternity and child welfare was not aroused until the beginning of the 20th century when the Notification of Births Act was passed in 1907 and in 1915 this was extended to give local authorities the right to levy rates for infant welfare work. The first welfare centre was opened in 1906 in the London borough of Marylebone by Dr Eric Pritchard and the next in St Pancras came to be known as 'the school for mothers' since instruction was given in infant care, sewing and mending, cookery, etc. By 1910, 90 Maternity and Child Welfare centres were in existence, but these and the maternity hospitals were largely supported by voluntary work and subscriptions thus demonstrating the general rule that in Britain individual action precedes government legislation. By 1939 there were 2,300 centres in England and Wales, three-quarters of which were supported by the local authorities and the rest by voluntary subscription and voluntary work. In 1918 the Maternity and Child

Welfare Act was passed empowering local authorities to give assistance, subject to the approval of the Minister of Health, to expectant mothers and children below the age of 5; provisions were made towards a grant in aid of centres whether voluntary or municipal. The standard of midwifery was raised by the passing of the Midwives' Act of 1902, and maternity homes were caused to be registered, maternity benefit being paid at the rate of 40s. under the National Insurance Act of 1911. Under the National Insurance (No. 2) Act of 1957 the following financial benefits were provided: (a) a maternity grant of £12 10s. and additional grants if more than one child is born; (b) a confinement grant of £5 if the confinement takes place at home or elsewhere at the mother's expense; (c) a maternity allowance of 50s. weekly for 18 weeks beginning 11 weeks before the expected date of confinement, payable, in addition to (a) and (b), to a woman who normally goes out to work and pays full National Insurance contributions. Schemes of the same sort operate in other countries such as Sweden, New Zealand, and some provinces of Canada.

Under the National Health Service Act of 1946 fresh provision was made for Maternity and Child Welfare as follows:

(1) *Maternity medical services.* The expectant mother who is having her baby at home can obtain without charge maternity care from her own doctor or from a general practitioner obstetrician; this includes ante-natal and post-natal examinations and attendance at confinement if necessary.

(2) *Local Health Authority Services.* Responsibility for the local Maternity and Child Welfare services is now vested in county and county borough councils who provide the maternal and child welfare centres in which ante-natal and post-natal and child welfare clinics are held, as well as services for immunisation, vaccination, etc. Dental treatment is free for expectant mothers, mothers with a child under 1 year, and for young children.

Hospital and specialist services. Maternity homes and hospitals and medical staff, are provided without charge. When for medical or social reasons a confinement is booked at hospital the mother's ante- and post-natal care is given at a clinic at the hospital. (About 4 out of 6 mothers are confined at hospital).

377

Provision of a health visiting service is the duty of the local health authorities who also provide the welfare food service for extra milk and vitamin supplements at reduced cost; the unmarried mother has the same rights as the married one and special provision for her particular needs. Also provided for are day nurseries and child minding, a home help service, and a home nursing service. Birth control clinics are not provided for as such but information regarding birth control may be given at the centres or at special clinics for women suffering from gynaecological conditions; it is given only when further pregnancy would be detrimental to health, but there are voluntary staffed birth control clinics in most towns.

Maternal mortality in 1954 was 0.59 per 1,000 births, the corresponding figure in 1938 being 2.7. The birth rate in England and Wales in 1955 was 15 per 100 persons and the infant mortality under one year 24.9 per 1,000; in 1938 the corresponding figures were 15.1 and 53 per 1,000.

Measles: in spite of the fact that measles has the highest infantile mortality of all the acute fevers, it is ordinarily thought of by the layman as being of no great moment. Being a virus disease it has a long incubation period (10–15 days) and one attack confers immunity for life. The first sign is the appearance of symptoms rather like an acute cold. The eyes become red and exposure to light is unpleasant (but not, as some seem to suppose, dangerous), the nose runs, the throat is inflamed, and a dry harsh cough develops. There may be headache and the temperature rises to 102 degrees or more. Usually the patient is a child between the ages of 8 months and 5 years and especially typical is the appearance before the rash of the so-called Koplik's spots (q.v.) which are small bluish-white raised papules on the inside of the cheek. The rash begins on the fourth day and shows on the forehead and behind the ears, spreading within a day downwards over the whole body; in another two days it starts to disappear but often leaves behind a brownish staining which may last for one or two weeks. Measles, when properly looked after, is not usually serious, but it has to be taken seriously; the complications such as bronchopneumonia and middle ear diseases are now preventable or curable by suitable treatment with antibiotics although, of course, these drugs have no effect whatever upon the virus itself but only upon the secondary invaders. The only other treatment is symptomatic to alleviate what symptoms may arise in the course of the disease. Quarantine period for contacts is three weeks, isolation period three weks. A live vaccine is under trial.

Meatus: any passage or opening, especially the external auditory meatus of the ear.

Mecholyl: acetyl-beta-mathylcholine is a drug which stimulates the para-sympathetic nerves, thus producing a fall in blood-pressure, stimulation of the gastro-intestinal tract and bladder, and slowing of the heart. It is used in paroxysmal tachycardia to slow down the heart and in abdominal distension or for glaucoma. It may also be administered locally by ionisation for Raynaud's disease and varicose ulceration where it dilates the blood-vessels.

Meckel's Diverticulum: a hollow and blind appendage sometimes attached to the small intestine about 3–4 feet away from its junction with the large intestine. It is a minor congenital abnormality and may become inflamed (diverticulitis) or cause intestinal obstruction if attached at the free end to some other organ or to the umbilicus.

Meconium: the brown semi-fluid material consisting of bile and debris discharged from the infant's bowels at birth or immediately afterwards.

Mediastinum: the space in the chest between the two lungs containing the heart and great vessels, the oesophagus, and the lower end of the trachea or windpipe, etc.

Medinal: barbitone sodium (*see* Barbiturates).

Mediterranean Fever: (*see* Malta Fever).

Medulla: (1) the marrow of bones; (2) the spinal medulla (i.e. the spinal cord); (3) the medulla oblongata, the part of the brain which adjoins the spinal cord and contains the centres for breathing, swallowing, heart-beat, etc., which are vital to life.

Megacolon: (*see* Hirschsprung's Disease).

Meibomian Cyst: a cyst caused by blockage of the Meibomian glands on the eyelids where styes also frequently arise. It is treated simply by an incision on the inner surface of the eyelid which relieves the small external bulge instantly.

Melaena: blackness of the motions caused by bleeding into the stomach or the upper part of the intestinal tract where the blood is digested and converted into iron sulphide that gives rise to the dark colour. Iron-containing medicines and bismuth also cause the motions to be black.

Melancholia: (*see* Mental Illness).

Melanotic: a term applied to certain black or dark-coloured tumours which are usually malignant in nature.

Melanuria: dark-coloured urine from jaundice, blood or haemoglobin in the urine, melanotic growths, and alcaptonuria or haematoporphinuria.

Memory: defects of memory result from (1) faulty taking-in of perceptions during preoccupation with other matters as in neurosis; (2) structural damage to the brain as in senility and cerebral arteriosclerosis or poisoning from bacterial or other toxins, e.g. syphilis, carbon monoxide, alcohol (*see* Korsakof's Psychosis); (3) massive amnesia for whole blocks of memory sometimes amounting to double personality as in hysteria. There is nothing wrong with the memory of a neurotic person, but he possesses to an abnormal degree the common ability for forgetting what it does not suit him to remember and of becoming panic-stricken at his 'poor memory' when his obsession with himself has in fact prevented him from making proper contact with his environment; his retention or power of recall in the latter case is not at fault – his ability to take in impressions is. The vast majority of cases of 'poor memory' in younger people are of this type which has nothing to do with memory and is really lack of attention. The type of memory defect common in organic conditions is described under Korsakof's Psychosis and ordinarily consists in clear recollections of the distant past combined with very poor ones of recent events; the patient recalls long-distant times and 'remembers not the events of today.' So-called 'loss of memory' is a form of hysterical dissociation, unconsciously produced, which nevertheless enables the individual to forget what he basically chooses to forget, e.g. when we read of the famous case of dual personality of the Reverend Ansell Bourne quoted by William James and how the respectable clergyman disappeared from a town in Rhode Island only to turn up two months later as the owner of a small sweet shop in Pennsylvania with the name of A. J. Brown who 'came to' in a state of terror asking who and where he was we do not for an instant doubt that the reverend gentleman was genuine in his lapse but we do wonder what Mrs Bourne was like and whether the financial affairs of his church were quite in order. Patchy defects of memory may result from some diseases and occurs after electro-convulsant treatment (q.v.) in a few cases; it is usually transient. Brain cells once destroyed cannot be replaced, but some kinds of organic memory defect are benefited or prevented from getting worse by the use of concentrated vitamin B1 or Parentrovite which also contains vitamin C.

Menarche: the first appearance of the menstrual periods.

Mendelism: (*see* Heredity).

Menière's Syndrome: is due to haemorrhage into or inflammation of the eighth cranial or auditory nerve. It is characterised by attacks of severe giddiness with buzzing in the affected ear and the patient may actually fall down. The attack passes in a few minutes and is commonly followed by vomiting. There is progressive deafness. Various drugs help in mitigating the giddiness and noises in the head but are unlikely to affect the deafness, the cause of which should be investigated.

Meninges: the membranes surrounding the brain and spinal cord including the tough fibrous dura mater attached to the inside of the skull, the more delicate arachnoid which surrounds the brain but is separated from it by spaces containing fluid, and the pia mater which is thin, transparent and closely applied to the surface of the brain. The arachnoid and pia mater are regarded as one membrane for practical purposes and this, the pia-arachnoid, contains the blood-vessels which supply the surface of the brain and the inside of the skull generally.

Meningism: irritation of the meninges due to some relatively minor condition or an acute fever which produces symptoms similar in many respects to those of meningitis.

Meningitis: meningitis may be of two main types: *pachymeningitis* or inflammation of the dura mater (*see* Meninges) is not common and only occurs in injury to the skull, middle-ear disease, or haemorrhage within the skull, *leptomeningitis* is the common type and there are numerous varieties according to the organisms present. These are meningococcal, which is the common variety; tuberculous, pneumococcal, pyogenic, and syphilitic; and the others associated with influenza, typhoid, scarlet fever, mumps, etc. The symptoms of meningitis are usually described in three stages the first of which may be quite mild including fever, headache, vomiting, and constipation; occasionally there are convulsions in young children but these may usher in any acute fever. In the second stage the headache becomes more severe and the sudden screaming or 'meningeal cry' may appear, the temperature reaches a high level and may show marked remissions. Signs of irritation appear, e.g. twitching of the muscles, stiffness of the neck and spine and generally rigidity of the muscles throughout the body. Typical of this stage are Kernig's sign (q.v.) in which when the thigh is bent up against the body extension of the leg produces great pain, and Brudzinski's sign in which when the neck is bent forward the knees are automatically raised. The third is the paralytic stage in which paralysis results from compression of the brain by the exuded pus and discharge from obstruction to the flow of the cerebro-spinal fluid. There may be any type of paralysis depending on the part of the brain affected, e.g. squint, blindness, deafness, facial paralysis, paralysis of one limb, both limbs, or one half of the body. In the last stages the opisthotonus position appears with the head drawn back and the body arched forwards and the temperature is very high. The cerebro-spinal fluid must be examined by lumbar puncture (q.v.) in order to discover what type of infection is present. *Tuberculosis meningitis* is always secondary to tuberculosis elsewhere although this may often be unrecognised. Characteristic are the three symptoms of headache, vomiting, and constipation. Once invariably fatal, t.b. meningitis now responds to streptomycin given as early as possible in the course of the disease. *Pneumococcal meningitis* caused by the pneumococcus (the organism responsible for the lobar pneumonia) is usually secondary to this disease or to middle ear disease, and *pyogenic meningitis* is caused by the staphylococcus or streptococcus; both respond well to penicillin and the sulpha drugs. *Meningococcal meningitis* is also known as epidemic cerebro-spinal meningitis, spotted fever, and cerebro-spinal fever or posterior basic meningitis, the latter type occurring nearly always in the first year of life and often within the first few weeks, the staring appearance and retraction of the head being very marked. Meningococcal meningitis occurs in epidemics especially in war-time but also sporadically and is sometimes but not always accompanied by the rash which gives it its name of 'spotted fever;' it, too, responds extremely well to the sulpha drugs and antibiotics. Young children are much more susceptible than adults and the infection, which probably takes place through the nose, is often conveyed by carriers who harbour the disease without suffering from it themselves. Quarantine of contacts is useless, but they may sometimes be given sulpha drugs as a precaution; patients are isolated and preferably treated in hospital with antibiotics.

Meniscus: a crescentic fibro-cartilage in a joint, especially the semi-lunar cartilages of the knee.

Menopause: many women are troubled at the prospect of the change of life or menopause which may begin at any time from the late thirties to the late forties or early fifties although ordinarily about the age of 45. At this time the menstrual periods cease, sometimes abruptly, but more frequently gradually with increasing intervals between. There is no necessary reason why any symptoms should arise but women often resign themeslves to a longer or shorter period of 'hot flushes,' excessive bleeding, depression, and general unwellness and there is no doubt that the expectation sometimes plays a part in bringing them on. It is advisable that a doctor should be seen if such symptoms appear, for they are usually capable of being treated and if anything more serious be present this is the best time to deal with it. In particular *bleeding after the periods have ceased should be reported immediately at whatever age it may happen.* Most menopausal symptoms respond satisfactorily to sex hormones and sometimes sedatives or tranquillisers may be necessary. It is worthwhile pointing out that although the period of fertility comes to an end, sexual activity and desire are unaffected or may even be increased; the woman who has passed the menopause does not cease to be a woman even if she is no longer capable of being a mother. Normally the post-menopausal age should be one of comparative peace of mind in which depression is not natural so its appearance to any disturbing degree should be mentioned to the doctor. Putting up with such symptoms is not being stoical but simply giving in to foolish and unnecessary suffering and if other worries be present, however absurd, the woman will be wise if she unburdens herself of them to her medical adviser. The folk-lore of the change is so extensive and for the most part so ill-advised that exploding of old wives' tales is both helpful and therapeutic to those burdened by them.

Menorrhagia: excessive menstrual flow. Common in general causes are such blood diseases as pernicious anaemia and purpura, chronic kidney disease and high blood-pressure, nervous tension, excessive alcohol, hot climates and disturbances of the glands. Local causes are infections of the womb, Fallopian tubes, or ovaries, cysts in the ovaries, fibroids in the womb, displacements of the womb and tumours. The cause must be looked for before treatment is considered.

Menstruation: is a normal function of the female in man and the higher apes which consists in the monthly loss of blood by the vagina when pregnancy has not taken place. The lining of the womb or endometrium is a soft velvety covering in which the fertilised ovum embeds itself and this is grown monthly in the expectation of pregnancy only to be discharged with a varying amount of blood if this does not occur. The cycle is divided into four: the stage of quiescence, the constructive stage, the destructive stage, and the stage of repair. During the constructive stage the endometrium becomes greatly thickened partly by increase in the number of cells, partly by engorgement of the glands and blood-vessels. This is followed by a destructive stage during which the endometrium breaks down, blood leaks into the cavity of the womb and soon the discharge of endometrial tissue and blood appears outside as the period. As soon as the menstrual flow has ceased, the repair of the endometrium begins; the remains of the blood is absorbed and the broken-down tissues replaced. Of the usual twenty-eight days of the cycle about five are taken up by premenstrual congestion, four by the menstrual flow, seven by the period of repair, and twelve in a state of quiescence, the whole being controlled by the hormones of the ovary and the pituitary gland at the base of the brain. Ovulation occurs at some time about the mid-period, usually in a twenty-eight day cycle on the fourteenth day before the beginning of the next period. Since fertilisation can occur whilst the ovum is passing down the Fallopian tubes, there are about three days in the month during the midperiod when pregnancy can take place; it is unlikely (but not impossible) for it to occur in the week before, the week after, or during the period. It is important that girls should be given full information about the menstrual periods before they start and that no feelings of disgust or guilt should be associated with them for there is no doubt that a major cause of dysmenorrhea (painful periods) is the individual's attitude towards this perfectly normal function. A great deal of nonsense has come to be associated with the menstrual flow originating in its apparently mysterious nature and the supposed connection (which is wholly imaginary) with the phases of the moon. Thus superstition and religion have combined to suggest that women are 'unclean' at this time and amongst primitive (and not so primitive) people it is believed that contact with a woman at this time is fraught with dire results or even that the woman herself is in some mysterious condition such that she ought not to wash her hair or have it waved during her periods. This, of course, is absurd and the periods should occasion as little upset as possible and no change of any kind in the daily routine. A mentally normal girl looks forward to the time when her periods will begin as the age when she is sexually mature; to ill-informed women it remains 'the curse.' Menstruation is very much under glandular control from the pituitary and this, in turn, under the control of the hypothalamus in the base of the brain; since the hypothalamus is also the centre for the emotions it happens that emotions have a potent influence upon the periods. The association between painful menstruation and one's feelings about the function has already been mentioned and it is possible for the periods to be stopped by fear or hope. A common cause of *amenorrhea* (stopping of the periods) is the fear of being pregnant in those who have been in a position to become so or, in childless women, the hope that pregnancy has occurred. In fact in pseudo-pregnancy the woman may show all the symptoms of pregnancy and even go through a stage of imitated labour or have a distended abdomen from purely psychological causes. As is well known, amenorrhea is normally present before puberty, during pregnancy and lactation, and after the menopause (contrary to general belief, pregnancy can occur whilst the periods are absent, e.g. just before puberty, during lactation, and just after the menopause). Other causes of amenorrhea are anaemia, debilitating diseases, change of environment and nervous strain. The periods may fail to *begin* in girls with an undeveloped

385

womb or anaemia or in an unsuitable environment; this is known as primary amenorrhea, the other types being secondary amenorrhea. Another fallacy about the periods is that when they occur something 'bad' is being expelled from the body and that consequently when they do not occur the 'bad' is being retained. This is untrue because the absence of periods nearly always implies that the material usually excreted has not been formed. The only circumstance when menstrual blood is actually retained is the form of primary amenorrhea due to the blocking of the opening of the vagina by an imperforate hymen, i.e. the membrane that usually partially obstructs the opening and is (wrongly) regarded as an infallible sign of virginity. *Menorrhagia* or excessive menstrual flow is dealt with under that heading, and *metrorrhagia* which means bleeding between the periods may be due to: a threatened abortion or miscarriage, a pregnancy in the Fallopian tubes, various tumours of the womb or fibroids, high blood-presure, chronic inflammation of the lining of the womb following pregnancy, or polypi (i.e. small protuberances containing blood-vessels). *Premenstrual tension* is common and many women feel uncomfortable just before the period with pain, irritability, and a feeling of fullness. This can be dealt with either by hormones or, preferably, by one of the new diuretics, e.g. hydrochlorothiazide since oedema or congestion of the tissues with fluid seems to play a major part in premenstrual tension. Tranquillisers and vitamin A have also been used. Ordinary *dysmenorrhea* resulting in painful periods may be due to an under-developed womb, displacements of the womb, clotting of menstrual blood (which does not usually clot), glandular defects, and from psychological causes, e.g. feelings of resentment or anxiety about the menstrual function, inculcated by a stupid mother.

Mental Defect: means lack of intellectual development and is not to be regarded as a synonym for mental illness in general. Those whose intellectual development has been inadequate from the start are said to be suffering from *amentia* whereas *dementia* results from such chronic mental illness as schizophrenia or general paralysis when a formerly normally equipped individual loses his intellect as the result of a disease process. There are certain well-defined types of mental deficiency but others which come into no special category other than the legal ones of idiocy, imbecility, and feeble-mindedness or moral deficiency which apply to all categories. Although primary amentia is present from birth, it would be wrong to think that all such cases are inherited and we now know that many result from damage done within the womb as when the mother develops German measles during her pregnancy and yet others appear to be due to glandular defects in the mother or child, metabolic defects, disease of the child, birth injury, and other causes. Thus the belief that mental defect was caused by the child being injured on the head in early life, although largely a fable, carried a grain of truth in its implication that inheritance was not necessarily at fault. By and large it is true to say that, whilst dull or feeble-minded children are the offspring of dull or feeble-minded parents, the grosser forms of idiocy and imbecility may occur in any family no matter how intelligent the parents may be and are sometimes the result of recessive genes carried by both parents, or sometimes wholly unrelated to heredity. Minor degrees of backwardness become apparent only in delay in reaching the ordinary landmarks of growth, e.g. sitting up at 6 months, standing at 1 year, but the grosser forms are fairly obvious from the earliest months. There is general apathy to the surroundings combined with restlessness and repeated purposeless movements; inability to learn bowel and bladder control, dribbling, and constant protrusion of the tongue; the inability to utter sensible syllables at the end of the first year whilst making strange noises is suggestive of idiocy but may result from deafness and mutism. Fits are often associated with mental deficiency being a sign of damage to, or malformation of, the brain.

The legal categories of mental deficiency are:

(1) An *idiot* is one who is 'unable to avoid common physical dangers' and they are quite unable to exist unprotected.

(2) An *imbecile* is one who is unable to manage himself or his affairs.

(3) A *feeble-minded person* is one who in protected circumstances is able to provide for himself; he is, however, unable to compete with the normal person in most types of work and in life.

(4) A *moral imbecile* is not a medical category at all but refers to those people who, in spite of training, require to be

controlled for the protection of others, i.e. they are anti-social psychopaths who (let us admit) have become this way often *because* of faulty training. Particular types of mental deficiency are *mongolism, cretinism, microcephaly, hydrocephaly, tuberose sclerosis,* and *amaurotic family idiocy*. Most mongols are above the idiot class and are likely to be imbecile or feeble-minded. They are often attractive and friendly with allegedly mongoloid features, slant eyes, and reddish-yellow skin; the cause of mongolism is genetic but it is often found that they tend to come at the end of a large family or as the child of a mother over the age of forty. Breathing is often difficult owing to the narrowness of the space at the back of the nose and respiratory disease together with congenital heart disease are common causes of death. Mongols do not often live long and even when they outgrow childhood early senility is their lot. Cretinism, if discovered in time, can be completely compensated for with thyroid hormone used throughout life. The microcephalic idiot has an abnormally small head and is of low mental development; the limbs tend to be spastic and there is a tendency to fits. Few outlive the period of childhood. In hydrocephalus the head is too large and various surgical operations have been devised to deal with the condition with varying success; the syphilitic type requires special treatment, but generally the outlook is not good. Tuberose sclerosis is character-ised by small sebaceous swellings about the face, connective tissue (neuroglial) nodules throughout the brain, and congenital tumours elsewhere, in the heart, kidneys, or skin. There is nearly always epilepsy and the outlook is poor. Amaurotic family idiocy or Tay-Sachs disease is allegedly found only in Jewish children, although since few anthropologists believe in the existence of a Jewish race and a similar type of condition has been described in non-Jews one may reasonably doubt this claim. Progress is normal until the sixth month when blindness and spastic paralysis set in leading to death before the third year. Typical of this condition is the cherry-red spot in the retina of the eye. Mongolism is now known to be caused by an extra chromosome.

Mental Health Act: the Mental Health Bill passed in July 1959 was based on the recommendations in the Report of the Royal Commission on Law relating to Mental Illness and Mental Deficiency 1954-7 and briefly changes the emphasis in the treatment of the mentally ill from the old one of primarily custodial care in mental hospitals to a more optimistic one of dealing with mental sickness in the same way as any other form of disease as far as is possible. It recommended the repeal of the Lunacy and Mental Treatment Acts and the Mental Deficiency Acts which had formerly laid down rigid regulations for administration and treatment.

Mental cases are to be treated as other hospital patients with the exception of a few who may require to be taken to hospital without their consent for the protection of themselves or others but even for these improved legal safeguards were proposed. Three categories of disease are mentioned: (1) mental illness, (2) severe subnormality, (3) psychopathy, the latter referring to cases whose abnormality is mainly in the social sphere. In place of the Board of Control regional appeal tribunals were proposed to deal with patients' complaints of unjust detention and in place of Ministry of Health authority the Royal Commission advised increased control by the local authorities.

Mental Illness: mental illnesses are not illnesses in the usually accepted sense of the word, being forms of social maladaptation predisposed to in a greater or lesser degree by heredity and influenced by such factors as upbringing and physical disease. They are not usefully regarded as diseases of the 'mind' since, without entering into philosophical discussions, modern psychology and psychiatry are not concerned with metaphysical entities but with behaviour and inter-personal relations. 'Mind' is the totality of an individual's socially-acquired traits as they have been impressed upon an inherited nervous system and particular constitution and 'insanity' or 'mental disease' is the state of affairs when the traits which have been so impressed through the medium of the family result in a personality which (a) is troublesome to the individual himself, or (b) is troublesome to society in general. Insanity is largely a legal concept, not a medical one. Thus, if a man believes himself to have been harmed from a distance by one who intends his death and has pointed a bone at him he is quite normal in Australia amongst the aborigines and

389

quite abnormal in England – but even in England one might take a different view of the case if one knew that he was a peasant to whom this belief was natural or on the other hand a highly sophisticated ass who was a member of a modern witch 'coven.' Insanity is also a social and cultural concept. Thus, during the war, the writer was somewhat amused to find that a simple country boy from South Africa who whilst sitting in the desert had heard God call him by his Christian name of 'Willy' was regarded by the priests attached to the hospital as insane whilst he, an agnostic, found the boy wholly normal. Nevertheless, there is something inconsistent about psychotic or insane beliefs. Most people are elated or depressed almost regardless of circumstances; true, we should think it abnormal if a person were to be depressed after hearing that he had won a football pool, but even the most normal person is sometimes depressed without obvious reason. However if a man is depressed all the time for a period of months and feels that he has committed 'the unforgivable sin' when we know that, so far from being worse than other people, he is a highly moral individual, we should regard him as suffering from severe depression requiring medical treatment and if he remained unduly elated over an appreciable period of time he would be a case of mania. If we further knew that he was liable to swing without obvious cause from one extreme to the other we should diagnose him as a case of manic-depressive insanity although we ourselves may be prone to moods. Violent swings of mood without apparent cause are typical of this type of functional insanity (i.e. insanity in which no physical disease has been found) and delusions, auditory hallucinations, with strange social behaviour are typical of of schizophrenia, the other type. A man who believes that the police are broadcasting obscene statements to himself which he can hear – and we can even watch him 'listening' to them – is abnormal even when we realise that the 'broadcasts' are coming from his own unconsciousness which he refuses to recognise and we recall a maiden aunt who always looked under the bed at night to see if a man were concealed there – the wish being father to the thought. The real issue is that a man who believes that he is being persecuted is dangerous, objectively wrong, and shares his conviction with no other group of people, whereas a man who believes that the earth is flat may be a primitive, inadequately educated, a member of the Flat Earth Society, and in and case is harming no one, nor is he aware of harming himself. A major difference between the neurotic sufferer from 'nerves' and the insane is that the neurotic is very aware of his abnormality whilst the other is not; neurotic people go to doctors, psychotic people do not or go for the wrong reason as did one patient who kept coming to his doctor for treatment for stomach trouble brought on, as he believed, by poisoned milk from a hostile dairy company. The neurotic patient has insight, the psychotic has none. Some psychiatrists believe that heredity is important in mental disease, others do not. The most that can be said is that no definite hereditary influence has ever been proved and it is difficult to see how it could, e.g. patients suffering from an obsessional neurosis are said to have obsessional children but no tendency is more readily *learned* than the obsessional one so the demonstration is not conclusive. *That* heredity may have an influence is more than likely, *how much* influence nobody knows but it is unlikely that a specific disease is inherited although the tendency may well be. The real cause of mental illness is faulty upbringing leading to mental conflicts; 'there are no problem children, only problem parents,' and what we impress upon our children is not, alas, what we consciously wish to impress, but our own unconscious conflicts within ourselves and the conflicts within the family. Some types of insanity are associated with physical disease and even with specific types of physical disease but these are due to brain damage and, even so, the type of symptom produced is as typical of the person as it is typical of the disease. The most usual classification of mental disorders is as follows:

(1) *Organic Psychoses* caused by bacterial toxins in the acute fevers (delirium); infections of the brain (as in general paralysis due to syphilis); poisons such as alcohol, carbon monoxide, lead, etc.; disease of the arteries of the brain as in arteriosclerosis; the changes of senility or premature senility. Typical symptoms are disorientation for time, place, and person, loss of memory for recent events, hallucinations and delusions, poor control over the emotions (*see* Korsakof's Psychosis).

(2) *Functional Psychoses* or true insanity in which no organic disease has been found.

391

(a) Manic-depressive psychosis in which there are alternating moods of elation and depression, sometimes happening alone as in the case of mania without apparent depression following or depression without following elation.

(b) Involutional depression or depression occurring at the change of life.

(c) Schizophrenia, characterised by many varied symptoms but usually by delusions, foolish behaviour, and general deterioration sometimes leading to dementia. Hallucinations are usually of hearing rather than of sight as is common with the organic psychoses. Paraphrenia and paranoia (persecution mania) are forms of schizophrenia coming on later in life so that there is less deterioration and the delusions are more integrated and less irrational than in the type with an early onset which used to be called dementia praecox.

(3) *Psychopathic Personality* is an ill-assorted group of which it would not be unfair to say that it includes all the people one happens to dislike, e.g. the abnormally aggressive, the sexually perverse, the inadequate, the brilliant, the drug-addict. There is no such disease as psychopathic personality; these are basically people who, whilst not being psychotic, hurt society more than they hurt themselves.

(4) *Neuroses* are divided into three groups:

(a) anxiety neurosis in which anxiety and its physical accompaniments are the main symptom.

(b) hysteria which mimics physical disease.

(c) obsessional neurosis in which obsessions are the main feature, i.e. the compulsion to do or say or think certain things.

Treatment has been revolutionised in recent years both with the discovery of new drugs and physical methods of therapy and with the greater understanding of mental illness due to the work of Freud and others. Insulin therapy and drugs such as chlorpromazine (Largactil) have completely changed the outlook in schizophrenia and even the apparently hopeless case can be helped in some instances by the operation of leucotomy (q.v.). Depression is treated by electroconvulsant therapy and the typical case clears up in 10–14 days; this treatment is, indeed, almost specific for involutional depression and for less typical or milder cases such drugs as phenelzine, iproniazid, and nialamide (Nardil, Marsilid, and Niamid) seem to be effective. General paralysis of the insane is treatable with anti-syphilitic remedies and malarial therapy and the tranquillising drugs and monoamine-oxidase inhibitors are used in the neurosis. In the latter, however, the treatment of choice is psychotherapy (q.v.) with or without special methods such as L.S.D. (lysergic acid) and pentothal to aid it. Psychoanalysis is reserved for the neuroses and is suitable for relatively few of these; also the time and cost involved put it out of the reach of most people. The most important change has been in the attitude of the psychiatrist and the staffs of mental hospitals who, in the last thirty years have ceased to regard their work as largely one of diagnosis followed by the custodial function of a jailer and adopted an active and optimistic rôle in treatment which has a turnover as rapid as that in a general hospital.

Menthol: crystals of menthol are obtained from peppermint oil when it is cooled. They are mildly antiseptic and have a local anaesthetic effect, their commonest uses being in a lotion or ointment to stop itching, to relieve headache when painted or rubbed on the skin, to ease breathing either as an inhalation or when a crystal is inserted in the tip of a cigarette.

Mepacrine Hydrochloride: or atebrin is a synthetic anti-malarial drug much used both for prophylaxis and treatment during the last war when quinine was in short supply.

Mephenesin: proprietary name Myanesin, is a muscle relaxant drug used in the treatment of spastic conditions of organic origin and in states where the muscle tension is secondary to emotional tension, e.g. in anxiety states and obsessional neuroses.

Meprobamate: proprietary names Equanil, Mepavlon, Miltown, is a tranquilliser which produces relaxation without sedation.

Mercaptopurine: one of the antimetabolite drugs which seem to act by depriving rapidly-dividing (e.g. cancerous) cells of materials needed for growth. Hence their use in leukaemia (q.v.).

Mercury: is much less used in medicine than formerly when it was a major standby for physicians with the salts as powerful antiseptics, ammoniated mercury ointment for use in septic skin conditions, the yellow oxide of mercury ointment for use on the eyelids, calomel as an aperient, and the wide use of mercury in the treatment of syphilis. Mersalyl, a complex organic salt, was until recently the most powerful diuretic. Many of these are being replaced, the antiseptic applications by the antibiotics and the diuretics by chlorothiazide, syphilis is treated by penicillin, and purgatives are, by preference, not used at all.

Mercury Poisoning: may be acute or chronic, the former usually from corrosive sublimate, the latter as a side-effect of the (now obsolete) treatment of syphilis with mercury or any condition where mercury has been used over a long period. Workers with the metal (e.g. mirror and barometer makers) may be poisoned by the fumes. In acute poisoning with corrosive sublimate there is burning pain in the mouth and stomach, the lips and mouth being burned white, followed by diarrhoea and vomiting. The patient becomes very collapsed and death may occur quite rapidly. An emetic such as sodium bicarbonate in warm water should be given and when the stomach is cleared white of egg or milk must be swallowed in order to precipitate the salt. In chronic poisoning the most striking feature is inflammation of the mouth (stomatitis) with bleeding of the gums, swelling of the tongue, foul breath, loss of the teeth, and disease of the jaw-bone. There is also tremor and paralysis with severe anaemia. The treatment is to stop the drug and give a good full diet; in more serious cases injections of dimercaprol may be used to speed elimination.

Mersalyl: or Salyrgan (*see* Mercury).

Mesencephalon: the mid-brain joining the cerebrum with the cerebellum and pons.

Mesentery: the double layer of peritoneum supporting the small intestine by its attachment to the back of the abdominal wall.

Mesmerism: named after Anton Mesmer (*see* Hypnosis).

Metabolism: the total of building-up (anabolic) and breaking down (katabolic) processes in the body; i.e. the 'speed' at which the body runs. The *basal metabolic rate* is a measure of the rapidity of these processes in the resting body and is raised, e.g. in some types of thyroid disease. Since the basal metabolic rate is a useful guide to diagnosis it is taken by measuring the amounts of oxygen and carbon dioxide exchanged during breathing under certain fixed conditions. The apparatus the patient has to breathe into is known as a Douglas bag.

Metacarpal Bones: (*see* Hand).

Metastases: the secondary growths to which a cancer gives rise elsewhere in the body.

Metatarsal Bones: (*see* Foot).

Metatarsalgia: one of those words meaning pain in a specific part and very little else (c.f. pleurodynia – pain in the chest). Pain in the metatarsal region is usually due to flat-foot but may be 'rheumatic' (another blanket word) or gouty.

Meteorism: gas in the intestines which produces distension (*see* Flatulence).

Methadone: methadone hydrochloride is Physeptone, a powerful pain-killer only obtainable on prescription which may also cause addiction.

Methedrene: a synthetic compound closely related to ephedrene and amphetamine (q.v.). It is given by mouth as a nerve stimulant in depression and by injection in psychiatry or to maintain the blood-pressure during an operation.

Methonium Compounds: are quaternary ammonium compounds used in medicine to block the ganglia of the autonomic nervous system (*see* Nervous System) and thus cause reduced blood-pressure and stomach activity. They are used in duodenal ulcer and high blood-pressure in such forms as hexamethonium (Vegolysen) and pentolinium tartrate (Ansolysen).

Methylpentynol: a relatively safe but short-acting sedative often given in capsules to those who fear a dental appointment; its use in medicine is limited by its very brief period of action although methylpentynol carbamate (Oblivon C) has a more prolonged effect. Other (proprietary) names are Atempol, Insomnol, Oblivon, Somnesin. These are useful for insomnia only when the primary difficulty is getting to sleep, for they do not last long enough to maintain sleep. The main action is the rapid relief of fear and apprehension.

Methylphenobarbitone: or Prominal is a barbiturate used in the treatment of epilepsy.

Methyl Testosterone: (*see* Testosterone).

Metritis: inflammation of the womb.

Metropathia Haemorrhagica: a condition due to excessive and

395

prolonged action of oestrogens, i.e. ovarian hormone or the hormone from the anterior pituitary which stimulates the ovary to produce oestrin. The lining of the womb is thickened and there is irregular bleeding with cysts in the ovaries. The symptoms appear most commonly between the ages of 35–45 and the irregular bleeding comes on usually after a period of amenorrhoea. Treatment is curettage (i.e. scraping-out the womb in a minor operation), hormones which have an anti-oestrin effect such as progesterone and testosterone, radium or X-ray therapy, rarely removal of the womb.

Metrorrhagia: irregular bleeding between the periods (*see* Menstruation).

Microbe: (*see* Bacteria).

Microcephaly: (*see* Mental Defect).

Microsporon: (*see* Ringworm).

Micturition: the act of passing water or urine.

Middle Ear Disease: or Otitis media (*see* Ear, Mastoiditis).

Migraine: 'sick headache' is quite a specific condition although the term is often wrongly used for severe headaches of any sort. The headache is usually one-sided, accompanied by feelings of nausea and vomiting and great sensitivity to light or sound. Often there are feelings of tingling or numbness in various parts of the body, a family history of the condition (which begins between the ages of 5–20), and a particular type of personality which might be described as intelligent and fussy. An attack is preceded by feelings of tiredness and abdominal discomfort and begins with nausea, vomiting, black spots before the eyes, yawning, noises in the ears and intolerance to bright light. Odd figures may be seen (the fortification spectra) which resemble jagged or zig-zag lines and the characteristic headache begins over one or other frontal region and later spreads over the whole head. The face may be paler or more flushed on one side than the other. Migraine, however, is not serious and the condition dies out at the age of 50 or so. Theories as to its origin have ranged from the belief that it is caused by spasm of the blood-vessels of the brain (as it almost certainly is) to the idea that it is allergic like hay-fever or a nerosis; doubtless both may be true and produce their effect by inducing cerebral spasm. Treatment is, so far, with drugs to alleviate symptoms and these include ergotamine tartrate, cortisone, Phenergan (promezathine), hormones, Stemetil (prochlorperazine), and Ronicol (nicotinyl alchol). These have differing effects in each case so several may have to be tried until a suitable one is found. The attack usually lasts for one day but occasionally lasts for two, three, or more.

Miliary: the size of a millet seed (e.g. miliary tuberculosis, miliary aneurisms). Reference to the size of the lesions.

Millilitre: or mil, is the 1000th part of 1 litre; practically speaking, 1 cubic centimetre (1 c.c.).

Miscarriage: or abortion which in medical terms has no necessary criminal implications and means simply expulsion of the foetus before the child is capable of life (i.e. the 28th week); later expulsion is described as premature labour. About one in five pregnancies end in miscarriage and 37% of child-bearing women miscarry before thirty years of age, most commonly before the end of the fourth month. The symptoms of miscarriage are unmistakable and the appearance of vaginal bleeding with periodic pains in the lower abdomen in a woman known to be pregnant should receive immediate attention from the doctor; prior to the doctor coming all she can do is to rest in order to discourage further bleeding. There are many possible causes of miscarriage, some certain, others more doubtful. It is doubtful for example whether a normal pregnancy is terminated by a fall or even lack of food in the mother, for many experiences during the war show the resistance of the foetus to expulsion even in the most unfavourable circumstances. In habitual abortion there is an endocrine defect with deficiency of progestin and thyroid, and, of course, Rh negative blood (q.v.) is liable to bring about a miscarriage. Again, displacements of the womb, especially backward tilting or retroversion, fibroids or other causes of local congestion in the womb are important causes as, if more rarely, are drugs and internal toxins. Even here, as in criminal abortion, one knows that, short of seriously endangering the life of the mother, very few drugs have the slightest effect on pregnancy. The treatment of a threatened miscarriage is a matter for the doctor who will use hormones and sedatives and in incomplete but inevitable abortion the remains of the pregnancy will have to be removed by a minor operation. Habitual abortion requires prolonged treatment, but the outlook is quite good.

The great dangers of a miscarriage, whether accidental or deliberate are haemorrhage and sepsis; these are very considerable risks and no unprofessional interference with pregnancy is ever justifiable.

Mitral Stenosis: (*see* Valvular Disease).

Mole: a pigmented spot on the skin, usually raised above the surrounding level, and sometimes hairy. These should not be interfered with except by an expert as there is a real risk of malignancy developing in later life (*see* also Hydatidiform Mole).

Molluscum Contagiosum: a skin condition usually seen in children and caused by a virus. The small nodules are each about the size of a split pea with a small dent at the top and are contagious, sometimes spreading to the mother's breast from a child with the disease. They are unsightly but not dangerous and are best dealt with by squeezing out the contents and cauterising.

Molluscum Fibrosum: or von Recklinghausens's disease is a generalised neurofibromatosis in which numerous nodules of varying sizes appear throughout the skin; these are growths on the connective tissue which are believed to arise from the nerve sheaths and may cause considerable deformity although the disease is not dangerous to life and its cause is unknown. There is no treatment, but the larger or more inconvenient nodules may be surgically removed.

Mongolism: (*see* Mental Defect).

Moniliasis: an infection caused by the fungus candida albicans, the organism found in thrush. Similar fungi cause infection of the skin, lungs, and the vagina in women.

Monoamine-oxidase Inhibitors: a group of drugs used in the treatment of depression in psychiatry which have also been found useful for other purposes, e.g. in inhibiting the pain over the heart in angina pectoris. Amongst the best-known are iproniazid (Marsilid), phenelzine (Nardil), isocarboxazid (Marplan).

Moron: a feeble-minded individual (*see* Mental Defect).

Morphine: (*see* Opium).

Mouth, Diseases of: (*see* Gumboil, Lips, Teeth, Tongue, Thrush, Vincent's Angina).

Mucomembranous Colitis: a type of colitis largely brought on by the excessive use of purgatives in neurotic people (*see* Colitis).

Multipara: a woman who has borne several children.

Mumps: (epidemic parotitis) is not very common in infants but quite frequent among older children by whom it is spread directly from case to case. The incubation period is 14–21 days and isolation should be maintained for three weeks whilst the period of quarantine is 4 weeks. The earliest symptom is usually a pain behind the angle of the jaw and in 2–3 days the swelling of the gland in front of the ear becomes visible and opening the mouth is painful. The temperature is generally slightly raised but many remain normal or on the other hand become quite high. Later the gland on the other side enlarges, but this may not happen and after 4–5 days the swelling starts to go down. The other salivary glands below the jaw or under the tongue may be enlarged and the lymphocytes (*see* Leucocytes) increase in number in the blood-stream. Possible complications are orchitis with swelling of the testicles in boys or there may be pelvic pains in girls and pain in the breasts; occasionally there is inflammation of the pancreas. Mumps is unlikely to be mistaken for any other common disease but sometimes the gland is swollen when ordinary sepsis in the mouth is present leading to a simple parotitis. The disease is caused by a virus and no specific treatment exists, all that is necessary being treatment of any troublesome symptoms; mouth washes and hot applications over a painful swelling are helpful.

Munchausen Syndrome: a condition named after the famous Baron Munchausen, the notorious liar of German folk-lore, in which the patient deliberately seeks unnecessary surgical treatment in one hospital after another and to this end learns the symptoms of the disease he is pretending to suffer from and elaborately plans means of deceiving the surgeons concerned. It is an example of malingering carried to the degree at which one realises how grossly abnormal such behaviour really is (*see* Malingering). The Ganser syndrome is one in which insanity is simulated.

Murmur: the sound heard through a stethoscope over the heart when valvular disease is present, due to the flowing of the blood over loose and roughened valves or through narrowed ones usually resulting from rheumatic fever. Murmurs vary greatly in the significance to be attached to them, the greater number being of negligible importance (*see* Valvular Disease).

Muscle: there are three types of muscle in the human body differing both in structure and function. These are striate or striped which is the type found in the ordinary voluntary muscles of the body (i.e. the ones over which we have voluntary control), the smooth or involuntary muscles of the intestines, bladder, and the muscles lining the larger blood-vessels over which we have no control, and the muscle of the heart, or cardiac muscle which is in a category of its own. Striped muscle is seen under the microscope to be composed of a large number of fibres held together by the loose connective tissue which also surrounds the whole muscle and these fibres (which are about an inch in length) are built up from even more minute fibrils embedded in a semi-fluid substance and also surrounded by a delicate sheath. The fibres are seen to be marked with alternate bands of dark and light which give them their name. As each end of a muscle is attached to a bone, contraction will draw the two ends together thus producing either flexion (bending) or extension (straightening) of a limb. The process which causes a muscle to contract is very complex and it must suffice to say that under the influence of nervous impulses from the brain the substance within the fibrils (glycogen) is broken down to a sugar and then still further to lactic acid which, occupying a smaller space, causes the muscle to contract. After contraction the glycogen is built up again and the process is ready to be repeated, but if not enough oxygen is present lactic acid accumulates and fatigue (q.v.) results. But even when a muscle is at rest it remains slightly contracted and, since all such movements give off heat, this normal 'tone' of the muscles plays a large part in maintaining the body heat as well as enabling movements to take place more rapidly than would otherwise be the case.

The plain or unstriped muscle of the alimentary canal, the respiratory and urinary tracts, and the pupil of the eye also supplies fibres to the skin which cause the involuntary phenomenon of 'gooseflesh.' These muscles are without stripes and receive their nervous supply from a different source; for whilst the voluntary muscles are supplied by the brain and spinal cord the involuntary ones are supplied by the autonomic nervous system. Their normal stimulus is to pressure or stretching both of which give rise to a feeling of pain if carried to excess, but cutting produces no effect on plain muscle and it is therefore possible to operate under local anaesthesia on the internal organs only the skin and muscles of the abdominal wall being anaesthetised. Cardiac muscle in the heart is partly striped but differs from voluntary muscle in not being under voluntary control and in not being able to go into constant (tetanic) contraction.

The attachment of a muscle to the less movable bone is known as its origin, its attachment to the more movable one is its insertion. Thus the deltoid muscle of the top of the shoulder arises from the collar-bone and shoulder blade and is inserted into the humerus. When it contracts the arm is raised from the side of the body (abduction). For diseases of muscle *see* Myositis, Myasthenia, Rheumatism, Cramp, and Myopathy.

Mustine: a form of nitrogen mustard which, with others, has an action inhibiting cell division; it is therefore used in the treatment of chronic leukaemia and Hodgkin's disease.

Myalgia: muscular pain.

Myasthenia Gravis: a muscular disease characterised by rapid exhaustion of the voluntary muscles when repeatedly contracted. Although serious, myasthenia is not a common disease. It affects young adults and the voluntary muscles, especially those of the face, eyes, and neck, become infiltrated with lymphocytes (*see* Leucocytes) and progressively weakened but without any very obvious wasting. The involuntary muscles concerned with swallowing and breathing are similarly affected with the result that there is difficulty in breathing and eating and speech is soon exhausted whilst the eyelids droop, the face becomes expressionless, and the head tends to fall forward. Sometimes squint is present. The symptoms are due to lack of the substance called acetylcholine necessary for muscular contraction and this can be in part replaced by injections of prostigmine which enables the muscles to move and in some cases seems to have a curative effect. Thymectomy or removal of the thymus gland has led to some good results. All cases of this disease should have a chest X-ray to exclude tumour of the thymus.

Mycotic Diseases: those diseases caused by fungi or moulds, e.g. ringworm, thrush, actinomycosis, some lung and ear infections, Madura foot in the tropics.

Mydriatics: drugs such as belladonna which cause dilation of the pupil.

Myelemia: another name for spleno-medullary leukaemia (q.v.).

Myelin: the substance forming a sheath around myelinated nerve-fibres.

Myelitis: inflammation and degeneration of an area in the spinal cord which may result from exposure to cold, syphilis, the extension of inflammation from surrounding parts, compression of the cord by a tumour or collapse of a vertebra as in Pott's disease (i.e. tubercular infection of bone), from fracture-dislocations, or following certain acute illnesses, e.g. influenza, typhoid, measles, infective endocarditis, poliomyelitis. First of all there is a flaccid paralysis with loss of knee and ankle-jerks and retention of urine and faeces, numbness and tingling, weakness and pain in the legs usually coming on suddenly. Later there is spastic paralysis when the limbs affected are jerky owing to being out of control of the higher centres and involuntary movements take place. Treatment varies with the cause but the general outlook is not good.

Myelocyte: the cells in the bone-marrow which give rise to the granular white cells of the blood. In leukaemia and other conditions they may be found in the blood.

Myeloma: a tumour composed of bone-marrow cells. In *multiple myelomatosis* or Kahler's disease the tumours occur throughout the marrow leading to spontaneous fracture and anaemia. The latter disease is invariably fatal.

Myocarditis: in myocarditis the heart muscle itself is affected, the commonest form being a process which leads to the muscle degenerating into fatty material or fibrous tissue. This may result from two conditions dealt with elsewhere, *angina pectoris* where the coronary vessels periodically go into spasm and *coronary thrombosis* where they become blocked by a thrombosis, but old age, acute fevers, excessive alcohol, anaemias, e.g. pernicious anaemia, can all have the same effect as indeed may overweight although here the fat does not involve destruction of the heart muscle but only infiltration around it. Rheumatic carditis following a history of rheumatic fever, tonsillitis, joint pains, or even with no abnormal history at all is a less common cause than formerly but common enough nevertheless (*see* Heart Diseases).

Myoma: is a tumour, nearly always non-malignant, which consists mainly of muscle fibres. These are common in the uterus where they are known as fibromyomas or fibroids.

Myopathy: a group of diseases in which no change has been found other than in the muscles themselves which begin to atrophy with or without previous increase in bulk; the nerves appear to be unaffected. The following types are described according to the muscles affected and the age of onset: (1) the *pseudo-hypertrophic type of Duchenne* in which upper parts of the lower limbs of children of about 6 are affected. In these cases the buttocks, thighs, and calves seem excessively well-developed but there is difficulty in walking and the gait becomes waddling. (2) The *juvenile type of Erb* in which the muscles of the shoulder and upper arm first begin to waste about the age of 14. (3) The *facio-scapulo-humeral type of Landouzy-Dejerine* beginning about the same age shows wasting of the muscles of the upper arm and face. In all cases the affected muscles completely lose their power to contract and in the first the patient seldom reaches the age of 20, but the others may stop and remain stationary for the rest of life. The treatment is largely symptomatic, movement being encouraged and rest in bed on the whole avoided as far as possible. Amongst drugs given have been pituitary extract, glycine and ephedrene, which appear in some instances to improve the symptoms.

Myopia: short-sight (*see* Spectacles).

Myosis: narrowing of the pupil by *myotic* drugs such as eserine and opium, or resulting from the normal effect of light or paralysis of the sympathetic nerve fibres supplying the pupil.

Myositis: inflammation of a muscle as in *myositis ossificans* where bone is formed in the muscles which lose their power to contract and become completely rigid, or *myositis fibrosa* where a similar condition arises from fibrosis of the muscles. No treatment is known, although the latter condition may become arrested with physiotherapy.

Myotonia Congenita: or Thomsen's disease is characterised by stiffness of the muscles which decreases on exercise, e.g. on shaking hands it is at first difficult to leave go. The disease appears shortly after birth, is harmless, and perfectly compatible with a long life.

Myringotomy: the operation of cutting the ear-drum in cases of acute middle-ear disease.

Myxoedema: the condition resulting from failure of function of the thyroid gland in later life once common in those areas where the iodine content of the water is low (the Derbyshire dales and many Swiss and Himalayan valleys) but now resulting most frequently from failure of the gland occurring sporadically from unknown causes. Myxoedema is about seven times more common in women than in men and generally occurs in the 40–55 age group resulting in a degeneration of the tissues beneath the skin and the connective tissues throughout the body. The appearance is typical, the face being swollen and coarse-looking with almost complete loss of any emotional expression; the skin is dry and yellowish although the cheeks tend to be red; the hair falls out and sometimes complete baldness may result, the outer part of the eyebrows being conspicuously lacking in hair. Mentally the patient is dull, unresponsive, drowsy, and deaf, and although usually placid to begin with, irritability and sometimes actual delusions of persecution may develop later. The treatment of this unpleasant condition is the administration of thyroid extract which clears it up completely but must continue to be taken throughout life.

Naevus: the term applied to birth-marks consisting of a tangled mass of blood-vessels. These commonly take the form of the so-called 'port-wine stain' most noticeable on the face but may be more restricted in size and capable of being dealt with by removal of the area of skin affected or by electrolysis.

Nails, Diseases of: comparatively few diseases affect the nails and here it is only necessary to mention four. *Ringworm of the nails* which causes them to be blackish and grooved was once very intractable but can now be treated orally by an antibiotic; infection at the base of the nail or *paronychia* is often rather resistant to treatment and needs expert care and abscesses or *whitlows* may occur here or at the edge of the nails, usually requiring a small incision to relieve the inflammation by letting out pus; sometimes a blow causes a *haematoma* to form beneath the nail at its base giving rise to considerable pain from the accumulation of blood but this is immediately relieved by drilling a small hole to allow it to escape. *Ingrowing toe-nail* affects only the nails of the foot and results (like most foot problems) primarily from ill-fitting footwear or from lack of care of the nails. The treatment is best carried out by a chiropodist but consists in wearing properly-fitting shoes, packing the side of the nail-bed affected with boric lint, and cutting the toe-nails square across the top in future. The nails are strongly indicative of a person's state of health (*see* also Hand) and the bluish nails with clubbed finger-tips of heart or lung disease, the spoonshaped nails of anaemia, the ragged finger-nails of the neurotic given to biting them, the groove across the nail indicating a serious illness recently recovered from (the date can be calculated from the distance from the tip of the nail since it takes about six months for the groove to reach there from the base), are all well-known to the doctor.

Narcissism: love of self, usually regarded as a normal stage of development which is abnormal when carried on to excess in later life.

Narcolepsy: is a condition in which the patient finds it impossible to resist a tendency to fall asleep. In children the condition is nearly always a result of encephalitis (q.v.) but in adults it appears to arise spontaneously, the cause being unknown. Amphetamine (benzedrene) with or without a barbiturate is helpful in these cases.

Narcotics: is a term applied in the legal sense to certain drugs, e.g. opium and its derivatives which produce in sufficient amounts a deep sleep (in the U.S. the term is used loosely to refer to almost any drugs of addiction). Medically speaking, narcotics are a motley group of drugs ranging from the hypnotics which produce more or less natural-seeming sleep to the general anaesthetics. The former can produce sleep if given in large doses, the latter produce complete unconsciousness. The term is therefore not a scientific one, and the 'narcotic squad' is a legal or fictional not a medical concept.

Nasal Disorders: (*see* Nose, Diseases of).

Naso-pharynx: the part of the back of the throat which lies behind the rear part of the nose.

National Health Service: this was inaugurated in July of 1948 under the National Health Service Act of 1946. Separate Acts provide for Scotland and Northern Ireland. The service is open to everyone regardless of insurance qualifications and is planned 'to promote the establishment in England and Wales of a comprehensive health service designed to secure improvement in the mental and physical health of the people 'by the prevention, treatment, and diagnosis of illness. Its main heads are: (1) the general medical and dental services, pharmaceutical and supplementary ophthalmic services; (2) hospital and consultant services; (3) local health authority services.

(1) *General Medical Services* the family doctor, the dentist, and the pharmaceutical and supplementary service are organised by regional executive councils whose members serve in a voluntary capacity. Any doctor is entitled to take part in the family doctor service and in doing so they are not prevented from having private fee-paying patients as well. Payment is on a capitation basis, i.e. so much a year (at present £1) per head, the maximum number of patients allowed to a single-handed doctor being 3,500. Everyone over the age of 16 may choose his or her own doctor and people away from home can be treated by another doctor as 'temporary residents'. These doctors who joined the Service at the beginning were free to continue practising where they already were but those joining later must first get the permission of the Medical Practices Committee who will grant it provided that the area is not already over-supplied with doctors. Drugs and medicines are free. Nearly all pharmacists in Britain have joined the service. Dentists, like doctors, are free to join this service or not and, unlike doctors, are paid for each item of treatment rather than by a capitation fee; patients do not need to register with a particular dentist as they must do with a doctor. Conservative treatment is carried out at a charge of £1. Mothers who have borne children within the previous 12 months, or those expectant mothers, children under the age of 16, or attending school full time are exempt from any charge. Those under the age of 21 are exempt from charges except dentures. Maximum payment for any one course of treatment, including dentures, is £5. Those requiring ophthalmic treatment must first obtain a certificate stating their need from the family doctor but are entitled to go to any optician or ophthalmic medical practitioner they please. Formerly the only charge was to patients who chose more expensive frames but now various payments have to be made except by the needy and children who accept the standard type of frame.

(2) *The Hospital and Consultant Services* are described under the heading of Hospitals.

(3) *Local Health Authority Services* are the responsibility of county councils and county borough councils. They provide midwifery, child-welfare, and ante- and post-natal services which are described under the heading of Maternity and Child Welfare in addition to health visiting, home nursing, ambulances, local mental health services, vaccination and immunisation, and domestic help on health grounds, all but the last being free except for the use of day nurseries. Their work also includes the provision of special foods and special accommodation for invalids and convalescents and the making of grants to voluntary organisations doing work of this sort.

In addition to the capitation fee doctors receive a basic practice allowance of £925 yearly; an initial practice allowance for the first three years to those setting up in practice single-handed: mileage allowances for visiting distant patients; payment for the treatment of temporary patients; payments to encourage doctors to practice in unpopular areas; and maternity, vaccination, and immunisation fees. The goodwill of a practice is no longer saleable but those who were practising prior to the commencement of the Service are entitled to compensation for this loss payable on retirement or death; in the meantime they receive interest on the unpaid compensation money. There are special tribunals to deal with doctors, dentists, chemists, or opticians who are alleged to have failed to give efficient service. These have a legal chairman appointed by the Lord Chancellor and include a person of the same profession as the one whose case is being investigated and one other, both of these being appointed by the Minister of Health.

Natural Childbirth: just as it was difficult in Queen Victoria's time to persuade doctors and the public of the value of chloroform in childbirth, so it is now equally difficult to persuade them of the value of natural childbirth. There are various reasons other than natural human aversion to change for this: presumably anaesthetists do not like being done out of a job, many doctors and nurses in hospital are extremely busy and understandably prefer their patients to be passively under their control, the antenatal teaching of natural methods is time-consuming and in some clinics might require space and trained staff which are not available, but mainly – so far as doctors are concerned – the reason has been that the method

407

first introduced here was by no means always, or even often, effective. This method was that of Grantly Dick Read which was based on teaching mothers that childbirth was a natural process, explaining what went on, and exercises in relaxation. However, four years ago, Erna Wright brought a new method to this country known as psychoprophylaxis now recommended by the National Childbirth Trust and being taught to midwives all over the country. In the Charing Cross Hospital in London 150 women are taught the method every month and of the 4,000 taught at the National Childbirth 35% reported that their labours were completely painless whilst the rest say that their labours were never unmanageable. Psychoprophylaxis originated in Russia where it is the official method and is very widely spread in France; it is based on active control rather than relaxation and mothers have to learn firstly, that uterine contractions which force the baby out of the womb are not, in themselves, painful; secondly, that most of the pain comes from bringing into use other muscles in the abdomen and elsewhere which not only does not help but causes distress – they must learn to isolate the uterus and let it get on with its work; thirdly, breathing exercises are necessary in order to supply adequate oxygen and prevent exhaustion, to prevent the diaphragm from pressing on the uterus, and to distract the mother's attention from its automatic activity. There can be no doubt that this method is spreading rapidly and that if mothers can obtain the training and are prepared to co-operate they themselves and certainly their babies will be the better for it.

Naturopathy or Nature Cure: this refers to a varied group of people who believe that 'natural' cures are possible by such methods as eating 'natural' foods which may simply mean a largely vegetarian diet or (in the case of extreme purists) food which is not only vegetarian but 'compost-grown,' i.e. on which modern artificial fertilisers, insecticides, or methods of cultivation have not been used. Amongst other methods employed are exercise and massage or, even colonic lavage. For convenience we will also include those ordinarily known as 'herbalists' who believe that 'natural' medicines from herbs are better or healthier or safer than those used by orthodox medicine. It has already been admitted (*see* Fringe Medicine) that it is not only likely but beyond doubt that overfed executives and many others suffering from a surfeit of high living and low thinking are likely to be benefited by such a régime from time to time, but that any sort of diet in itself – except in such conditions as diabetes and other conditions where the diet necessary needs to be *scientifically* worked out by a skilled dietician – is likely to cure a disease, is improbable in the extreme. It is also true that some of the food we eat has been spoilt or even made dangerous by modern methods of farming such as the use of poisonous fertilisers and insecticides or the giving or sex-hormones to animals to fatten them up for killing. This, of course, is a matter which requires stricter legal control. But that, with the exceptions mentioned, naturopathy accomplishes anything worth while is incredible and its beliefs often verge on the ridiculous.

In the first place, we must ask ourselves what is meant by 'natural' food or methods? The Eskimoes 'naturally' live on blubber for the simple reason that there is very little else to eat, hunting tribes in many cases exist almost wholly on lean meat – what we can say with certainty is that no known tribe has ever been exclusively vegetarian. Indeed, man's teeth show that they were designed for a mixed diet, so it is vegetarianism which is unnatural. Again, it is one of the major mysteries of life why the consumer of 'herbal' medicines should go to the trouble of buying senna pods; boiling, stewing, and infusing (or whatever one does with senna pods) all night, and then drinking the nauseous mixture which is full of impurities and contains a wholly unknown amount of the active substance, when he could walk into a chemist's and buy senna pills prepared in the same way, but standardised so that he knows exactly what dose he is taking, and purified so that he is not swallowing dust and unnecessary derivatives. Then there is the argument that we live an 'unnatural life' and that we should turn to one which is closer to nature; but, if this is so, why is it that it is precisely those who live closest to nature whose lives are, in the words of Hobbes, 'nasty, brutish, and short'? Nobody nowadays believes in the noble savage, but what we do know is that amongst primitive peoples the average expectation of life is something like 30 years whilst in our 'unnatural' civilisation it has advanced to more than 70 years! We have seen elsewhere that within 7 years the death-rate of Ceylon has been halved by modern medicine plus DDT which

409

together have practically wiped out malaria. How does a herbalist or naturopath cure malaria or syphilis, how does he deal with a hole-in-the-heart baby? Even G. B. Shaw as an enthusiastic vegetarian only lived to the great age he did with the aid of injections of liver extract for his pernicious anaemia. Finally there is the odd argument that herbs are not only more natural than, say, arsenic used in the treatment of syphilis but that they are safer, that even when they do not cure they at least do no harm. This is plain nonsense, because everybody with a smattering of knowledge about drugs knows that the most deadly poisons in existence are the vegetable ones – strychnine, prussic acid, and the alkaloids in general. In so far as naturopathy or the art of the herbalist claim to be a complete system of medicine in opposition to orthodox medicine – and doubtless it is only the extremists who would make this claim – to that degree the public is being deceived. Helpful or at least usually harmless to the sort of case described above, yes, a cure-all, no.

Nausea: (*see* Vomiting).

Navel: the umbilicus or scar on the abdomen where the umbilical cord joined the body to the mother's placenta in the womb.

Near Sight: (*see* Spectacles).

Neck: the part of the body joining the upper part of the chest to the base of the skull. Its main contents are the thyroid gland, the tubes for air and food (i.e. the trachea or windpipe and the gullet or pharynx and oesophagus), the great blood-vessels going to and from the head and brain, the muscles in front and behind the seven cervical vertebrae which support the neck. The cervical nerves which leave the cord in this area supply the muscles and skin of the neck and arms. The pharynx or throat-cavity lies in front of the spinal column from the base of the skull above to the sixth cervical vetebra below at which point the oesophagus continues it below and the larynx opens out in front where the thyroid cartilage can be felt just beneath the skin. The larynx is continued below by the trachea which is crossed by the narrow part of the thyroid gland, the lobes of the gland being easily felt on either side. The main muscle is the sterno-mastoid passing from the mastoid process behind the ear to the top of the sternum or breast-bone and the inner end of the clavicle or collar-bone. This covers the sheath containing the carotid artery, the internal jugular vein, and the vagus nerve (q.v.) and also a chain of lymph glands. More superficially lie the external jugular vein passing from the angle of the jaw almost straight downwards and the smaller anterior jugular vein which passes down near the midline on either side. The apex of each lung just manages to project a short distance above the collar bone.

Necropsy: an autopsy or post-mortem examination.

Necrosis: the death of a small part of the tissues, usually bone, e.g. in gangrene.

Needling: the old operation for cataract still performed in India where the lens was torn by a needle in order that the opaque material could escape to be absorbed by the fluid of the anterior chamber and subsequently dissolved (*see* Eye, Cataract).

Negativism: in psychiatry the refusal of a patient to attend to stimuli or even, as in schizophrenia, his tendency to do the opposite of what he is asked.

Nematode: a round-worm (*see* Worms).

Neoarsphenamine (Neosalvarsan): an arsenical compound used in the treatment of syphilis and other diseases due to spirochaetes; it is more soluble and less toxic than the original salvarsan.

Neomycin: an antibiotic derived from the *streptomyces fradiae* which being too toxic to be given by injection is mainly employed for skin, eye, and other local conditions as an ointment or lotion. It is sometimes given by mouth for bacillus coli infections of the bowels.

Neoplasm: a tumour.

Nephrectomy: the operation for removal of the kidney,

Nephritis: inflammation of the kidney is classified in many different ways but it is simplest to regard all types of nephritis as a single disease which may (*a*) heal completely (possibly after relapsing occasionally), (*b*) smoulder for a time to clear up later, or (*c*) become chronic after (*b*) has gone on for some time. In childhood the first stage (acute haemorrhagic or glomerular nephritis) usually follows a streptococcal sore throat, often a mild one, or indeed no apparent one at all when the child's face and ankles suddenly swell up with oedema due to the increased permeability of the capillaries all over the body. Blood and albumen are found in the urine, the blood pressure is slightly raised, and there may be pain in the loins. But as in rheumatic heart disease although the streptococcus

411

seems to be responsible and is usually found in the child's throat, it is never found in the urine, its action being apparently from a distance, an allergy rather than a true inflammation. The outlook is extremely good so far as the immediate prospect is concerned, but about 5–10% of cases go on to become chronic and stage (b) may develop (subacute nephritis) with or more often without the earlier one. This too may recover or go on to chronic nephritis in adult life. Most cases of acute nephritis recover completely if the kidneys are rested and this is done as far as is possible in an everactive organ by starving the patient of protein and restricting his intake of salt and water. The usual result of this treatment is that the blood-pressure falls, the oedema or swelling disappears, and the albumen and blood leave the urine. In the majority of cases no trace of the disease is left behind but in the neglected or severe one the symptoms of oedema and raised blood-pressure may go but the albumen persists in the urine; a progressive process has been set in motion which, although the patient may be free of symptoms for many years, ultimately catches up with him. To begin with, the blood-pressure begins to rise in order to maintain the circulation through the kidneys, but in spite of this their ability to concentrate urea in the urine gradually begins to fail so that in time the urine itself becomes increasingly dilute while the amount of urea in the blood rises. Finally death from chronic nephritis may arise from the effects of raised blood-pressure and the over-taxing of the heart in its attempt to maintain the circulation through the kidneys, e.g. heart failure or a stroke, or the end-products of protein metabolism accumulating in the blood and producing a state of coma known as uraemia which is necessarily fatal.

A different state of affairs which some have thought to be a continuation of acute nephritis and others (now in the majority) consider to have no relationship with sore throats or nephritis whatever is nephrosis where the main damage is to the tubules (see Kidneys) rather than to the glomeruli as in the previous cases. Here the main system in the adolescent or young adult who is most commonly affected is oedema and the patient starts to notice that his face is getting white and puffy and soon his feet and ankles are swollen too. In this early stage there are no other symptoms but, on examination, the urine is found to be loaded with albumen which is derived from the blood plasma and treatment resolves itself into restoring lost protein by a protein high diet. The exact cause of this process which is described as nephr*osis* rather than nephr*itis* to indicate that it may be degenerative rather than inflammatory in origin is unknown but the outlook is never good. There is likely to be a period of indifferent health when the patient is liable to catch any minor infection that is going and sooner or later the blood-pressure starts to rise, the urea in the urine to go down whilst that in the blood rises, and the ultimate state is the same as that of the chronic nephritic with death from a stroke, heart-failure, or uraemia.

Nephrolithiasis: stones in the kidney.

Nephropexy: the operation of fixing a 'floating kidney' in its original position; the state of 'floating kidney' is known as *pephroptosis* which is an aspect of *viceroptosis* (q.v.).

Nephrostomy: the operation of making an opening into the kidney for the purpose of draining it.

Nephrotomy: the operation of cutting into a kidney for a stone or other reason.

Nervous System: the nervous system consists of the brain and spinal cord and the innumerable nerves to which these give rise. From the spinal cord housed within the vertebral column there issue thirty-one pairs of nerves which run to different parts of the body. The brain itself gives rise to twelve pairs of cranial nerves which are chiefly concerned with the special senses of sight, hearing, taste, and smell. The whole of the nervous system is made up of the spider-like cells of the neuroglia or support-tissues in which are embedded the star-shaped neurons or nerve cells proper which are smaller than the head of a pin but usually end in a long thin filament which may be several feet in length. These fibres form the nerves of the body which are formed from those of the nerve roots at the side of the spinal cord within which they are continued as columns each going to or coming from its particular destination in the brain, the posterior nerve roots passing into the cord are sensory in function bringing sensations from all parts of the body whilst those further forward are the motor roots bringing impulses of movement to the body muscles. After leaving the spinal cord the roots mingle to form the body nerves which are mostly both motor and

413

sensory. The brain is like a telephone exchange which receives and gives out messages from the rest of the body. Essentially it consists of two levels, the cerebral hemispheres which resemble the two halves of a walnut kernel when looked at from above and are the newest part of the brain in the evolutionary sense, being the seat of man's intellect and the lower centres or old brain where primitive emotions are felt (in a sense the part known as the hypothalamus could be described as the seat of the unconscious or instinctual mind), the viscera controlled, and simple actions initiated. The cerebral hemispheres spend a good part of their time in keeping the old brain in check but there are a great many processes which can take place without its help. Thus when a pin is jabbed into a limb the message of pain passes up the sensory fibres of the nerve to the part, reaches the lower centre in the spinal cord, and a motor message is immediately returned to order the limb to withdraw; this can be done without any interference from the brain and is what is known as an *ordinary reflex* which takes place in the lower animals even when the brain has been destroyed. Many actions are of this sort and it is only a later elaboration of evolution that enables learning in one of its forms to take place by the development of the *conditioned reflex* which necessitates the intervention of the higher (but not necessarily the highest) centres. Here the dog which used to salivate expectantly at the sight of food (simple reflex) soon learns to salivate equally well when a bell which has been constantly sounded when food was given is sounded alone (conditioned reflex). Most of the highest activities of the brain, and some think all, can be understood as conditioned reflexes which in man are complicated by the existense of symbolic and conceptual thought where one thing is made to stand for another (e.g. the word 'fire': causes us to behave as if a fire were present) or things are grouped together to form concepts, e.g. the concept of 'beauty' which is abstracted, as it were, from the numbers of beautiful objects experienced. When the lower centres are damaged no movements or feelings are possible at all over the area of the body supplied by the part affected; there is flaccid paralysis, e.g. of the legs with the limbs as helpless as those of a rag doll. Thus in a disease such as tabes dorsalis or locomotor ataxia where part of the spinal cord is affected by syphilis the knee and ankle jerks are absent, the individual's gait is stamping and he may fall down when his eyes are closed because the sensory messages are being gradually cut off and those which control the body's position in space do not reach their destination. In syphilis of the brain, on the other hand, the reflexes are exaggerated because the upper centres are being slowly destroyed and the lower ones are free to act in an uncontrolled way; in this case there is an increasing spastic paralysis with the muscles tense and ready to overact in an uncontrolled way. Similarly a haemorrhage into the brain or stroke causes exaggerated reflexes whereas one into the spinal cord leads to absent ones sometimes after a brief period of exaggerated responses. These are known as upper motor neuron and lower motor neuron lesions respectively. Whilst the main central nervous system is chiefly concerned with sensations and movements, the *autonomic nervous system* regulates the purely automatic functions of the body such as the activity of glands, the constriction and dilation of the blood-vessels, and the movements of the internal organs. Like the central nervous system it has two components known as the sympathetic and the parasympathetic, the former broadly speaking preparing the organism for fight or flight, the latter for rest. The centre of this part of the system is in the hypothalamus in the base of the brain and from here many fibres and nerve cells come and go to form a chain on either side of the spinal cord but separate from it, passing down the back of the chest and abdomen where it forms various ganglia or groups of nerve cells in 'centres' of which the solar plexus is one. The importance of this system will be realised when one recalls that the hypothalamus is also the seat of the emotions; for this reason the emotions have a considerable influence upon the behaviour of the internal organs in health and disease. This is the basis of what is described as 'psychosomatic medicine' (q.v.). Thus when an individual is *normally* preparing for fight his blood-pressure should rise to improve the supply of blood to the muscles and brain *and it goes down again when the emergency is past*. So with the animals, but man has the power, mentioned above, to form concepts and symbols and with him an emotion is not necessarily here today and gone tomorrow but long drawn out, e.g. his business worry raises his blood-pressure

415

but *his thought of it keeps the pressure up even when he has left the office* and some day may kill him. The autonomic nervous system can both cause diseases and cure them when they have arisen through the agency of what we usually call the mind; indeed it is now obvious that *all* diseases are psychosomatic, i.e. body-mind diseases, smallpox no less than anxiety neurosis. For a man's mental attitude is not irrelevant in considering whether or not he will develop smallpox after exposure and it is possible to cure symptomatically an anxiety neurosis by the use of drugs acting on the autonomic system.

Nervous Diseases: properly speaking, are the diseases *physically* affecting the nervous system although the word is often used in a confusing sense as a euphemism for psychological diseases which have as much (and no more) to do with the nervous system as they have to do with the intestines. A physician who specialises in nervous diseases in the former sense of the term is a *neurologist* whilst the one who deals with psychological ailments is a *psychiatrist*. By virtue of the unfortunate rule that material on the border-line between two large subjects is accepted by the practitioners of both who immediately talk rubbish when they depart from their own speciality, neurologists sometimes know very little about psychiatry and psychiatrists not as much as they might do about neurology, the reason being that each takes over into the other's field wholly unsuitable concepts from his own, e.g. one cannot explain a brain tumour in psychological terms nor can one explain writer's cramp or anxiety neurosis neurologically since, like most mental disorders, these are social rather than structural deviations. The more important nervous diseases are dealt with under appropriate headings throughout the book, psychological disorders are similarly dealt with under the headings of Mental Illness, Neuroses, etc.

Nettle-rash: or urticaria is an allergic condition associated with the appearance of an eruption similar to that found in nettle-stings, i.e. raised red or white patches either locally or spread over the whole body and accompanied by great irritation. The condition may be acute or chronic and is the response of the body to some substance to which it is allergic (*see* Allergy). This is likely to be a foodstuff and a search should be made to discover which in order that it may be avoided in future. Other types are caused by applications to the skin, the use of certain drugs, injections of sera, and the irritation caused by some plants. The use of the anti-histamine drugs immediately stops an attack in most cases but as many such are on the market it is necessary to find out which is most suitable for a particular case. Cortisone preparations rapidly relieve the itching.

Neuralgia: this is a nondescript term implying pain along a nerve-route whatever its cause. Usually no damage is found but there may be evidence of mild inflammation in a nerve-sheath or a ganglion. The types most frequently described are trigeminal neuralgia or tic douloureux, intercostal neuralgia with pain between the ribs, occipital neuralgia at the back of the head but sciatica and even migraine are sometimes in-cluded under this rather dubious heading. Trigeminal neu-ralgia is a clear-cut syndrome affecting the trigeminal nerve which supplies sensation to the face; this has three divisions roughly corresponding to the upper, middle, and lower parts of the face and one or more divisions may be affected. Those affected are most commonly elderly women often with a high blood-pressure and the attacks of very severe pain may be brought on by the slightest stimulus, e.g. cold air or a de-cayed tooth. When the first division is affected there may be watering of the eye with redness both of the eye and the sur-rounding skin and severe frontal headache which is usually one-sided. Similar redness and swelling appears in the upper or lower jaw when the second or third divisions of the nerve are affected and in time the skin may become coarsened, atrophied, and even show changes in the colour of the hair in the parts. The only medical treatment is symptomatic but if the pain is prolonged and very severe it may become neces-sary to operate or inject the ganglion with alcohol. Inter-costal neuralgia, too, is commoner in women and usually makes its appearance on the left side either at the point where the nerves leave the spinal column at the back or the area at the front where they break up into smaller branches. Such an attack often precedes or follows the advent of shingles or herpes zoster (q.v.). Sciatica is discussed under that heading, but of this, as of all the other types of neuralgia it may be said that there is no single cause and those generally given such as damp weather, septic foci in the body, and 'a rheumatic and gouty disposition' are the ones which have been adduced in most diseases of which the cause is either complex or wholly unknown.

Neurasthenia: an out-of-date term which, nevertheless, it is difficult to avoid using on medical certificates from time to time in order to cover a neurotic illness whilst avoiding the social implications of the latter term. Literally, neurasthenia means nerve weakness and is based on the wrong theory that 'nerves' (*a*) is an illness in the usually accepted sense of the term, and (*b*) that it is caused by exhaustion of the nerves in the body. Since neither of these assumptions is true the term is best avoided (*see* Neuroses).

Neurectomy: the operation of removing part of a nerve as in trigeminal neuralgia.

Neurilemma: the thin covering which surrounds every nerve-fibre.

Neuritis: usually this means inflammation of the lower motor neurone (*see* Nervous System) causing typical lower motor neurone symptoms, but degeneration from physical damage will produce the same result. Neuritis may be *local* as in Bell's palsy of the facial nerve or *general* as in neuritis due to alcohol. Since the lower motor neurone is affected the typical symptoms and signs will be: (*a*) loss of power, (*b*) loss of ordinary sensation combined with pain or 'pins and needles' sensations, (*c*) trophic changes in the skin supplied, i.e. the skin is bluish, cold, shiny, and ulcers sometimes develop, (*d*) changes in the muscles which tend to waste and lose their power owing to degeneration of the nerve. The causes in local neuritis are cold as in facial paralysis where the condition frequently arises after driving on a cold night at an open car window, pressure as in the case of fractures or tumours or that from a slipped disc between the 4th and 5th lumbar vertebrae, extension of local inflammation as in middle-ear disease, and, occasionally, there are the rather selective effects of generalised poisoning when lead may cause wrist-drop, and arsenic or alcohol foot-drop. Finally, there is the paralysis of the palate, eyes and legs found in diphtheria and the much commoner neuritis with 'pins and needles' feelings in the fingers due to dropping of the shoulder in housewives carrying too heavy burdens of groceries or even those who are over-fatigued.

In generalised neuritis the causes are the rare disease of acute febrile polyneuritis; the poisons of alcohol, lead, arsenic, typhoid, diphtheria, and leprosy; such metabolic diseases as gout, diabetes, and anaemia; and the deficiency diseases of beri-beri and pellagra resulting from lack of the B vitamins (*see* Vitamins). Most of these causes, it would seem produce the symptoms by the single factor of depriving the nerve of necessary nourishment and mainly of the vitamins of the B group which, therefore, play a large part in treatment in addition to rest, massage and removal of the cause. Heat and analgesics relieve the pain but no amount of heat will remove the cause which is the primary consideration.

Neuroglia: the supporting and connective tissue of the nervous system (q.v.).

Neurology: (*see* Nervous Diseases).

Neuroma: a tumour connected with a nerve which is usually painful and composed of fibrous tissue.

Neurone: (*see* Nervous System).

Neuroses: as pointed out under Mental Illness the so-called mental diseases are either (*a*) physical diseases with 'mental' symptoms, or (*b*) forms of social maladjustment especially in the sphere of interpersonal relations which, of course, may also produce real or apparent physical symptoms. Since this is the case, group (*a*) requires ordinary medical treatment, group (*b*) a prolonged process of adjustment and analysis which, however, can in some cases be avoided by drugs which suppress the symptoms although this is unlikely to lead to permanent results.

The neuroses, then, are caused by social maladjustment learned in the individual's early life with heredity as a negligible factor; for although neuroses often run in families they are generally agreed to be handed on by unconscious training rather than by heredity as such, e.g. it is hardly surprising that obsessional neurosis runs in families since no habit is more readily acquired than the obsessional one. Some of the factors causing neurosis may be briefly summarised as follows:

(1) In Freudian theory (*see* Psychoanalysis) the main cause is the difficulty in controlling primitive impulses by the more socialised ones, e.g. the neurosis manifesting itself as fear of the intentions of men who might even be found

419

    hiding under the bed is a clear indication of an unsatisfactorily repressed wish on the part of an elderly spinster.

(2) In the theory of Alfred Adler (as also in that of Freud) an important part is played by the individual's desire for significance or power and the fear of being shown up. A neurotic in this view is a person who, worried by his feelings of inferiority, tries to cover them up or use them as an 'illness' to get out of difficult situations.

(3) In more recent American schools of thought (Horney, Fromm, Sullivan, etc.) the neurotic's failures in personal relationships have been emphasised; the neurosis is simply the expression of a wrong attitude to such relationships.

All these theories are in part true, the neurotic is *never* a person who simply has 'bad nerves,' his physical nerves are *never* exhausted (although he may feel as if they were), he *cannot* be cured by 'nerve tonics' because no such thing exists, and he is *not* organically ill (although he may make himself so). He or she is a man or woman who has had an unsatisfactory training in his early personal relationships, whether this was neglecting or spoiling or simply anxiety-producing and such a thing can happen in the best-regulated homes. In fact, it usually does. *All* neurotics have difficulty in controlling their primitive instincts, especially if they have been over-controlled in early life and made to feel 'bad', *all* neurotics have feelings of insecurity or inferiority, and *all* make a mess of their relationships with others. That is why they are 'ill.'

The neuroses are divided into the following rough categories: *anxiety states* in which the main symptom is anxiety which takes the form of generalised apprehension without apparent cause, the appearance of the physical concomitants of fear, e.g. palpitation, nameless dread, attacks of breathlessness and sweating, the thought of going mad (which they never do), tremor of the hands and body, or the appearance of phobias which are irrational fears (claustrophobia in enclosed spaces, agoraphobia in open ones, fear of animals, heights, crossing the road, etc.). In *conversion hysteria* the main symptom is an apparently physical one without physical basis (e.g. paralysis, blindness, deafness, inability to write, etc.). This is now rather rare and furnishes an example of the unconscious duplicity of neurosis since these rather naïve physical manifestations have disappeared with an increasing knowledge of medicine and the realisation that paralyses and the rest are not popular when no physical disease is there to account for them. *Obsessional states* manifest themselves as the compulsion to carry out or think certain, usually absurd, actions or thoughts, e.g. touching the lamp-posts one passes, counting numbers which are invested with a magical significance. In all these there exists the idea 'if I do this then . . .' or 'if I don't do this then . . .' and some event is supposed to follow for better or worse. To these may be added the *personality disorders* in which relationships with others are disrupted to an extent which causes inconvenience to the individual or his associates (e.g. the sort of woman who always 'by fate' marries the wrong man) and the *psychosomatic diseases* (q.v.) where tension, perhaps at a much deeper level, leads finally to serious and sometimes fatal physical disease (e.g. duodenal ulcer, essential hypertension). The treatment of the neuroses or psychoneuroses is, by choice, psychotherapy (q.v.) which gives the patient a chance of looking himself in the face and understanding his problems with a view to dealing with them. He must also understand his problems in relation to those of others; for we are all neurotic in varying degrees and it is simply a medical convenience to describe as neurotic someone who is so to such a degree or in such a way as to trouble himself or others. Many gross neurotics are overlooked because their failing is in a direction approved of in general by society, e.g. it is neurotic and a nuisance for a housewife to keep on cleaning unnecessarily or for a man to think of nothing but money and his work, but although these types need a psychiatrist's help as much as anyone else who is neurotic, they are often commended for their behaviour. As already mentioned, there is no such thing as 'nerve tonics' for the excellent reason that there is nothing to build up and the neurotic (heaven knows!) does not need rest or a holiday unless the cruise so often recommended is of such a nature as to take him away from the task he is busy evading through his illness when he will naturally recover almost instantaneously until the day when he has to return. Sedatives and the tranquillising drugs have some effect upon symptoms but do not alter the fundamental state, yet, like the cruise, they too may be effective when the

421

unfulfilled task is one that disappears with time (*see* Mental Illness, Psychoanalysis, Psychotherapy).

Neutropenia: reduction in the number of the neutrophil leucocytes (*see* Leucocytes) in the blood to below 2,500 per cu. m.m. as in influenza, typhoid, measles, or resulting from the drugs chloramphenicol, chlorpromazine, and some of the sulpha group.

Nicotinamide: the amide of nicotinic acid (q.v.) sometimes used as a substitute.

Nicotine: (*see* Smoking).

Nicotinic Acid: or niacin is a member of the vitamin B complex which is essential to life and health. In pellagra, a defiency disease, nicotinic acid or nicotinamide is used in treatment and the drug by reason of its ability to dilate the capillaries is also used in diseases not due to vitamin deficiency but showing signs of vascular spasm, e.g. 'dead' fingers, chilblains.

Niehan's Cell Therapy: Dr Niehans is a qualified physician living near Montreaux in Switzerland. His particular form of treatment is based on the belief that, if any organ of the body is not functioning properly, it can be revitalised by the injection of fresh cells taken from the corresponding organ of a young or preferably unborn animal. The new healthy foetal cells, it is claimed, inevitably find their way to the affected part of the body. Thus there exists a natural affinity between the embryonic heart cells, for example, of a chicken, mouse, or man. In practice, the organs are collected at the local slaughter-house where the pregnant animal is killed, and the required parts extracted from the foetus. They are then rushed as quickly as possible to the patient, passed through a sieve to reduce them to a 'cellular state' and, suspended in a normal salt solution, injected into him. In spite of the many famous people who are said to have benefited from this method, it is rejected by most orthodox medical bodies in America and France; in Britain ampoules of dried cells which, it is said, can also be effective are on sale. Most medical men here believe that the whole rationale is highly dubious, and that sometimes the treatment may be dangerous.

Night Blindness: is caused by lack of vitamin A in the diet which shows itself in inability to see in dim light whilst seeing quite normally in bright sunlight. The visual purple of the retina is built up from the vitamin.

Nightmare: (*see* Sleep, Insomnia).

Night Sweats: used to be typical of tuberculosis and are found in many other conditions where there is a persistent low fever, e.g. rheumatic fever, undulant fever.

Nikethamide: the official name for nicotinic acid diethylamide with the proprietary name of Coramine which is used as a respiratory stimulant.

Nipples, Disease of: (*see* Breast).

Nitrites: are used in conditions where spasm has to be relieved and their most important action is in dilating the blood-vessels. Hence amyl nitrite is used in angina pectoris by inhalation, and the tablets of erythroltetrate and nitroglycerin have a similar but more prolonged action.

Nitrofurantoin: a synthetic drug effective against a wide range of organisms but used mainly in infections of the urinary tract. The proprietary name is Furadantin.

Nitroglycerin: (Trinitrin, glyceryl trinitrate) *see* Nitrites.

Nitrous Oxide Gas: laughing gas (*see* Anaesthetics).

Noradrenaline: the substance liberated at sympathetic nerve endings which helps transmission of the impulse.

Normoblast: the primitive red blood cell before it has discarded its nucleus.

Nose, Diseases of: Tonsils and Adenoids, and Sinusitis, are dealt with separately, and here it is only necessary to mention nose-bleeds, polypi, foreign bodies in the nose, and loss of the sense of smell or anosmia. *Bleeding from the nose* is never dangerous except in those who are suffering from a blood disease as haemophilia and it is extraordinary that those who would unhesitatingly donate a pint of blood to the Transfusion often become quite upset at the loss of less than a tenth of that amount by the nose and, of course, anxiety is the worst possible thing in haemorrhage since it causes the heart to beat harder and the blood-pressure to go up. Apart from direct violence the commonest cause of nose-bleeds is a vascular area in the lining of the nose like a small varicose vein which breaks down from time to time although bleeding also occurs in general diseases such as certain blood disorders, vitamin deficiencies (which are very rare in the West), high blood-pressure, and sometimes the so-called

423

'vicarious bleeding' which happens in women at the time of their period. The treatment is well known: keep quiet and lie down, loosen the collar, do not blow the nose or even touch it no matter how 'stuffy' it may feel, apply cold packs to the back of the neck. If these measures do not succeed the doctor may have to pack the nose with gauze soaked in adrenaline. *Polypi* are soft jelly-like masses usually in the area of the middle turbinate bone. They are shiny and greyish in colour and arise from an overgrowth of the mucous membrane due to chronic inflammation as with frequent colds and chronic sinusitis. The main symptom is an awareness that the nose is always blocked and the condition can only be diagnosed for certain after an examination by the doctor who will recommend the simple operation for removal. *Foreign bodies* are often found in the noses of children and sometimes adults. They should be removed by the doctor if blowing the nose will not dislodge them; poking in the nose should be strongly discouraged unless done by an expert. *Anosmia* or loss of the sense of smell is always present in any condition which causes blockage of the nose; it is also present in some cases of fracture of the skull affecting the olfactory nerves. It must be remembered that no sense is sooner tired than that of smell and the presence of a particular odour in a room very quickly leads to total unawareness of its existence after a short period of exposure; hence the danger of gas leaks where the gas may reach a dangerous concentration without the individual being aware of the fact.

A curious fact is the quite disproportionate concern attached to the nose and the sense of smell which can only be explained on psychological grounds since in fact hardly any serious diseases affect this area. Yet the doctor is constantly meeting those who complain bitterly of 'catarrh,' of perpetual bad smells, of loss of the sense of smell, or of nose-bleeds which as already noted are of no general grave significance. One of the earliest signs of mental disease is quite often the belief that particular smells are present or that other people behave towards the patient as if he smelled badly. This can partly be understood when we remember (*a*) that the nose has a sexual significance, and (*b*) that smell is developmentally one of the oldest of the senses and certainly the most primitive.

Nosology: the scientific classification of diseases.

Notifiable Diseases: those infectious diseases which are required by law to be notified to the Local Authorities.

Novarsenobenzol: is neosalvarsan or neoarsphenamine (q.v.).

Novocain: a proprietary name for procaine hydrochloride (*see* Anaesthetics).

Nuclein: a protein forming part of the nucleoprotein which enters into the formation of the cell nucleus. Medically it is used to stimulate the formation of leucocytes or white cells in a granulocytosis (q.v.)

Nucleus: the body in the centre of a cell which controls its function.

Nullipara: a woman who has no children.

Numbness: results either from damage to or inflammation of the sensory nerves or diseases of the arteries (*see* Arteries, Neuritis).

Nursing: as we know it today the profession of nursing dates from Florence Nightingale and the Crimean War although in quite early times there were hospitals (q.v.) for the sick poor in Egypt, India, Greece, and Rome. The nursing system as an organised state of affairs and a branch of medical treatment originated with the deacons and deaconesses of the early Christian Church and from the 4th century onwards hospitals were managed by the clergy and male and female nurses recruited from the various monastic orders; in England the oldest surviving institutions are St Thomas's and St Bartholomew's hospitals. It was not until the Reformation that nursing came to be separated in some measure from religion but properly trained nurses (as contrasted with those who simply learned their work by experience in the wards) are a creation of the mid-19th century. This system developed in Germany under Pastor Fliedner whose institute at Kaiserwerth was founded in 1836 and was the training-school of Florence Nightingale. Two years later an institute was founded in Philadelphia and in another two Elizabeth Fry had founded one in London, the nurses of which were trained at Guy's and St Thomas's hospitals. The appalling conditions of the Crimean war to which Florence Nightingale brought a band of trained nurses led to new reforms in nursing and played a large part in raising the profession in the public esteem. In 1860 the Nightingale Fund Training School for Nurses was founded at St Thomas's by public subscription, and soon similar schools were rising all over the Continent.

Nursing is usually thought of as a feminine profession but the number of male nurses has greatly increased in recent years. Information about training can be obtained from the Ministry of Health or the General Nursing Council for England and Wales.

Nuts: are one of the more nourishing forms of vegetable food containing not less than 50% of vegetable fats and oils. In a wholly vegetarian diet they form in part a useful substitute for meat.

Nux Vomica: is obtained from the seed of *strychnos nux-vomica*, a West Indian tree. Its actions (as in tincture of nux vomica) are due to those of its alkaloids, strychnine (q.v.) and brucine. It is used in small doses as a 'tonic' (q.v.).

Nyctalopia: night-blindness.

Nystagmus: the condition in which the eyeballs show an involuntary movement from side to side or, less frequently, up and down or rotary. It occurs in miners as a neurosis, in children with some defect of vision, and in certain nervous diseases, e.g. disseminated sclerosis.

Nystatin: an antibiotic obtained from the fungus *streptomyces noursei* and used internally in the treatment of other fungus diseases, e.g. moniliasis (q.v.). It is also used as an ointment for similar conditions.

Obesity: in the strict sense there is only one cause of being overweight: eating too much or eating too much of the wrong kind of food so that the intake of calories (q.v.) is greater than the output. This is not invalidated by the fact that glandular factors may play a part or that there are some people who can eat as much as they like without becoming overweight since their basal metabolic rate increases to deal with the excess; for the overweight person's diet is unsuitable for him or her in the circumstances. It is now recognised that a major factor in the production of obesity is the psychological one and that some individuals can be addicted to food (and especially to sweet and starchy foods) as others are addicted to drink and for this reason drugs which reduce the appetite such as dexedrene, diethylpropion (Tenuate), and others or thyroid extract which increases the metabolic rate are only occasionally successful although useful aids to dieting. In practice dieting means taking a low calory diet high in protein and low in fat and carbohydrate. Such a diet would be somewhat as follows: coffee or tea with milk but no sugar at breakfast accompanied by crispbread or Energen rolls and a small amount of butter but no jam or marmalade and no brown or white bread or toast. At lunch, grilled lean steak, grilled fish, or an egg dish and salad followed by jellies or fruit or crispbread and cheese – but no potatoes, peas or beans (with the exception of French beans). The evening meal may consist of grilled or steamed fish, clear soup, cheese and fruit, but there must be no fried food or sweets at any time. The basic principles of this diet are obvious: lean meat, non-fatty fish (i.e. no kippers or herring), eggs, fruit, crispbread or Energen rolls but no fried foods, fat meat or fish, bread, potatoes, sweets or cakes. However small amounts of butter and quite a lot of milk are permissible.

This is the conventional diet but of recent years a new theory has sprung up which takes the view that fat people are those who have some innate difficulty in dealing with carbohydrates and that therefore a diet which cuts out carbohydrates almost entirely and allows as much fats and protein as desired – in fact the more fat the better – is indicated. It is pointed out that people such as the Eskimos who live on a fat-high diet do not become overweight whereas those whose diet has a high carbohydrate content very well may unless their basal metabolic rate is capable of increasing to deal with it. A specimen diet of this type (which has proved very successful in suitable cases) is as follows: a large breakfast of bacon, eggs, kidneys, etc. fried in plenty of fat, or kippers, ham, or Continental sausage (no English sausages which contain cereal); Energen rolls (no crispbread), butter but no jam or marmalade. Midday meal of steak with fat or any other fat meat, omelette or Continental sausage, salad but no potatoes, tomatoes as desired, French beans or other green vegetables, high-fat cheese (cream, Camembert, Wensleydale etc.), apple or orange. Main evening meal as for breakfast and lunch combined. Cheese, tomato, water, is unrestricted and dry alcoholic drinks may be taken, e.g. dry sherry, dry white wine, gin and bitters, but no beer, rum or sweet wines or liqueurs. The great benefit of this diet is that it works, that it can be carried on without discomfort even after the weight has been reduced, and that it is safe – although it is not for people who are suffering from chronic illness or whose digestion is poor. According to this view the total intake of calories is less relevant than the form in which they are taken in and the conventional slimming diet is only a form of slow starvation. To be avoided are bread and root vegetables, potatoes, anything from the baker's or confectioner's, soups other than clear soups, beer and sweet drinks. Leading authorities on nutrition do not deny that this diet works but hold that it is, in fact, merely a low-calorie diet since those who eat much fat (*a*) do not eat a great deal of it and (*b*) do not desire carbohydrates. Theories involving polyunsaturated fats are nonsense.

Obsession: (*see* Neuroses).

Obstetrics: the study and practice of midwifery.

Obstruction of the Intestines: can be caused by a tumour, by a loop of intestine becoming twisted on itself (volvulus), by the bowel being caught in a hernial sac (*see* Hernia), or as a result of adhesions from a previous operation. Acute obstruction is a surgical emergency and if an operation is not performed death will result in a few days unless the cause of obstruction is such as to occasionally relieve itself. The symptoms are severe colic, profuse vomiting from progressively lower levels of the tract, distended abdomen, absolute constipation, and collapse. Chronic obstruction in which the blocking is gradual is usually due to a tumour; the symptoms in this case are periodic attacks of vomiting, loss of weight, and constipation alternating with diarrhoea. Initially the surgeon may by-pass the area by a colostomy or the entire affected area may be removed. In children intussusception (q.v.) is a not uncommon cause of obstruction, although in a few cases the condition unravels itself or is relieved by manipulation.

Occiput: the back of the head.

Occupational Diseases: few trades or even professions are free from the risk of specific diseases although until recently the main concern of the practitioner of industrial medicine has been with the manual worker. It was with the manual worker in mind that Paracelsus in 1567 published his monograph on *Miners' Sickness and Other Miners' Diseases* and possibly the first specialist in industrial medicine was the Italian Bernardino Ramazzini (1633–1714) who wrote the textbook *Diseases of Tradesmen*. But today, two hundred years after the beginning of the Industrial Revolution in England, the scope of the specialist is much wider with the realisation that the director's duodenal ulcer or coronary thrombosis is as much an occupational disease as caisson sickness (q.v.). Of course, one may play safe with the observation that many people may get a duodenal ulcer who have never worked at all whilst caisson disease can only be contracted in a diving bell but the modern industrial medical officer rarely takes this attitude; for the fact is that a better understanding of 'tradesmen's diseases' has played a large part in wiping them out. Some of the more obvious conditions may be mentioned here, taking the apparently safest professions first – and what could be safer and healthier than working on the land? The agricultural worker may develop epithelioma or cancer of the skin from exposure to sun and weather, actinomycosis (a serious fungus infection) from working with grain, anthrax from working with horses or hides, tuberculosis from cattle, spirochaetal jaundice from working in muddy ditches, and an endless number of aches and pains from physical stress. Pet-shop dealers may develop psittacosis, telegraphists cramps, workers with cosmetics dermatitis, musicians callosities and emphysema of the lungs (if their choice is the wind instrument), housewives housemaid's knee or prepatellar bursitis, clergymen and politicians laryngitis, doctors angina pectoris from prolonged mental stress (although the misguided will say that a diet rich in cholesterol is the main cause), and the more specifically industrial diseases include the following: anthrax or woolsorter's disease, caisson disease in divers, cataract in glass-blowers, spirochaetal jaundice in miners and sewer workers (who may also be affected with hook-worm or ankylostomiasis); poisons employed in various trades which may harm workers are arsenic, antimony, mercury, lead, nickel, and such non-metallic substances as phosphorus, carbon disulphide, carbon tetrachloride (in cleaners and dyers) and the coal-tar products. Other very important occupational diseases are silicosis, asbestosis, byssinosis, dermatitis, chrome ulceration, and cancer induced by irritant chemicals, and the dangers from radioactive substances in medical work and atomic research stations. Industrial diseases proper are governed by the Factories Acts the provisions of which are supervised by inspectors of the Ministry of Labour and by examining surgeons specially appointed for the purpose. Most large factories now have their own medical and welfare workers whose work extends from the prevention of physical hazards to the worker or hazards to the consumer (e.g. in food factories) and the possession and application of some knowledge of industrial psychology in respect of particular tasks in a given environment and morale in general, as well as examinations and treatment. The factory medical officer would be of little help if he restricted his work solely to the physical hazards facing workers, for at the best he should be a sort of liaison point between workers and management acting faithfully on his knowledge that nothing which harms the worker physically or psychologically can be good for either the firm or its customers in the long run. Many such diseases are subject to compulsory notification and compensation of diseases and injuries is regulated by the Workmen's Compensation Acts.

Ocupational Therapy: work in Occupational Therapy was first carried out in Britain during the First World War and mainly by those without a medical training but between the wars a group of people began to realise its importance as a specialised employment. Therefore in 1930 Dr Elizabeth Casson founded the Dorset House School in Oxford and other schools soon followed, the Association of Occupational Therapists being founded in 1936 with Sir Hubert Bond as first president and Mrs Glyn Owens as chairman. Membership is limited to those who hold the Association's diploma or that of an approved school obtained before the Association's examination system was established. A fully qualified occupational therapist must have a knowledge of at least 10 crafts as well as a knowledge of anatomy, physiology, psychology, first-aid, departmental management, general medicine and surgery, together with some knowledge (according to specialisation) of psychiatry, advanced anatomy and physiology, physical medicine, or orthopaedics.

Occupational therapy originated in mental hospitals as a means of taking the patient's mind off his own problems and rehabilating him into society but today it takes all forms from the physical aspect of designing work to exercise specific groups of muscles to the encouragment of free expression painting in psychiatric work which may give insights into the patient's problems. Much is being learned not only about specific skills but also about the emotional and social aspects of employment from hobbies to hard work.

Ochronosis: a rather rare condition associated with dark brown staining of the ears or face as melanin is deposited in the cartilage of the ears, nose, and eyelids. There may be associated osteoarthritis of the large joints and the urine darkens on standing and stains the clothes (alcaptonuria). This is sometimes an inborn error of metabolism but it frequently occurred when carbolic acid was used for dressings over long periods of time. Ochronosis does not shorten life.

Oculentum: an ointment for the eye.

Oedema: swelling due to the passage of fluid through the walls of the blood or lymph vessels as in heart and kidney disease, liver disease, anaemia, obstruction of the circulation, and allergy.

Oesophagus: the gullet. For diseases of this area *see* Throat.

Oestradiol: one of the hormones secreted by the ovaries and responsible for the development of the female sexual characteristics (*see* Ovaries).

Oestrogen: a collective name for the various forms of the female sex hormone whether natural or synthetic.

Oidium Albicans: the fungus causing thrush (q.v.).

Olfactory Nerve: the nerve of smell or first cranial nerve.

Oliguria: the passing of small amounts of urine.

Omentum: an apron of peritoneum usually loaded with fat which hangs down in front of the intestines.

Onchogryphosis: gross thickening and overgrowth of a toe nail due to chronic inflammation.

Oophorectomy: ovariotomy, the removal of an ovary, e.g. for a cyst.

Oophoritis: chronic single inflammation of an ovary due to defective metabolism, renal disease, or sexual problems. The symptoms are vague abdominal discomfort, low backache, pain before the periods, and heavy loss. The treatment is usually diathermy and if necessary removal (*see* Ovaries).

Ophthalmia: inflammation of the eye or conjunctivitis (*see* Eye).

Ophthalmoplegia: paralysis affecting one or both eyes due to brain disorders. It is *external* when the muscles moving the

431

OPHTHALMOSCOPE

eyes from outside the eyeball are affected, *internal* when there is interference with the dilating or contracting of the pupil and accommodation.

Ophthalmoscope: an instrument for examining the back of the eye.

Opisthotonus: the position assumed in certain forms of seizure where the tensed body, as in tetanus, rests only on the back of the head and the heels. It is also characteristic of strychnine poisoning.

Opium: the effects of opium in man are largely due to its morphine content and the two may be dealt with together. Opium is obtained from the capsules of the white poppy *papaver somniferum* which contains about 10% of morphine as well as codeine and 18 other alkaloids. It diminishes all the secretions of the body except sweat thus making the mouth dry, delays the emptying of the stomach thus relieving the sense of hunger whilst causing constipation; in some people opium and, in particular, morphine causes vomiting; the respiratory centre is depressed including the cough centre and death may occur from asphyxia; in the nervous system there may be initial excitement but eventually this leads to drowsiness and relief of pain without loss of intelligence. The pupil is contracted. Applied locally, opium is used, e.g. in lead and opium lotion on the fallacious assumption that it produces local anaesthesia, but internally it is one of the most useful drugs known to man; opium or morphine are used for the relief of severe pain, for diarrhoea, in congestive heart failure to stop the rapid shallow breathing and cause slower and deeper respirations, in grave internal or external haemorrhage, to suppress severe coughing, in Dover's powders (q.v.) to increase sweating, and to relieve anxiety prior to operation or labour. These are, of course, drugs of addiction (q.v.) and morphine and heroin are undoubtedly dangerous; nevertheless men have taken opium for many years without obvious ill-effect (Coleridge and De Quincey both lived to a ripe age) and in England up to the end of last century laudanum was as commonly used as aspirin today. Poisoning with opium or its derivatives necessitates the use of an emetic if the drug has been taken by mouth followed by strong stimulants, e.g. black coffee.

Opsonins: substances in the serum of the blood which so act on bacteria as to make them capable of being destroyed by the white blood cells or phagocytes.

Optic Nerve: the second cranial nerve connecting the eye with the brain (*see* Eye).

Orbit: the bony hollows of the skull containing the eyes, lacrimal glands, and various blood-vessels and nerves.

Orchitis: inflammation of the testicle (q.v.).

Organic Disease: means structural disease of the body such as can be demonstrated on ordinary examination or under the microscope. It is contrasted with *functional disease*, once almost a term of abuse, in which only the functions of the body are disordered without demonstrable structural change. This was once regarded as synonymous with 'neurotic' but we now know that one may readily, as in the psychosomatic diseases (q.v.), pass into the other.

Organic Substances: are essentially those derived from living matter or related to them. Organic chemistry is the study of the carbon compounds which play the major role in living tissues.

Orgasm: the climax of sexual pleasure accompanied in men by the emission of semen and in women by reaching a height of excitement with contractions of the vagina followed in both cases by a sudden decline in tension. In men failure to reach orgasm or reaching orgasm too soon (premature emission) is a sign of partial impotence (q.v.) which will either disappear in time as the couple become adjusted to each other or may need to be referred to a psychiatrist or the Marriage Guidance Council. But, on the whole, few men fail to reach orgasm on some occasion or another. In the case of women the situation is rather different and in Britain and America few women reach orgasm every time and some – perhaps as many as 60–70% – never do so at all. The main reason for mentioning this is that, whilst in Victorian days and even earlier, women were literally thought to be licentious if they showed any sign of sexual pleasure, in our own day the attitude has been entirely reversed and, as every doctor knows, many women literally worry themselves sick because they either obtain little pleasure or do not achieve orgasm. Complete frigidity should be referred to the bodies mentioned above, but the failure to reach orgasm whilst still obtaining some pleasure is perfectly compatible with a happy married relationship. It is society which

makes many women feel 'bad' in these circumstances by causing them to feel that there is something shameful about not
being completely sexually satisfied. Society is wrong, and it is
time we grew out of the silly idea derived from the early sex
reformers (many of whom, like Havelock Ellis and Marie
Stopes, themselves had serious marital difficulties) that sexual
technique is everything in a happy marriage. Many couples
who have orgasms every time have ended up by divorcing
each other, whilst the majority who do not achieve in most
cases perfectly satisfying relationships. Sex and affection can
never be entirely separated from each other in marriage, but
affection and mutual understanding are far more important
than sex (*see* Sex and Sexual Problems).

Oriental Plague: (*see* Plague).

Oriental Sore: (*see* Kala-azar).

Ornithosis: a virus infection of birds transferable to man.

Orthopaedics: the branch of medicine dealing with physical
deformities (usually of the bones and joints) both congenital
and acquired.

Orthoptic Treatment: the treatment of squint by giving special
exercises for the muscles of the eye.

Osteitis: inflammation of bone (q.v.).

Osteo-arthritis: (*see* Rheumatism).

Osteomalacia: a disease causing deformity of the pelvis, back,
and legs which is a form of adult rickets and therefore due to
lack of vitamin D and sunlight. The patient is generally a
woman of 20–30 in the poorer parts of the world suffering
from such deformities with weakness and aching of the back;
occasionally there may be attacks of tetany (q.v.). The treatment is to give a diet rich in the vitamin and surgery may be
necessary to correct the deformities which, of course, are not
reversed by medical treatment.

Osteomyelitis: (*see* Bone, Diseases of).

Osteopathy: 'a complete science of healing based on the nor-
malising of the body and its functions on the assumption that
a structural derangement of skeletal parts known as the
"osteopathic lesion" is the significant factor in all disease.'
Osteopathy has no connection whatever with manipulative
surgery although its procedures involve manipulation and its
theory that defect in structure is at the root of all pathological
conditions is not accepted by orthodox medicine which does

not believe that diseases are caused to any significant degree by obstruction of arteries or nerves by the pressure of mal-adjusted bones in the vertebrae of the spinal column. The system originated with the American physician Andrew Taylor Still in 1874 and numerous colleges teaching osteo-pathy exist in America. In London the British School of Osteopathy is at 16 Buckingham Gate, S.W.1. From the ortho-dox point of view the main fallacy of osteopathy is that of any similar branch of 'fringe medicine,' namely the assumption that diseases have any one basic cause or can be cured by a single basic method. But nobody doubts that most prac-titioners are sincere and capable men who may in many cases have a better knowledge of bones and joints than most general physicians (*see* Fringe Medicine).

Osteoporosis: increased porousness of bones due to lack of calcium.

Osteotomy: the operation of cutting a bone.

Otitis: inflammation of the ear (q.v.).

Otology: the branch of medicine dealing with diseases of the ears.

Otorrhoea: discharge from the ear.

Otosclerosis: a condition of hardening and bone formation in the inner ear leading to progressive deafness.

Ouabain: Ouabaine is G-Stropanthin obtained from a South African tree and used as an arrow poison in E. Africa. It is a diuretic and cardiac stimulant with a similar action to digitalis.

Ovaries: the two ovaries are almond-shaped, about 1½ inches long and 1 inch wide, and lie against the side walls of the pelvis close to the open ends of the Fallopian tubes which lead to the upper corners of the womb. They are the female sex glands and have a tremendous influence over a woman's life from the beginning of puberty to the end of the change of life and even after. The functions are of two main types, the first relating to the production of ova, the second to the production of hormones. Each month (except during preg-nancy) an ovum or egg is discharged from the ovary out of the many thousands of immature eggs embedded in its sub-stance; this matures more quickly than the rest, bursts through the capsule of the ovary, and is soon drawn into the Fallopian tube on that side by the motile hairs or cilia surrounding the tube's trumpet-like end. This process is called ovulation and if the egg is fertilised by a sperm as it passes down to the womb pregnancy begins and the production of ova temporarily ceases, if it does not ovulation (which happens at the mid-period) is followed in two weeks or so by menstruation (q.v.). During pregnancy the point at which the ovum escaped, a small yellow body or corpus luteum gives out a hormone that helps to maintain pregnancy. In the absence of pregnancy it shrivels up in a week or so. The sex hormones are two in number: oestrogen and progesterone the former being concerned with the production of the female sexual characters, the development of the breasts and body hair, etc., and the maintenance of the first two weeks of the menstrual cycle, the latter being secreted by the corpus luteum and stimulating the growth of the lining of the womb during the second two weeks of the menstrual cycle; if pregnancy begins the secretion of progesterone continues until birth. In a general way it might be said that oestrogen is a stimulant hormone, progesterone a relaxing one. Both are under the control of the anterior lobe of the pituitary gland at the base of the brain through the medium of the gonadotropic hormone it secretes. Because of this close relationship to the hypothalamus or emotional centre just above the pituitary the menstrual cycle is very responsive to emotions as when the periods stop when there is fear or hope of pregnancy. Only one ovary is necessary to carry on all the normal functions.

The conditions of the ovaries which require treatment are inflammation, cysts, benign tumours, hormone-producing tumours, cancer, and endometriosis. *Inflammation* is usually capable of being treated by the antibiotics but sometimes an abscess forms in association with the tube and this may require removal. The commonest cause of this is gonorrhea but other germs may be found and at one time tuberculosis was fairly frequent although this has greatly decreased. These conditions may be acute or chronic and the main symptoms are pain in the lower part of the abdomen during or just after menstruation, pain on passing water, sickness and vomiting with fever in the acute cases. Menstruation is often excessive and there may be a discharge between periods. Back pain in the lumbar region is usual as with most pelvic diseases.

Cysts are extremely common, and as noted above a tiny cyst is normally formed each month which ordinarily disappears after the egg is discharged from the ovary; if these persist and become large they may need to be removed but often they cause no trouble at all unless haemorrhage into a cyst occurs or it bursts into the abdomen when pain, fever, and tenderness suddenly develop. *Cystic ovaries* are present when the ovary is full of small cysts and sometimes severe symptoms arise if a cyst develops a stalk and twists on this, the blood-supply to the ovary being cut off.

Benign cystic tumours are sometimes dermoid cysts which contain hair and teeth and others (pseudomucinous cysts) become filled with a mucous substance and may become very large indeed. About 30% of cysts affect both ovaries and the cyst may be removed alone or the whole of one ovary and the cyst in the other. Less common are the hormone-producing tumours which can produce either male or female sex hormones, the former causing the development of male characteristics such as a deep voice and growth of hair on the face. *Cancer of the ovary* can be diagnosed early in those who have regular pelvic examination but otherwise they tend to develop silently without any notable symptoms. The treatment has to be radical and all the female pelvic organs are removed. Surgeons have often been criticised for unnecessary removal of the ovaries, but it must be remembered that removal of one ovary leads to no disability at all and in other cases factors to be taken into consideration are the nature of the disorder (e.g. no risks can be taken with cancer), the condition of the other ovary, the patient's attitude to further pregnancies, and her age. In neither case is sexual desire removed.

Endometriosis is a condition in which cells from the lining of the womb are found growing on the surface of other abdominal organs, e.g. the tubes, ovaries, and ligaments, the intestines, or the periotoneal lining of the abdomen. Typically there is lower abdominal pain beginning a week or ten days prior to the period, getting worse during menstruation, and passing off on about the second or third day. Sometimes cysts are formed. In older women radical removal of the womb and appendages will cure, but in younger women when cysts are absent injections of male sex hormone are often helpful.

Ovum: (*see* Ovaries).

Oxalic Acid: is an irritant poison although oxalates sometimes appear in the urine after eating rhubarb or strawberries and may give rise to pain on passing water. The treatment for poisoning by oxalic acid is to give large amounts of chalk mixed with water and followed by an emetic. When the stomach has been emptied milk may be given to soothe the lining.

Ox-Gall: is used in medicine as a cholagogue (q.v.) to stimulate the flow of bile and also to those who suffer from intestinal flatulence from faulty digestion of fats. It may be taken as Veracholate tablets which contain bile salts.

Oxophenarsine: (Mapharsen or Mapharside) an organic arsenical used in the treatment of syphilis.

Oxycephaly: the name given to 'steeple head' where the skull is highly domed with bulging of the eyes and sometimes deformity of the limbs with optic atrophy. The mentality of these patients is normal and it is sometimes necessary to operate to relieve the pressure within the head by decompression.

Oxygen: is a colourless odourless gas which forms more than one fifth of the atmosphere and is essential to life. It is administered to patients suffering from oxygen lack either through a mask or in an oxygen tent.

Oxymel: a home-made medicine used for coughs and colds or sore throats and made of vinegar and honey. Its effect is mildly soothing but little else although one of the dottier fads in the U.S. during the late 1950's has been the use of cider vinegar and honey as a cure-all.

Oxyphenonium: an anticholinergic for relieving spasm and excessive motility of the intestinal tract in peptic ulcer, etc. The proprietary form is Antrenyl (oxyphenonium bromide).

Oxytetracycline: the approved name for terramycin. Obtained from a soil mould, its range of action is comparable with that of aureomycin (q.v.).

Oxytocic: an agent which stimulates contractions of the pregnant womb at full time.

Oxytocin: (*see above*) an extract, also known as pitochin, which is obtained from the posterior lobe of the pituitary gland and has this effect.

Oxyuriasis: infestation with thread-worms, i.e. Oxyuris (*see* Worms).

Ozaena: a chronic disease of the nose in which there is atrophy of the lining with the formation of foul-smelling crusts inside.

Ozone: a gas is chemically O_3 in contrast to oxygen's O_2. It has a typical salty odour but is poisonous in large amounts and, although its existence has been publicised in travel pamphlets as appearing in the air of mountain and sea-side resorts, it is doubtful whether any large amount is really present or whether any benefit would arise if it were. Ozone is a powerful deodorant and germicide in suitable amounts and is probably found in the highest concentrations in the dynamo rooms of power-stations.

Pachymeningitis: (*see* Meningitis).

Pacinian Corpuscles: the bulbs at the ends of sensory nerve fibres which are scattered throughout the skin and form the end-organs for sensation.

Paediatrics: the branch of medicine dealing with the diseases of children.

Paget's Disease of Bone: or osteitis deformans is a disease of bone usually found amongst men of 40–60 years of age in which, whilst the central parts of the bone become rarified, new bone is constantly formed just under the surface. Eventually the bones become thick, heavy, and curved, pain develops in the limbs, and there is progressive enlargement of the skull, with loss of height and a gorilla-like appearance due to these changes and the bending of the long bones. Deafness is common. There is no treatment.

Pain: (*see* Analgesics, Anaesthetics).

Painter's Colic: (*see* Lead).

Palate: the roof of the mouth which is also the floor of the cavity of the nose lying above. It consists of the *hard palate* in front made of bone and covered by the mucous membrane of the mouth below and that of the nose on the upper side, and the *soft palate* behind which is composed of muscle similarly covered. When food or air is passing through the mouth the soft palate rises to shut off the nose, the prolongation which hangs down in the centre being known as the uvula. Harelip is a failure of development in which the parts forming the lips and hard and soft palates have failed to unite; these consist of a fronto-nasal process in front and two maxillary processes at the sides, the spaces between forming a Y-shaped gap. The upper part of the Y contains the fronto-nasal process and the two maxillary processes lie one on either side. Thus there may be complete cleft palate with gaps beneath each nostril running back to join the lower limb of the Y which cleaves the palate right in two, or there may simply be a gap in the soft palate at the back or a failure to develop on the part of one of the upper limbs of the Y opening on to the lip at one side. The condition occurs in about 1/1000 births and there is a tendency for it to run in families. Operation should be carried out as early as possible both because the best time to remedy harelip and cleft palate is in the first weeks or months and because sucking is often impossible until this is done. The possession of a harelip is quite an unpleasant deformity which, in addition to its effect on appearance, causes a difficulty in speaking but even so there are few cases which cannot be improved at any stage if early results are not satisfactory.

Palpation: the method of examining the surface of the body by touching gently with the hands.

Palpebrae: the eyelids.

Palpitation: the state in which the heart beats forcibly or irregularly so that the person becomes aware of its action. This is nearly always a nervous condition which has very little to do with the heart itself and it is extremely doubtful whether tobacco, alcohol, coffee and tea, or even 'excesses' (whatever these may be) have anything whatever to do with it as was formerly thought. Although palpitation does occur as one amongst other symptoms in serious heart disease, the vast majority of cases are due to repressed anxiety and have no direct connection with heart disease whatever. The treatment is that of an anxiety state: reassurance after a careful examination of the heart (usually more for the patient's than the doctor's benefit), tranquillisers and sedatives.

Palsy: a somewhat archaic word for paralysis (q.v.).

Paludrine, Pamaquin: (*see* Malaria). Both are anti-malarial drugs.

Panacea: a fabled remedy which cures all diseases.

Pancreas: the pancreas is a soft flat yellowish gland lying behind the stomach and shaped roughly like a large tadpole. It is about five inches long and two inches wide and throughout its entire length runs the pancreatic duct to collect the digestive juices manufactured in the substance of the gland and transport them into the duodenum. But the pancreas not only makes the juice used in the digestion of food; it also produces insulin which is passed directly into the blood and is essential to the burning-up and utilisation of sugar. If too little insulin is produced diabetes will result, if too much hyperinsulinism and hypoglycaemia occurs. The main conditions affecting the pancreas are: pancreatitis, cysts, benign tumours (adenomas), and cancer.

Acute pancreatitis: comes on suddenly and reveals itself by severe pain in the upper abdomen, nausea, and vomiting. It is commonest in men between the ages of 40–50 and is difficult to diagnose without an examination of the blood chemistry. Quite often there is a history of gall-bladder disease or of gross over-eating or drinking just before the onset of the symptoms. Chronic pancreatitis is usually found in association with disease of the gall-bladder or bile ducts. Rest and antibiotics may be used in the first instance to cause the inflammation to subside, but if haemorrhage is serious or an abscess develops an operation may be necessary. In chronic pancreatitis an operation with examination of the gall-bladder to correct any defects may have to be carried out.

Cysts of the pancreas are not common nor are adenomas or benign tumours which sometimes involve the insulin producing cells of the islets of Langerhans thus leading to hypoglycaemia with trembling, great hunger, fainting, and sometimes convulsions. Cancer most commonly arises in the head of the gland and is of course a very serious condition which leads by pressure on the bile-duct to jaundice; this may be relieved by a short-circuiting operation to by-pass the obstructed bile-duct or a removal of the whole pancreas with the nearby part of the duodenum may be attempted; the stomach is sutured to the small intestine in the region beyond the duodenum.

Pandemic: an epidemic affecting a large area, e.g. a continent as did the 1918–19 influenza pandemic.

Panhysterectomy: (*see* Hysterectomy). Complete removal of the womb and its appendages.

Pantothenic Acid: part of the vitamin B complex known as the 'chick anti-dermatitis factor' since without it dermatitis develops in chickens together with degeneration of the nerves of the spinal cord. The vitamin is found in milk, meat, liver, and cereals.

Papilloedema: is swelling and congestion of the optic disc at the back of the eye due to increased pressure within the skull as in brain tumour.

Papilloma: a tumour growing from the *papillae* of the skin or mucous membranes which may be either simple or malignant. Papilloma is found frequently in the bladder where the main symptom is painless expulsion of blood in the urine.

Para-aminosalicylic Acid: or P.A.S. is used in the treatment of tuberculosis when it is given in conjunction with streptomycin or isoniazid. The organisms tend to become resistant to P.A.S.

Paracentesis: puncturing with a hollow needle any body cavity in order to withdraw abnormal fluid either for relief of symptoms or pathological examination.

Paraesthesia: the presence of abnormal feelings in the absence of any adequate external cause, e.g. hot flushes, itching, and 'pins and needles' sensations which are due to internal disturbances.

Paraffin: a hydrocarbon used in medicine internally in the form of liquid paraffin for constipation and externally as a base for various ointments and sprays. Liquid paraffin is not a satisfactory treatment for constipation as it is messy, acts solely as a lubricant and is therefore not always effective, and since crude paraffin is a known carcinogenic substance such preparations taken internally are not above suspicion however slight the risk.

Paraganglioma: (chromaffinoma, phaechromacytoma) is a tumour made up of the chromaffin cells found normally in the medulla of the suprarenal glands. Its main symptom is periodic high blood-pressure.

Paragonismus: a kind of fluke found in the Asiatic countries and S. America which infects the lungs and causes spitting of blood.

Paraldehyde: a colourless liquid of ethereal odour and burning and nauseous taste used as a safe and powerful hypnotic. It is less frequently employed than formerly because of its unpleasant taste and the strong smell it leaves on the breath.

Paralysis: loss of muscular power due to some interference with the nervous system (*see* Nervous System, Apoplexy, Parkinson's disease, etc.).

Paraplegia: paralysis of both sides of the body below a certain level, e.g. from the waist down.

Paramnesia: distortion or falsification of memory or recognition.

Paranoia: a form of insanity characterised by delusions, usually of persecution, which are fixed and typically occur in the absence of any other signs of mental disorder. It is extremely resistant to treatment and is more in the nature of a character disorder than mental disease as ordinarily understood.

Paraphrenia: a form of schizophrenia midway between paranoid schizophrenia and paranoia. Unlike the former it does not tend to early dementia and is a disease of middle age, unlike the latter the delusions, usually of persecution, are associated with other symptoms such as hallucinations of hearing. Treatment is a specialist matter but the outlook for social improvement is not bad even if complete recovery is unlikely.

Parasites in Relation to Disease: these creatures which are said to infest rather than infect the body are most conveniently divided into what are ordinarily thought of as insects living on the surface of the body and worms and flukes living inside. Amongst the best-known of the former are lice, fleas, bedbugs, and the mite of scabies. Scabies is still sometimes treated with sulphur ointment but the best method is the application of benzyl benzoate as a 25% emulsion; the others are killed with applications of D.D.T. Treatment, however, is best carried out at a Disinfestation Centre since clothes, etc., may have to be dealt with. Lice are usually classified as the head louse (pediculus capitis), the body louse (pediculus corporis or vestimenti) and the crab louse found in the hair of the pubic region (pthirius pubis). In themselves these creatures are not dangerous but some can carry the germs of very dangerous conditions: the flea, plague; the louse, typhus; and another, the mosquito, malaria and yellow fever (q.v.). This, however, is unusual in Western Europe where these diseases are no longer common. Some forms of worm and fluke infestation are discussed under the heading of Infection (*see* Worms).

Parasympathetic Nervous System: the part of the autonomic nervous system antagonistic in action to the sympathetic, i.e. it prepares the body in general for rest and relaxation rather than fight or flight and consequently stimulates the digestive action of the stomach whilst slowing down the beat of the heart. The centres in the mid-brain, medulla, and at the lower end of the spinal cord give rise to fibres which are carried in and 4th sacral nerves.

Parathormone: the hormone secreted by the parathyroid glands the 3rd, 7th, 9th, and 10th cranial nerves, and the 2nd, 3rd, (q.v.).

Parathyroid Glands: four small glands lying behind the thyroid gland which are primarily concerned with the metabolism of calcium and phosphorus. Deficiency of their secretion leads to tetany (q.v.) in which there is extreme restlessness and muscular spasms with a rise in the blood phosphorus and a fall in calcium; excess secretion causes an increase of calcium in the blood which is taken from the bones with consequent cyst formation and the development of the disease known as generalised osteitis fibrosa cystica.

Paratyphoid Fever: (*see* Typhoid Fever).

Paregoric: the camphorated tincture of opium used in cough mixtures.

Parenchyma: the secreting cells of the glandular organs.

Parenteral: a method of administering drugs other than by the mouth or bowel, e.g. injection, inunction.

Paresis: slight or temporary paralysis.

Parietal: concerned with the walls of a cavity, e.g. parietal pleura the layer which lies against the chest wall or the parietal bones which form walls on either side of the skull.

Parkinson's Disease: or paralysis agitans is a disease of older people caused by degeneration of the basal ganglia of the brain although a similar condition occurs after encephalitis lethargica in the younger age-groups. Its onset is gradual and a coarse tremor of the hands, fingers, and head develops together with a typical appearance in which there is stooping and rigidity of the muscles, an expressionless face, and a characteristic gait. The patient looks as if he were 'trying to catch up with himself,' the legs moving as if trying to prevent the head from overbalancing the body which is bent forward. The hands are in constant motion with the thumb and middle finger rubbing together in 'pill-rolling' movements. Treatment of this condition is with hyoscyamus and stramonium or the many other drugs available and in selected cases a surgical operation often gives good results. In general Parkinsonism is slowly progressive.

Paronychia: inflammation in the region of the nails and nail-bed (q.v.).

Parotid Gland: the largest of the salivary glands which is situated just in front of the ear and has a duct which enters the mouth opposite the second last tooth of the upper jaw. The gland may be enlarged in mumps (which is sometimes described as epidemic parotitis) or from simple inflammation.

Patella: the knee-cap.

Pathogenic: capable of producing disease.

Pathognomonic: characteristic of a certain disease.

Pathology: the study of the changes brought about in the body by disease.

Pectoral: relating to the chest.

Pediculus, Pediculosis: lice and lice-infestation (*see* Parasites).

Pellagra: is a deficiency disease which is commonest in the maize-eating parts of the world especially in the Far East, the Americas, and around the shores of the Mediterranean. The symptoms are characteristic and readily recognised with the sore tongue and diarrhoea, the chronic inflammation of the skin of the head and neck, and the mental changes which include those ordinarily found in the organic psychoses, namely, loss of memory for recent events, intellectual deterioration, and disorientation in time and space. The cause of pellagra is not entirely clear since although it is obviously due to lack of vitamins of the B2 group it cannot be produced experimentally by feeding human beings on a B2-free diet. It is probable that, because vitamins such as nicotinic acid and riboflavine are normally produced in the human colon by the action of bacteria, maize contains a substance which antagonises or destroys them and that therefore maize as such is the villain of the piece. This is confirmed by the fact that patients on certain antibiotics (chloramphenicol and aureomycin) which kill the vitamin-producing germs develop pellagra-like symptoms unless B2 vitamins are given at the same time.

Pelvis: the pelvis is a basin-like structure connecting the legs with the spine and consisting of the haunch-bones on either side and the sacrum and coccyx behind. The haunches are made up of three bones, separate in the child, but fused together in the adult, the illium the crest of which can be felt when one puts one's hands on one's hips, the ischium with a rounded tuberosity upon which one sits, and the pubis in front. The opening at the lower part of the pelvis is closed in life by the two levator ani muscles and behind by sacro-iliac ligaments leaving openings only for the urinary and genital passages and the rectum. Within the pelvis are the urinary bladder and rectum in both sexes, the seminal vesicles and prostate gland surrounding the bladder's neck in the male, and the womb, ovaries, and their appendages in the female.

Pemphigus: a skin eruption characterised by the appearance of large blebs, bullae, or blisters either in newly-born children (pemphigus neonatorum, Ritter's disease) or in older ones in whom it is occasionally fatal. The causes are various but include syphilis and lack of cleanliness in handling young children. Treatment depends on the cause but the non-syphilitic types respond well to the sulpha drugs and antibiotics such as penicillin.

Penicillin: the original antibiotic discovered in 1929 by Sir Alexander Fleming in the mould *penicillium notatum* first described by a Scandinavian in 1911 without its healing properties being known. Florey and Chain who shared the Nobel prize with Fleming in 1945 showed how penicillin could be produced in bulk, a discovery without which it might have been useless. Penicillin (apart from allergic reactions) is practically non-toxic to human beings but capable of killing a large number of disease-producing organisms. It is now supplied in many different forms, e.g. benzylpenicillin, procaine benzylpenicillin, phenoxymethylpenicillin and benzathine penicillin, and under many proprietary names including the new types which are capable of dealing with formerly resistant organisms; some, unlike the original, can be taken by mouth and there are variations in the length of time during which a given preparation acts.

Penis: the male sex organ through which both semen and urine are discharged by way of the urethra. The body of the penis contains spongy tissue which is capable of filling with blood in order to produce erection so that the organ becomes capable of sexual intercourse when excited (*see* Circumcision, Sex).

Pentolinium Tartrate: a methonium compound used in the treatment of high blood pressure in which it is longer acting than the other drugs.

Pentothal: (*see* Barbiturates).

Pepsin: a gastric ferment or enzyme which partially digests proteins into peptones. It has been given in medicine, as have peptonised foods, to people with 'weak digestions' but this has a distinctly Victorian flavour and there is little place in modern medicine for the digestive enzymes and partially digested foods.

Peptones and Peptonized Foods: (*see* Pepsin).

Peptic Ulcer: (*see* Stomach, Diseases of).

Percussion: the procedure of 'thumping' the chest or other parts with the fingers which is carried out by doctors in order to find out what is going on beneath. The principle behind percussion is simple being a matter of resonance; thus if a cigar-box filled with sand be percussed a dull 'flat' note will be given out but if it be empty the note will be hollow and resonant. Similarly the lung filled with exudate in pneumonia will give a dull note and the enlarged liver gives dull sounds farther down the abdomen than normally. What is distinguished is the difference between hollow and solid or semi-solid organs, whether they are normally so or by disease have become so.

Perforation: a perforation is a surgical emergency attaching to any condition of the stomach or intestines where ulceration into the abdominal cavity has occurred or when penetration has happened through a wound. The symptoms are those of peritonitis which is set up by the escape of infected material into the abdominal cavity, i.e. collapse, generalised pain over the abdomen, and evidence of gas and fluid set loose within it (*see* Peritonitis).

Pericarditis: inflammation of the pericardium, the cellophane-like sac which surrounds the heart in two layers. Its most common causes are acute rheumatism, acute fevers and pneumonia, tuberculosis, and blood-poisoning, although spread may occur from local disease, e.g. pleurisy, and pericarditis is common in anyone who is dying from another cause, e.g. diabetes, chronic nephritis. In the dry type the membranes are covered by a layer of fibrin which causes a to-and-fro friction sound through the stethoscope but later pericarditis with an effusion is likely to develop when the layers are separated by fluid. Here the pain over the heart which was originally present disappears but the patient becomes more breathless and the doctor will note that the area of heart dullness (*see*

Percussion) increases and the sounds heard are muffled. Treatment depends on the cause and on what symptoms are present but absolute rest in bed is essential. Sometimes the fluid becomes infected and turns into pus or it may become necessary to remove excess fluid through a needle. Ordinarily the outlook is good but adhesions between the pericardium and surrounding structures may give trouble later.

Perineum: the fork or region between the genitals in front and the anus behind.

Periods: (*see* Menstruation).

Periosteum: the thin membrane surrounding a bone which carries the blood-vessels and nerves necessary to its nutrition.

Periostitis: inflammation on the surface of a bone.

Peripheral Neuritis: neuritis (q.v.) of the nerves in the arms and legs at the periphery of the body.

Peristalsis: the alternate movements of contraction and relaxation by which the intestines and stomach propel their contents along.

Peritoneum: the cellophane-like membrane which cover all the internal organs of the abdomen and its walls; as the mesentery it hangs the intestines from the back of the abdominal wall and as the omentum it hangs down like an apron over the front of the large intestine.

Peritonitis: when a hole exists in the stomach or intestines or any other hollow organ in the abdomen the germs which are ordinarily helpful in the digestion of food or exist in the excretions escape and cause serious infection together with more or less haemorrhage. This may occur from a perforated ulcer, from a wound, a ruptured appendix, or a ruptured ectopic pregnancy when the fertilised ovum has continued to grow in the Fallopian tube. Sometimes, too, abscesses or cysts may burst. There is severe pain and tenderness all over the abdomen, signs of fluid and gas, vomiting, and a state of shock with low blood-pressure, high temperature, and rapid pulse. Immediate operation is necessary to close the ruptured or injured area and blood-transfusions and antibiotics will be given as necessary. Sometimes the peritonitis, instead of being generalised, is localised by adhesions to one area, and tuberculosis may give rise to a chronic peritonitis with pain, distension, and alternate diarrhoea and constipation over a period of time associated with the signs of tubercular infection elsewhere. Treatment is with P.A.S. and other drugs but a surgical operation may be necessary to let the fluid escape.

Peritonsillar Abscess: or quinsy is an infection with abscess formation in the region of the tonsils and usually secondary to acute tonsilitis. The abscess is likely to point and burst through the soft palate or may have to be opened in a slight operation. Antibiotics or sulpha drugs are given as in acute tonsillitis.

Pernicious Anaemia: (Addison's anaemia) is a severe anaemia with a typical picture in the blood, a progressive course, and cured by extracts of liver and stomach. It is brought about by the failure of the bone-marrow to produce red blood-corpuscles because it is not supplied with sufficient amounts of the P.A. factor; this is composed of an extrinsic factor taken in with the food and an intrinsic one secreted by the glands of the stomach which together are stored in the liver. Most types of pernicious anaemia are idiopathic (i.e. are not secondary to other causes) but cancer of the stomach or the after-results of gastrectomy when the lower part of the stomach has been removed may lead to similar results as also may intestinal disease which interferes with absorption, e.g. sprue. The onset is gradual with tiredness, weakness, and fainting attacks and the skin develops a characteristic lemon tint. The tongue is likely to be red and sore and loss of appetite, nausea, and indigestion are common. In more advanced cases the nervous system is involved with numbness, pins and needles sensations, and finally spastic paralysis. The patient is usually an adult over the age of 36 years. Under the microscope the red blood-cells are seen to be greatly reduced in number but each cell is larger than normal and contains relatively more pigment (this puts pernicious anaemia in the category of megaloblastic hyperchromic anaemias – *see* article on Anaemia). The hydrochloric acid in the stomach is great reduced or absent. Formerly this disease was incurable but in 1924 Dr Minot of Boston in the U.S. found that raw liver cured his patients and later it was shown that stomach extract had the same effect. Today pernicious anaemia is treated by injections of liver extract and vitamin B12. If, however, the condition has gone on for a long time prior to treatment there may be residual nervous symptoms due to damage to the spinal cord.

Peroneal: the name given to the nerves, vessels, and muscles on the outer side of the leg.

Peroxide of Hydrogen: or H_2O_2 is a colourless and odourless liquid the antiseptic properties of which are due to its ability to give up oxygen and turn into water in the process. It is therefore very safe and the strength of a solution is measured in terms of the amount of oxygen it is capable of releasing, e.g. the usual 10 volume strength is capable of releasing 10 times its bulk in oxygen. Hydrogen peroxide is most commonly used in cleaning wounds (but not as a dressing), in extracting wax from the ears – when it should be washed out by water subsequently as impurities in the solution may cause irritation, as a mouth-wash, and as a bleach for the hair. A solution in warm water is very useful for removing dressings that have stuck without disturbing the wound.

Perspiration: or sweat is secreted by the tiny sweat glands scattered over the surface of the body; over a pint a day is imperceptibly lost through evaporation from the pores but when the internal or external temperature rises or during exercise much more sweat appears and can then be seen on the surface of the skin. Sweat is an excretion which contains only about 2% of solids these including salts together with minute amounts of fat and urea (the bulk of which is excreted by the kidneys) although in kidney disease the skin to some extent takes over the lost function and excretes quite large amounts of urea. The openings of the sweat-glands can be seen quite easily through a hand lens on the tops of the ridges on the surface of the skin and the chief function of sweating is to regulate the body temperature which is controlled by centres in the medulla (the point at which the brain joins the spinal cord) and the spinal cord itself; these are connected to the vasodilator nerves controlling the size of the blood-vessels but also directly to the sweat glands causing them to secrete. Apart from excretion and temperature regulation sweat seems to have a sexual significance since its odour must at one time have been sexually stimulating and probably is so still to a greater extent than we care to recognise in a repressed function. The odour is in fact altered to a quite recognisable degree in various diseases: there is the sour odour of rheumatism, the typical smell of fear in neurotics, the unpleasant odour of dyspepsia, and doubtless many others which partly explain our 'intuitive' awareness of illness. Sweat may be coloured blue from taking indigo and red in certain blood conditions when it may be said that the individual is 'sweating blood.' The parts of the body where the glands are most numerous are the soles of the feet, the palms of the hands, the groin and the arm-pits, but bromidrosis or bad-smelling sweat, apart from those conditions already mentioned, seems to be in part due to bacterial decomposition, so frequent baths are indicated in addition to the usual toilet preparations sold for this purpose. It is extremely doubtful whether chlorophyll taken by mouth has any effect on body sweat although it undoubtedly reduces odour when applied locally, e.g. in the mouth. Sweaty feet should be similarly treated and it is useful to wring the socks out in boric acid solution before drying and to dust the inside of the shoes with antiseptic powder. Fungus infections if present must, of course, be treated. There is no evidence that antiseptic soap is any better than any other kind for excessive perspiration since soap is by its nature antiseptic.

Perthes's Disease: or pseudo-coxalgia is a disease of the hip-joint in children due to flattening and occasionally fragmentation of the head of the thigh-bone or femur. The cause is unknown but there is no constitutional disturbance and, although there is a limp and pain over the hip, little interference with movement except in abduction (i.e. movement away from the mid-line). Diagnosis is by X-ray and rest and extension are all that is necessary to recovery; for there is usually little permanent damage. Similar conditions occur in the tibia and in the vertebrae.

Pertussis: (*see* Whooping Cough).

Pessaries: (*a*) instruments in ring or other form designed to support a displaced womb from inside the vagina; (*b*) bullet-shaped bodies, usually with a glycerine base, designed to treat disease in the vagina where they dissolve to release a drug which varies according to the pessary.

Petechiae: small spots, usually reddish or brownish in colour, in the skin forming a rash which may be due to inflammation or tiny haemorrhages.

Pethidine: the official name for a very useful pain-killing and antispasmodic drug which to some extent takes the place of combined morphine and atropine usually given in such conditions as renal or biliary colic. Like the others, it is a drug of addiction.

Petit Mal: the minor type of epileptic attack which may take the form of altered states of consciousness without convulsions (*see* Epilepsy).

Phagocytosis: the process whereby the phagocites amongst the white corpuscles of the blood destroy and absorb invading germs (*see* Infection).

Phalanx, Phalanges: the small bones of the fingers and toes.

Phantasy, Fantasy: a day-dream in which images and the trains of imagery are divided and controlled by the emotions of the moment.

Phantom Limb: the impression often following an amputation that pain is coming from the removed area. The condition departs with the passing of time in the vast majority of cases.

Pharmacology: the branch of medicine dealing with the action of drugs.

Pharmacopoeia: the official list of approved drugs which gives their names, doses, the preparations made from them, and tests of purity, etc. The Pharmacopoeia for Great Britain and Ireland is issued under the supervision of the General Council on Medical Education, but many large hospitals issue their own list of drugs and standard prescriptions for the sake of convenience.

Pharmacy: the technique of preparing medicines or the place where it is carried out.

Pharyngitis: (*see* Throat, Diseases of) the name means inflammation of the pharynx which is the channel where the air and food passages meet with the base of the skull above, the upper six cervical vertebrae behind, the larynx and the gullet or oesophagus below, and the nose, mouth and larynx in succession from above down. In the upper part the Eustacian tubes from the middle ear open on either side, adenoids which are masses of lymphoid tissue may develop on the back wall, and the part is controlled by the three constrictor muscles. The complex act of swallowing entails the closing off of the nasopharynx so that food does not enter the nose and the shutting of the epiglottis so that it does not go down the breathing tubes.

Phenacetin: or acetphenetidin is a coal-tar product with an action similar to that of aspirin with which it is often combined.

Phenazone: or antipyrin has a similar action to that of aspirin and phenacetin. It is, however, much more dangerous and during one influenza epidemic in Vienna seventeen people were killed by this drug. Neither phenazone, phenacetin, or amidopyrine have any advantage over aspirin and there are many disadvantages which furnish an excellent reason for not employing them alone although there is no reason to think that phenacetin combined with aspirin is harmful if it is unlikely that the combination together with codeine or caffeine is more potent than aspirin alone.

Phenindione: (Dindevan) is an anticoagulant taken by mouth which, although slower in action than heparin, produces much the same effects.

Pheniodol: a drug which, when excreted by the liver, renders the gall-bladder opaque to X-rays; it is taken by mouth.

Phenobarbitone: (Gardenal, Luminal) is a barbiturate used in the treatment of epilepsy and as a sedative (*see* Barbiturates).

Phenol: carbolic acid.

Phensuximide: (Milontin) a drug used in the treatment of petit mal epilepsy attacks.

Phenylbutazone: (Butazolidin) a drug used in the treatment of chronic rheumatic disorders, especially rheumatoid arthritis, in which it relieves pain whilst producing toxic side-effects in certain cases.

Phenytoin Sodium: (Diphenylhydantoin sodium, Epanutin, Eptoin) is used in the treatment of epilepsy and produces its effects without the undue sleepiness resulting from phenobarbitone.

Phimosis: a tight foreskin which is the usual excuse for circumcision.

Phlebitis: (*see* Varicose Veins).

Phosphorus, Phosphates, Phosphoric Acid: *phosphorus* was at one time the cause of the dread condition known as 'phossy jaw' when poisoning in chemical or match works led to necrosis of the lower jaw. This is almost unknown today but illness and death still occasionally occurs from rat poison where the typical symptoms are those of an irritant substance followed by grave liver damage. *Phosphoric acid* is a constituent of many tonics where, like tonics in general, it has no effect whatever; the idea that it had, as in the case of the *glycerophosphates* (q.v.), arose from the assumptions that since nervous tissue contains phosphorus and neurosis is due to exhaustion of these tissues therefore they need phosphorus as food. Only the first of these statements is true. Phosphates constantly appear in the urine since this is one of the commoner elements in the body and in food; they have no particular significance but the cloudy appearance caused by them when the urine becomes alkaline often causes much needless anxiety to chronic urine-examiners. *Acid phosphatase* is a substance secreted into the blood in cases of prostatic cancer.

Photophobia: fear of light which is a symptom of many eye diseases and of measles in the early stages.

Phrenic Nerve: the nerve supplying the diaphragm which arises from the 3rd, 4th, and 5th cervical nerves. It may be divided or crushed in the treatment of tuberculosis (q.v.) in order to rest the lung.

Phrenology: the psuedo-science founded about 1800 by Gall and Spurzheim and based on the notion that the 'bumps' on the skull can be read to give an analysis of the individual's character, e.g. his 'amative' or 'possessive' propensities. This is based on the dual fallacy that such faculties are located in the brain when they are not and that the shape of the brain influences the shape of the skull when it does not (unfortunately the reverse is more often true). Today phrenology is limited to cranks or the uneducated but it had a considerable influence in its time and aided the development of the study of personality by more scientific means.

Phthisis: the wasting which used to accompany pulmonary tuberculosis and was often used as a synonym for that disease. The main function of the word today is to act as a spelling trap for the unwary student.

Physeptone: (*see* Methadone).

Physiology: the science which deals with the normal workings of the human body or, if preceded by an adjective, those of animals or plants.

Physostigmine: an alkaloid obtained from Calabar bean which produces the same effect as stimulation of the parasympathetic nervous system (q.v.). It therefore stimulates the gut, constricts the pupil, and increases the flow of urine and saliva. The drug is used in eye diseases to contract the pupil and reduce the tension within the eyeball when it is given in lamellae (q.v.) or eye-drops; injections are given to stimulate the intestines when they are paralysed or atonic.

Pia Mater: (*see* Meninges).

Pica: a perversion of appetite supposed to be typical of neurotic children or pregnant women when unusual substances such as coal are eaten. Dirt eating is common in mentally defective children but in others, and in pregnant women, it is more likely to be due to the desire to attract attention. Ordinarily no treatment is necessary.

Picric Acid: an explosive used in solution in order to produce a protective coat over a burn or injury by its capacity for coagulating proteins.

Picrotoxin: a respiratory stimulant used as an anecdote in barbiturate poisoning.

Piles: or haemorrhoids are varicose veins of the lower end of the rectum where they may be external or internal. External piles are outside the bowel and are therefore covered by skin, being brown or dark purple in colour, whereas internal piles, being covered by mucous membrane, are bright red and extend up the bowel as far as the top of the inch-wide sphincter muscle. The former may exist without any symptoms whatever but if large or inflamed can be extremely painful and cause chafing and irritation, the latter often cause no discomfort but are liable to lead to bleeding of dark blood when motions are passed. The causes of piles are both local and general; amongst local causes must be listed the fact that these veins have no valves and are liable to become distended and that constipation is likely to increase the interference with circulation, general causes are a sedentary way of life, overweight, pregnancy, interference with the portal circulation as in heart disease or cirrhosis of the liver, or any bowel disease. In treatment, constipation should be avoided and simple food with plenty of bulk and liquids taken; exercise is important and weight should be brought down if excessive. Local applications have no effect other than soothing irritation and itching. The doctor should be consulted and operation or a course of injections to thrombose the piles may be recommended. The main effect of suppositories is to relieve pain and itching and to some extent to prevent bleeding but, since all cases of piles do not require more radical treatment, this may in many cases be enough.

Pilocarpine: an alkaloid contained in the leaves of jaborandi which has an action similar to that of the parasympathetic

455

nervous system. Its only function in medicine is in hair-tonics for which purpose it is entirely useless.

Pineal Body: a small gland with no known function lying in the upper part of the mid-brain. It has evolutionary connections with the 'third eye' of certain lizards.

Pink Disease: or erythroedema is a disease of young children of between 6 months and 3 years in which a mild feverish illness leads in about five weeks to redness and swelling of the hands and feet. Redness also occurs on the nose, ears, and cheeks and the child in general is extremely miserable with sweating, itching, loss of appetite, and photophobia (distaste for light). The cause is unknown and pink disease has been regarded as a vitamin deficiency, a vasomotor disorder akin to chilblains, an infection, and as related to the use of mercury in teething powders. There is no specific treatment, but vitimin B complex is usually given. Most cases recover, but the disease may last for many months.

Piperazine: (Antepar) a drug used in the treatment of threadworm and roundworm infestations. Formerly used for gout, it is not now considered to be helpful in rheumatic conditions.

Pituitary Gland: the pituitary is the most important of all the ductless glands because although it produces its own secretions it also exercises control over the other glands. For this reason it has been called 'the conductor of the endocrine orchestra.' The gland is about the size of a large pea and lies at the base of the brain enclosed in a deep depression in the skull (the sella turcica); it is joined to the brain by a stalk and its connections with the emotional centres of the hypothalamus are important. The anterior and posterior lobes of the pituitary have different functions, the posterior lobe simply producing two hormones, vasopressin which raises the blood-pressure and controls the output of urine, and oxytocin which stimulates contractions in the pregnant uterus at full time, whilst the anterior lobe has a great variety of functions concerned with the most fundamental aspects of body-build and character in addition to producing the hormones which stimulate the other glands to action or inaction. Amongst the latter group are the thyrotrophic hormone which stimulates the other gland, the gonadotrophic hormone, the sex glands, and the adrenocorticotrophic hormone (better known as A.C.T.H.) which stimulates the cortex of the adrenal glands. Removal or underdevelopment of the anterior pituitary produces dwarfism whilst increased activity, as from a tumour, leads to gigantism or, if the bones have already 'set,' to the condition of acromegaly. Other disturbances of this part can cause premature senility, sexual immaturity and gross overweight (Frölich's syndrome), great wasting (Simmond's disease), diabetes insipidus (q.v.), Dercum's disease with great masses of painful fat, Lorrain dwarfism, and the type of individual who rejoices in the name of 'Fearnside's pudding-faced boy.'

Pityriasis: a skin disease characterised by the development of large brownish-red patches which desquamate with the production of larger quantities of bran-like scales. It is caused by a microscopic fungus.

Placebo: a drug given, not for its real pharmacological effect, but, as the name indicates, to please the patient. It is therefore usually inert. Two points must be made about the doctor's occasional use of placebos which no doubt many laymen may regard as a deceitful practice and would doubtless feel highly indignant if they knew that they were receiving one. The first is that, as medicine now is, the patient comes to the doctor in a frame of mind which positively demands 'a bottle' (in fact, in some parts 'a bottle' is the only *real* medicine and the patient may feel that mere pills or tablets are fobbing him off the genuine article). This is all wrong; for the doctor's real function is to give *advice* or carry out procedures which will be curative, but it can well be imagined in what frame of mind most people would leave their doctor's surgery if they were simply given advice as to diet and health regulations. People hate advice which is, by implication, a criticism of the way they have been leading their life, they love to feel that the doctor is like a watch-repairer to whom they take the offending part and demand that it be fixed as if it had nothing at all to do with their real self. Since the doctor cannot re-educate everyone, he must in some cases comply with his patient's often unspoken wishes so long as these do not go too much against the grain. Secondly, placebos are really little doses and symbols of faith. It does in fact have a remarkable effect on a man when he knows that regularly three times a day, in water, after meals, he must take a particular dose, and even the most intelligent amongst us is the better of this symbol of the persisting influence of the

457

doctor in our home. Many tests have shown what extraordinary effects can be produced by the inert pill plus belief and, indeed, the effect may be so potent as to nullify trials of a new drug when the patient's enthusiasm or that of the physician enter the field to relieve even the most deadly complaints. Placebos are the mark of the physicians' care and (in St. Paul's sense of the word) love; which is, after all, his chief weapon. 'Though I have the gift of prophesy, and understand all mysteries, and all knowledge . . . and have not love, I am nothing.'

Plague: or bubonic plague is caused by the bacillus *Pasteurella pestis* common in Europe at one time but now largely restricted to Asia. Nevertheless it caused millions of deaths in Europe during the years 1348 and 1668 and was the 'Black Death' which changed the course of history. Plague is carried by the bite of the rat flea but once people become infected spread may occur from one to the other by droplet infection, i.e. by coughing and sneezing. After an incubation period of 2–10 days a fever develops rather like severe influenza and in a day or two the glands in the groin begin to swell followed perhaps by swelling of the glands elsewhere. It is the glands in the groin which are known as buboes and give the disease its name. This is the usual type of plague but it is also possible to get disease of the lungs from droplet infection or blood-poisoning with the germ in the bloodstream. Both the latter types are almost invariably fatal and even the glandular type has a normal mortality of 80%. There is a vaccine to prevent plague and a serum to be used in the sick but the modern treatment is with the sulpha drugs combined with streptomycin. The vaccine affords only partial protection and therefore in the case of outbreaks the sulpha drugs are administered to contacts.

Plasma: the fluid part of the blood when the corpuscles have been separated out. It is composed of serum and fibrinogen (*see* Coagulation). Plasma transfusion is useful in the treatment of shock and as plasma can be prepared in powder form and testing for blood-grouping is unnecessary it is convenient as a temporary substitute for blood-transfusion. It cannot, of course, carry out all the functions of a whole-blood transfusion.

Plasmoquine: (*see* Malaria).

Plaster of Paris: is calcium sulphate which, after mixing with water, sets hard and is used in the treatment of fractures.

Pleurisy: inflammation of the pleura or covering of the lungs is most commonly secondary to pneumonia or other disease of the lungs, e.g. a tumour, or a chest injury. There develops between the layers of pleura a sticky exudate of lymph and fibrin with the appearance of buttered bread when two slices have been separated and this roughness causes the pain and the friction rub heard through the stethoscope. Later pleurisy with effusion may develop when the fibrin is replaced by lymph and the pain which is typical of the first stage departs but breathing becomes more difficult. The two most obvious symptoms in the early stages, apart from those due to the primary condition, are stabbing pain in the chest made worse on deep breathing or coughing, and breathlessness. If too much fluid develops it may be necessary to withdraw it with a syringe. Treatment depends on the cause but most cases respond to antibiotics and sulpha preparations with streptomycin and other drugs for the tuberculous cases. Iodine and other counter-irritants may be applied to the chest and in pleurisy with effusion diuretics and purgatives are used to reduce the amount of fluid in the body. Whether they help is doubtful.

Pleurodynia: pain in the chest of a non-specific character.

Plombières Douche: colonic lavage or washing out of the lower bowel usually carried out by cranks for cranks; for, although there may be a few cases where lavage is helpful they are certainly not very many and not nearly as numerous as the addicts who allow their bowel to be maltreated on the false belief that 'auto-intoxication' is the root of all evil. Excessive lavage is positively harmful to the mucus membrane of the intestines.

Plumbism: lead poisoning.

Pneumoconiosis: this is the general name for a group of diseases caused by the inhalation of dust at work and leading to fibrosis of the lungs. The following types may occur: anthracosis (from coal); silicosis (from inhalation of sand-particles in gold, tin, zinc, iron, and coal mining, in sand-blasting, metal grinding, slate quarrying, granite, sandstone and pottery work); siderosis (from tin, copper, lead or iron particles); lithosis (from stone particles); asbestosis (from

459

asbestos); byssinosis (from cotton). Anthracosis is not necessarily harmful, but silicosis predisposed to pulmonary tuberculosis, and in asbestosis the so-called 'asbestosis bodies' containing iron silicate may be found in the sputum. The general symptoms of this group of diseases which tends to be progressive are: cough with copious amounts of sputum, breathlessness, tiredness and loss of weight. X-rays show fibrosis, i.e. scar tissue formation, in the lungs with nodules of varying size especially in the central parts of the lungs. The patient must, of course, be removed from his work and the subsequent treatment is as for chronic bronchitis and emphysema which are the main features of these diseases. Prevention is more important than cure and there are now regulations in force regarding the use of respiratory sprays and extractor fans to prevent inhalation of dust in such trades in which workers should be X-rayed every six months.

Pneumonectomy: the operation of removing the whole of a lung, e.g. for tuberculosis or bronchiectasis.

Pneumonia: consolidation of one or more lobes of the lung is usually caused by the pneumococcus of which there are at least 32 types. Types I and II account for nearly 70% of all cases. Less frequently the germ responsible may be that of typhoid fever, plague, or tuberculosis, and other organisms are found such as the streptococcus or staphylococcus or a virus. The condition may occur in healthy young adults and begins suddenly with shivering and a stabbing pain in the chest in this way differing from broncho-pneumonia (q.v.) which is a disease of unhealthy infants or old people coming on gradually as a complication of bronchitis or a childhood fever or in conditions where food or vomit has gone down the wrong way. In broncho-pneumonia, too, the consolidation is patchy, not affecting a whole lobe at a time. The pathological stages in lobar pneumonia are described as *hyperaemia* when the part becomes congested with blood, *red hepatisation* when as exudate fills the alveoli (*see* Lungs) the lobe soon develops the consistency of liver and thus cannot be used for breathing, *grey hepatisation*, and *resolution*. Typically the temperature rises rapidly to 102–3 degrees, the pulse to 110–120, and the respiration rate to 30–40 and falls on the seventh or ninth day by crisis or gradually by lysis, but since the use of the sulpha drugs and the antibiotics these typical stages are now rarely seen. The doctor will note shallow breathing with grunting expiration, the blood-stained 'rusty' sputum on the 2nd or 3rd day, and later the signs of consolidation (dullness on percussion and loss of the breath sounds over the affected area). Various subtypes of pneumonia are described but need not be mentioned here with the exception of *virus pneumonia* (primary atypical pneumonia) which has only recently been identified as a separate condition. Here the onset tends to be in winter, the incubation period 2–21 days, the onset insidious rather than sudden, the temperature from 100–103 degrees, the pulse slow in relation to the temperature, and the main symptom cough. The outlook is good although progress may be slow and take a matter of several weeks in place of the single week of pneumococcal pneumonia. The new antibiotics chloramphenicol, aureomycin, and oxytetracycline (terramycin) are used successfully. In chronic *interstitial pneumonia* the parts between the air cells are affected and there is fibrosis; this type is virtually synonymous with pneumoconiosis (q.v.) but may arise in the course of any chronic disease of the lungs. Pulmonary tuberculosis is a form of (usually) chronic pneumonia.

Pneumoperitoneum: means the introduction of air into the peritoneal cavity, i.e. the abdomen, with the intention of collapsing the lung by raising the diaphragm in the treatment of pulmonary tuberculosis. It is an alternative to pneumothorax (*see* below).

Pneumothorax: may be intentional or unintentional. The former is a procedure carried out to collapse and rest a diseased lung as in tuberculosis or bronchiectasis, the latter may result from an injury to the chest wall, a tumour, or from an inhaled foreign body blocking the bronchial tubes. In either case the air is soon absorbed and the lung fills out again.

Podagra: Gout (q.v.).

Poisons: most of these are described under separate headings but the following is a summary. There is no satisfactory definition of poison but it is usually taken to mean a substance which in relatively small amounts is dangerous to life or at any rate injures health, its effect being produced chemically and through absorption into the blood-stream (ground glass, for example, which produces any result it might produce by physical means is not a poison). There is hardly any substance which could not, in sufficient amounts, produce poisonous effects and it is well-known that in allergy (q.v.) comparatively innocuous foods may prove deadly to those who are sensitised to them. Two of the many possible classifications of poisons are: (1) according to source we may describe them as animal, vegetable, or mineral, or to chemical type as organic, inorganic, acid, alkaloid. (2) According to effect they may be classified as narcotic, corrosive, convulsant, and irritant. Narcotics cause giddiness, headache, drowsiness, and weakness of the muscles by acting directly upon the brain and spinal cord and often produce initial excitement, e.g. opium and its derivatives, hyoscine, chloral and chloroform, the barbiturates, etc. Corrosives include the strong acids and alkalies, carbolic acid, lysol, and corrosive sublimate; they stain and blister the mouth and the area surrounding it, damage the gullet and the stomach lining, and thus affect swallowing and breathing. There is vomiting, diarrhoea, intense colic, and subsequently perforation or gangrene of the intestinal tract. Irritants are many and include oxalic acid, arsenic preparations, copper sulphate, phosphorus, zinc and lead salts, croton oil, cantharides, etc. There is indigestion when these substances are given in continued small doses, wasting, and many of the appearances of a chronic infection of the intestines (hence their appeal to the poisoner who does not realise how easily most of them can be traced after or before death). Convulsant poisons like strychnine produce fits and the symptoms of strychnine poisoning are very similar to those of tetanus. Death is due to suffocation or exhaustion but consciousness is ordinarily unaffected. Food poisoning is usually caused by infection of the individual with germs which continue to multiply in his body causing gastro-enteritis (inflammation of the stomach and intestines) but the rare condition of botulism is caused by the actual toxins of a specific germ which has reproduced itself in canned food. Poisons which exert their effect over a long time and are not taken with (conscious) suicidal intent are the drugs of addiction and alcohol which are described elsewhere. The principles of treating cases of poisoning are fairly simple. When a caustic poison has been taken (this will be observed by noting signs of burning around the mouth and lips) an emetic should *not* be used but large amounts of milk can be given, water, or liquid paraffin whilst sending for the doctor; alkalies can be dealt with by giving lime or lemon juice, acids by alkaline substances such as baking soda. All other cases such as poisoning by pain-relieving or sleep-producing drugs must be given an emetic. Lay the patient on his face and, if conscious, tickle the back of his throat and administer two tablespoonfuls of salt in a tumbler of warm water. Later strong coffee or tea may be given but in all cases the prime need is to send for urgent medical attention.

Poliomyelitis: is one of the two virus diseases affecting the nerve roots. One, herpes zoster or shingles affects the sensory roots as they enter the cord, poliomyelitis is an infection of the anterior horn cells where they leave the cord to pass to the voluntary muscles. Fortunately all motor roots are never affected and the muscles picked out depend upon where the infection is located; these may be the roots supplying the respiratory muscles, a serious event which may necessitate a longer or shorter stay in an iron lung, but it is uncommon for the cranial nerves to be influenced with disturbance of swallowing and facial movement. Infection may be by droplets, by food, or from carriers and the epidemics usually occur in summer or autumn, young and otherwise healthy people being most often affected. The onset is comparatively sudden with headache, vomiting, and muscular pains, fever, and at times convulsions. There is rigidity of the neck and after this constitutional disturbance one or more muscle groups suddenly get weak, the legs being more commonly concerned than the arms. The paralysis, like lower motor neurone paralyses in general, is flaccid with depression of the reflexes and no sensory involvement. There is no specific remedy for poliomyelitis but the muscles recover to a varying degree with proper nursing, some weakness usually being left behind. Thus, although poliomyelitis is not so very common nor as killing as many other diseases, it is often very disabling and it is important that it should be protected against by inoculations before the risk of infection arises. The disease is particularly difficult to prevent since only a small proportion of all cases are recognised there being no paralysis in the others, although it is such cases that spread the disease about and account for it appearing in often widely separated areas.

The prophylactic injections give a high degree of protection at least two, and preferably three, being required: live oral vaccines are also in use and parents should be guided by their doctors in this choice. During epidemics crowded buildings and swimming pools should be avoided, foods protected from flies and treated with attention to hygiene (as, of course they should be at all times), and other forms of protective inoculation postponed. In cases where severe paralysis and wasting of limbs has occurred which shows no further sign of improvement, surgery may help to reduce the deformity to a considerable degree. The usual treatment of the paralysed muscles has been complete immobilisation in splints but the Sister Kenny treatment is based on the application of hot wet strips of blanket hourly so long as the pain persists. This is followed by gentle passive movements and the patient is encouraged to concentrate on movement of the unparalysed opposing muscles. Splints are not used and the incidence of deformities afterwards is said to be small. In America where this system has been extensively tried out special instruction centres for nurses have been established, the disease being much more common there than here.

Pollantin: a serum made from pollen and used in the prevention of hay-fever.

Polycythaemia: (Erythraemia or Osler's Disease). A condition in which there is an increase in the number of red cells in the blood together with enlargement of the spleen. The red cells may be twice the normal and the haemoglobin as much as 180%. There is blueness of the skin, headache, and giddiness, the disease being due to overactivity of the bone-marrow where the cells are normally created. Treatment is a matter for the specialist, but bleeding gives temporary relief.

Polymorph: (*see* Leucocytes).

Polymyxin: a mixture of several antibiotic substances obtained from a soil bacterium. It is mainly effective against Gram-negative organisms and notably so against the pyocynanea bacteria which produce blue pus. Polymyxin is not absorbed from the intestine and hence is safe to give by mouth being used for certain types of dysentery; but by injection it is somewhat toxic to the kidneys.

Polyneuritis: (*see* Neuritis).

Polypus: a tumour of whatever type (malignant or more often benign), arising from various types of tissue (the name referring to its shape only) which possesses a stalk and is usually composed of a thin fibrous core surrounded by the tissue from which it springs. Polypi may arise from the mucous lining of the bladder or bowel, the inside of the nose, or outer ear, the womb, etc., and are usually treated by cutting off with a snare or burning with a cautery. The usual symptom in the first two types is the appearance of blood painlessly in the urine or motions.

Polyuria: the passage of large amounts of urine as after drinking quantities of fluid, using a diuretic drug, or in diabetes, some kinds of kidney disease, and in states of anxiety.

Popliteal Space: the space behind the knee.

Population Explosion: this is the popular term for the well-known fact that the population of the world is increasing to an unprecedented degree, and, like a runaway train, the rate of increase is greater with every year that passes. This has a number of significant implications: (a) that the great benefits made possible by science of better health, better nutrition, and higher standards of living are being nullified as quickly as they are being developed; (b) that population pressure is not only a serious problem in itself but a major cause of war (the basic cause of the Sino–Japanese war was the desperate attempt of the grossly overcrowded islands of Japan to find an outlet for their excess population); (c) in the words of Julian Huxley, one of the foremost world experts, '. . . beyond his material requirements, man needs space and beauty, recreation and enjoyment. Excessive population can erode all these things. The rapid population increase has already created cities so big that they are beginning to defeat their own ends (and) even in the less densely inhabited regions of the world open spaces are shrinking and the despoiling of nature is going on at an appalling rate. Wildlife is being exterminated; forests are being cut down, mountains gashed by hydroelectric projects, wildernesses plastered with mine shafts and tourist camps; fields and meadows stripped away for roads and airports.'

A century and a half ago, the Reverend Thomas Malthus pointed out that population always increased more rapidly than the available food supply, and consequently that there was likely to be widespread misery and starvation in some parts of the world for any foreseeable time to come. Expressed more scientifically, population increase is based on a geometrical or compound-interest progression, whereas food production only increases by arithmetical progression. Now, during the late 19th century and the early 20th, this was shown to be not entirely true; for at that time food production increased in more than arithmetical progression. But we now realise that there is an inevitable limit to this rate of increase, and that Malthus was basically right. Briefly, the population of this planet has accelerated from a very slow beginning until it has now become explosive, each phase of increase following some major invention or discovery. Before hunting gave way to an agricultural way of life, about 6,000 B.C., the number of people in the world was about 22 million, and each new technological revolution – the building of the first cities, the harnessing of wind and water to do the work of man, the Industrial Revolution, and in our own time the revolution in medical techniques – has led to a fresh burst. In Shakespeare's day the world population was 500 million, but by the middle of the 18th century it had become 1,000 million and in the early 1920s 2,000 million. That is to say, it doubled itself twice over between 1650 and 1920, but the first doubling took two centuries, the second less than one. Consider the following figures: when the essay by Julian Huxley which was quoted above was written in 1955, there were more than 2,500 million people on the earth and this was being added to at the rate of 34 million people every year, i.e. 4,000 per hour and more than one every second. But today 135,000 babies are being born daily and 50 million babies will be born into the world this year. Those who believe that 'natural' treatments for illness are best and the closer man lives to nature the healthier he will be (see Naturopathy) will have difficulty in explaining the facts that in primitive civilisations the average expectation of life is something like 30 years, and as late as 1880 the average expectation of life in civilised Massachusetts was only 40 years; today all technically advanced societies have life expectancies of about 70 years. In the brief period since the last war the introduction of modern medicine and hygiene to Ceylon has halved the death-rate, largely by virtually wiping out malaria with drugs and D.D.T.; it was reduced from 22 to 11 per thousand in less than ten years – but the birth-rate remains the same and, at the present rate, the population will more than double every 25 years. The same is true of such countries as India, Malaya, and Thailand together with many others where death-rates have been reduced by a third.

Lastly, it is precisely in the poorest and most backward countries that people have the largest families: European couples average 2·3 children, but most Asiatic countries average about 6 and some as many as 8. The basic reason for this decrease in the technically advanced countries is industrialisation and the spread of knowledge. Agricultural societies tend to have more children, partly out of ignorance, but also because children are an economic asset as they help their parents on the land from a very early age; but in industrial society children are unable to work until 15 and often much later and, being an economic liability, families become smaller. Yet we cannot hope that industrialisation will have any significant effect in the near future, and at the rate of population increase in Ceylon and many other countries the inevitable result, without interference, would be a 64-fold increase in less than two centuries. The tragic fact is that, the more help we give to under-developed countries and the more their production increases a rising population will eat up almost all of these gains as fast as they are made.

The main cause of the present predicament is death-control without birth-control, and whether we like it or not the introduction of a birth-control plan such as is already in operation in Japan and India is the only possible solution. This solution is opposed, of course, by the Roman Catholic Church and, oddly enough, by many Communists, but few experts indeed believe that there is any other way out.

Porencephaly: a condition associated with mental defect resulting from cysts in the brain which arise from developmental errors or damage at birth.

Portal Vein: the large vein carrying blood from the abdominal organs and especially the intestines to the liver.

Porto-Caval Shunt or Anastomosis: an operation devised for cases of cirrhosis of the liver where there is a great congestion of the portal system due to fibrosis blocking the liver itself. By this manoeuvre a great deal of blood which normally enters the liver through the portal vein goes instead into the vena cava, the main vein of the body through an artificial junction between the two. This relieves the pressure upon the liver and in the portal system and reduces the chance of sudden death from haemorrhage of the varicose veins (varices) which tend to form at the end of the oesophagus and mouth of the stomach in this condition.

Post-partum: after childbirth.

Potassium: the salts of potassium have a damping-down effect upon the nervous system and their reduction through loss in the urine is one of the dangers of cirrhosis of the liver or cases in which modern diuretics are being used. This is known as hypotassaemia. Some potassium salts (e.g. potassium chlorate and potassium permanganate) are used in medicine as gargles or antiseptics.

Pott's Disease: curvature of the spine due to tuberculous disease from infected milk causing the collapse of a vertebra. Fortunately this is now rare since pasteurisation was introduced. Formerly these victims spent years in bed and wore disfiguring braces for their whole lives but the use of the new drugs and remedial surgical operations has changed all this even for the few cases who develop the disease.

Pott's Fracture: a fracture near the lower end of the fibula named, like Pott's disease, after Percival Pott the 18th century surgeon who first described the fracture having sustained it himself.

Precordial Region: the region in front of the heart, i.e. in the centre and slightly to the left side of the chest.

Prednisolone: a cortisone derivative, given by mouth, and active in such conditions as arthritic diseases, allergic states, bursitis, sprue and ulcerative colitis. It is several times stronger than cortisone itself.

Pre-frontal Leucotomy: (*see* Leucotomy).

Pregnancy: the average duration of pregnancy in the human being is from 274–280 days, the commonest early signs of its existence being amenorrhea or cessation of the periods, enlargement of the breasts, and occasionally nausea in the mornings or evenings and frequency in passing urine. The nipples and the surrounding area begin to get darker about the 3rd month, and 'quickening' or movements of the foetus may be felt from about the 18th week. From the 3rd month onwards the pregnant womb begins to rise out of the pelvis and can be felt through the abdominal wall. None of these signs is absolutely diagnostic of pregnancy, however, and it is even possible for a woman to have them together with progressive enlargement of the abdomen without being pregnant at all. Positive signs are the hearing of the heart-beat at about the 6th month, agreement on the part of experienced doctors from vaginal examination that a pregnancy has occurred, and positive results from one or other of the biological tests. These are the Ascheim-Zondek test which consists in injecting the patient's urine into immature female mice when, if pregnancy has occurred, premature maturation of the animal's ovarian follicles is found, and the Hogben or Xenopus test in which urine is injected into the back of a species of African toad which will lay six or more eggs within 4–12 hours if the patient be pregnant. These results are produced by the presence of an excess of gonadotrophic hormone in the urine of pregnant women.

Although pregnancy is a normal state of affairs, it is important that regular ante-natal examinations should be carried out so that if any abnormalities be present they can be corrected in time. Amongst data collected during the first examination will be the patient's family, personal, and obstetric history; her general medical condition; measurements of the pelvis and blood-pressure; urine tests and blood-tests for kidney disease and the presence of Rh antibodies (*see* Rh factor); in addition, the Wassermann reaction for syphilis will be done and the blood-group ascertained. The mother is advised too, as to health and diet and may be put in touch with an ante-natal clinic or a hospital where arrangements regarding confinement can be made. Subsequent examinations enable the doctor to find whether the head fits the pelvis and continue to reassure himself as to the patient's general condition (*see* Foetus, Labour).

Premature Birth: (*see* Birth, Miscarriage).

Presbyopia: the changes occurring in the eye with the onset of old age beginning about the age of 40 and largely caused by decreasing elasticity of the lens.

Prickly Heat: a skin condition affecting Europeans in tropical countries, usually in the period before they have become acclimatised, and characterised by the appearance of multiple tiny blisters accompanied by severe itching; the rash occurs most frequently in the areas (around the waist, etc.) where clothes are tightest. The probable cause is a blockage of the sweat glands in areas where the skin has become sodden with sweat and all that is necessary is to take frequent baths and use one of the dusting powders supplied for the purpose to absorb the perspiration and keep the surface of the skin as dry as possible. If the itching is severe a doctor will be able to supply one or other of the extremely potent modern antipruritics.

Primidone: Mysoline is a drug used for the control of epilepsy of the grand mal type.

Primipara: a woman who has given birth, or is in the process of giving birth, to her first child.

Probenecid: (Benemid) a drug used in gout, mainly for taking between attacks, or for gouty arthritis. An important effect is that it is capable of blocking the excretion of certain drugs through the kidneys, e.g. penicillin and P.A.S. and is therefore used to raise the blood levels of these drugs in people taking them.

Procaine Hydrochloride: a synthetic drug with a cocaine-like action used as a local anaesthetic both by injection and in eye drops to anaesthetise the surface of the eye for minor operations. It can also be used as a spinal anaesthetic (*see* Anaesthetics), and is commonly known by its proprietary name of Novocain.

Procaine Amide: (Pronestyl) is a drug used in the correction of irregular heart beat, particularly during anaesthesia.

Proctalgia: pain in the rectum without discoverable cause.

Proctitis: inflammation in the region of the rectum or anus.

Progesterone: the hormone secreted by the corpus luteum (*see* Ovaries). It is used to prevent abortion and for other purposes, having a generally sedative effect on the womb.

Prognosis: the outlook for an illness.

Progressive Muscular Atrophy: this is also called chronic anterior poliomyelitis although it has no relationship with that disease save the degeneration that occurs in the anterior horn cells where the motor nerves to the muscles leave the spinal column. It is threfore different from the myopathies (q.v.) in which no such changes have been found. The muscles in a particular area become flabby and wasted, e.g. the peroneal muscles with resultant foot-drop, the small muscles of the hand, or the muscles of the shoulder, according to the type of the disease. The peroneal type (Charcot-Marie-Tooth) occurs in young children, the others tend to begin from 25–40 years. There is no specific treatment and the cause is unknown but the disease, which often runs in families, is sometimes arrested of its own accord. Massage and exercises are important.

Proguanil Hydrochloride: a synthetic anti-malarial drug (*see* Malaria).

Prolactin: an anterior pituitary hormone which stimulates the flow of milk in nursing mothers.

Prolapse: the falling-down of a part, usually used of the rectum, which may prolapse in small children, or of the womb which sometimes prolapses after injuries caused by childbirth. One may also speak of a prolapsed disc referring to a slipped intervertebral disc (q.v.).

Prominal: methyl phenobarbitone (*see* Barbiturates).

Pronation: the movement of turning the hand palm down. The opposite movement is known as supination.

Propamidine Cream: a useful antiseptic used in the treatment of fresh burns, wounds, and abrasions: the ophthalmic solution is used in the treatment of chronic conjunctivitis of the eyes, especially that due to the Morax-Axenfeld bacillus.

Prophylaxis: treatment adopted in the prevention of a disease.

Proptosis: prominence of the eyeballs.

Prostate Gland: the prostate is a gland surrounding the neck of the urinary bladder in males; it is about the shape and size of a small horse chestnut and the beginning of the urethra passes through its three lobes. Its function is the production of the major part of the fluid in the semen and sterility usually follows its removal. The four commonest disorders to which it is subject are infection and abscess formation, simple or benign enlargement, cancer, and stones. Infections lead to fever, low back pain, and frequent and painful passing of water. Many of them were at one time due to gonorrhoea but this is less common today. Most types respond to antibiotics but if an abscess forms a slight operation to open it may be necessary either through the urethra or by an incision in the perineum. The majority of men have some degree of enlargement of the prostate from the forties onwards and the main significance of this is that it can interfere with the passing of water and the ability of the bladder to empty itself resulting in difficulty in urination and possible urinary infections. There may initially be no symptoms at all and often the enlargement is never sufficient to give trouble but in other cases there is frequency during the day and the need to get up at night; later there is difficulty in starting the act (hesitancy) and some dribbling afterwards. The increase in bladder pressure may finally tell upon the kidneys leading to failure or ureamia. Every now and then the patient may find that he is unable to pass any urine and there is complete urinary retention which requires to be dealt with immediately. Broadly speaking three-quarters of all men have some enlargement after 60 but only about one quarter of these require surgical treatment. The operation for removal of the gland may be carried out through the abdomen or the perineum and in one or two stages; sometimes no incision is made but the gland is removed through the urethra with an electrically-charged wire loop. The symptoms of cancer of the prostate are the same as those of benign enlargement and when discovered early the prospects of complete cure are excellent. In inoperable conditions or in extreme old age when prostatectomy is inadvisable the growth is controlled by the administration of female sex hormones such as stilboestrol sometimes accompanied by removal of the testicles which stimulate its growth. Prostatic stones usually go with enlargement and are not in themselves an indication for surgery but other circumstances may make prostatectomy advisable.

Prosthesis: any artificial part used to replace one which has been removed, e.g. an artificial eye, denture, or leg.

Prostigmin: a synthetic drug with actions similar to physostigmine in producing contractions of voluntary muscle. It is used in the treatment of myasthenia gravis (q.v.).

Protamines: a type of protein substance used in medicine in combination with insulin to prolong its effect or as an antidote to heparin.

Proteins: (*see* Diet); *Protein Shock* is the injection of foreign proteins to produce a body reaction in certain diseases.

Protoplasm: the material of living tissues.

Proximal: the part of a limb nearer the centre of the body as distinguished from *distal*, the part farther away, e.g. the foot is distal to the knee but the knee is proximal to the foot so far as the leg is concerned.

Pruritis: or itching is a symptom found in many widely different conditions which may be summarised as: (a) bites from insects or parasites as in ant bites or scabies and lice (*see* Bites, Parasites); (b) in allergic states (*see* Allergy, Nettle-rash); (c) in many skin diseases which are too numerous to mention and have to be diagnosed by the doctor; (d) in old age as the skin becomes dry or after an attack of herpes zoster (q.v.) where the temporary itching felt in all cases tends to persist; (e) in generalised diseases such as chronic nephritis (*see* Nephritis), liver diseases or other conditions accompanied by jaundice (q.v.), and diabetes (q.v.); (f) in the tropics in the form of prickly heat (q.v.); and (g) in those who apparently have no organic disease at all and the itching appears to be the result of neurosis (q.v.). Other causes are blood diseases such as leukaemia and Hodgin's disease. Pruritis of the anus and vulva (i.e. the female external genital organs) come in a separate category.

Obviously, in all these conditions the treatment is the treatment of the underlying cause, and except in those cases where the cause is known the doctor should be consulted. However, localised itching can usually be controlled by (amongst older remedies) calamine lotion, or an ointment containing benzocaine; the more effective modern applications are anti-histamine creams or creams containing cortisone or its derivatives. Allergic itching can be helped by anti-histamine pills and most kinds of itching by other anti-pruritic drugs such as trimeprazine or Vallergan, etc. Pruritis of the vulva or anus may be the result of vaginal infection in the first case or threadworms in the second and these should always be excluded, but it must be noted that in a very high percentage of such cases no organic disease is found and the cause is psychological. Generalised itching around the genitals in either sex is a common symptom of diabetes, so the urine should immediately be examined for sugar.

Pseudocyesis: false pregnancy in which the signs of pregnancy may be imitated by the presence of a tumour or by flatulence in hysterical women.

Psittacosis: (parrot fever) a virus disease of birds transmissible to man. In the main it is communicated by imported birds kept as pets, e.g. parrots and love-birds, but pigeons can also transmit the disease. Essentially the symptoms are similar to those of bronchitis or pneumonia and the condition, although serious, usually responds to such antibiotics as terramycin, aureomycin, and chloromycetin in this respect differing from most virus diseases which are unaffected.

Psoriasis: a skin disease characterised by the formation of dry, silvery scales over the affected parts. It is commonest in middle and old age but may occur in children over the age of 8 or 9. The commonest sites are the elbows and knees but almost any part of the body can be affected, the distribution being usually symetrical. There is no constitutional disturbance nor much itching and the cause is unknown but the disease appears to run in families. The most popular applications are tar ointment, salicylic acid, crysarobin, and ammoniated mercury. These usually cause the condition to disappear temporarily but it is very chronic in most cases.

Psychiatry: the branch of medicine dealing with the study and treatment of mental illness (q.v.).

Psycho-analysis: refers (*a*) to the theories of Sigmund Freud and (*b*) to the method of treatment based thereon. Freud showed that mental illness (and normal behaviour too) can be explained in terms of the conflict between primitive emotions in the unconscious mind and the more civilised and learned tendencies in the conscious mind. The personality is divided into the id which is the unconscious containing primitive and repressed impulses, the conscious ego, and the half-conscious, half-unconscious superego which may be roughly equated with the conscience. Thus all behaviour is the result of a three-cornered struggle between the ego (representing reality), the super-ego (representing the social impulses) and the id (representing the primitive desires). Initially the child is entirely primitive but his growing up is a process of slowly putting away childish ways and learning to repress unsuitable behaviour or sublimate it into something more useful; if this process fails, neurosis may develop in later life and the individual's relationships with others suffer. The first persons with whom the child has to relate himself are, of course, the parents, and psychoanalysis attaches great importance to this as the prototoype of all later relationships, e.g. a child who hates his father may grow up with an unreasoning hatred of all authority, or a child who is unloved will be unable to form any genuine love relationships later. The main instincts are the sexual and aggressive ones from which all the others arise, the word sexual being used in the widest possible sense to include, for instance, the infant's pleasure in sucking or in its bowel motions. Psychoanalysis is a form of psychotherapy (q.v.) but refers only to the Freudian method which is suitable in certain selected cases only, i.e. in those whose personality is on the whole good, who are young and of high intelligence, and who are capable of affording the time and money for treatment which takes about an hour on five days a week during which the patient's problems are analysed by the method of free association. The patient lies on a couch and says whatever comes into his head and this enables the analyst to unravel the sources of his troubles. Although free treatment can be obtained at the various Institutes throughout the great cities of the world it is ordinarily necessary to obtain private therapy which can be quite costly. Psychoanalysts must be trained in an Institute and only such are reputable psycho-analysts from the orthodox standpoint.

Psychology: the branch of science which deals with the work-ings of the mind or, more loosely, with the study of normal behaviour.

Psychoneurosis: is synonymous with neurosis.

Psychopathic: the adjective applied to any form of abnormal behaviour but a *psychopath* (*see* Mental Illness) is one who is in some respect at odds with society, i.e. his illness takes the form of social or anti-social actions. In this way he is a trouble to others rather than to himself.

Psychoprophylaxis: (*see* Natural Childbirth).

Psychosis: insanity as ordinarily understood (*see* Mental Ill-ness).

Psychosomatic Diseases: are physical diseases in which a major factor in causation is psychological. The mind acts through the autonomic nervous system (*see* Nervous System) by means of its sympathetic and parasympathetic divisions and by hormones to produce effects which may ultimately influence the structure of the body and lead to such con-ditions as peptic ulcer, essential hypertension, many skin diseases, and other conditions. This happens by way of the centre of the hypothalamus at the base of the brain and doubtless by the hormones of the anterior pituitary which are controlled by it. Of course, the major discovery of 20th century medicine has been that all diseases are in some degree psychosomatic, i.e. they happen to persons, not to inanimate objects and what the person thinks and feels will have an immense influence upon his health. To take a single example, the blood-pressure normally rises when a man or woman is annoyed only to return to normal when the occasion passes, but one who is constantly in a state of repressed rage will some day have a permanently raised blood-pressure with changes in the arteries and elsewhere. It is incorrect, except in a very loose sense to speak of this as 'mind over matter' because the individual is one and it was only the medicine and science of the 19th century that thought of him as a 'ghost in a machine.'

Psychotherapy: the general term used for any kind of mental healing. This may take many forms which can be described briefly under the headings of autosuggestion, heterosuggestion, and analysis. Autosuggestion was much popularised in the early years of this century by Emil Coué whose 'every day and in every way I am getting better and better' became famous and it is, in fact, true that some results can be obtained in this way which amounts to a sort of self-hypnosis but the results are unlikely to be lasting and only comparatively trivial conditions could be so treated. Heterosuggestion either in the form of persuasion, telling with authority, or hypnosis is a good deal more potent but the disadvantages of hypnosis have been dealt with under that heading and briefly are that every symptom has a cause and can only be removed permanently by the removal of that cause. If someone has a fear of closed spaces there must be a reason why this is so which will not be moved by telling him even under the deepest hypnosis that he has no such fear; the symptom may certainly go but another will take its place or it will return. Most schools of analytical psychotherapy today are under the influence of Freud (*see* Psychoanalysis) and depend upon a rational examination of the causes of the trouble but it is impossible to assess the part played by faith and the personality of the therapist.

Ptosis: drooping of the upper eyelid caused by paralysis of the 3rd cranial nerve.

Ptyalin: the enzyme contained in saliva which breaks starches down into sugars prior to further digestion in the stomach and intestines.

Puberty: (*see* Menstruation, Sex).

Puerperal Fever: or child-bed fever was at one time the great scourge of mothers but the state of affairs has been revolutionised since the original discovery of its germ origins in the 19th century and the advent of antiseptics followed by that of the sulpha drugs and antibiotics.

Puerperium: the period after child-birth until normal health is regained. It is usually regarded as lasting a month.

Purgatives: (*see* Constipation).

Purpura: a group of diseases in which purple spots appear under the skin due to extravasations of blood sometimes accompanied by haemorrhages from the mucous membranes. Purpura may be secondary to many other diseases such as infections or septicaemia, any sort of fever, blood diseases such as leukaemia, vitamin deficiencies as in scurvy, mechanical causes as in whooping cough, some drugs, and the last stages of certain diseases. Primary types are *essential thrombocytopenia* associated with a reduction in the number of blood platelets, and *Henoch's purpura* in which abdominal pain and blood and mucus passed in the motions is believed to be due to allergy (q.v.) Those types which are secondary are dealt with by treating the cause, the others are treated with rest and a high vitamin diet (especially of vitamins C and K). Chronic cases respond to removal of the spleen.

Pyaemia: a form of blood-poisoning in which abscesses develop in various parts of the body.

Pyelitis: is an inflammation of the pelvis of the kidney due to infection with the bacillus coli or streptococci, the germs reaching the kidneys either through the blood-stream or up the urethra from the exterior. The patient has aching or tenderness in the loins, passes water frequently and develops a fever often with rigors or shivering attacks. It is treated with urinary antiseptics such as mandelic acid, the sulpha drugs, or an antibiotic. In chronic cases there is usually some other condition maintaining the infection and an investigation must be carried out for stones or kidney disease.

Pyelography: the process whereby the kidneys are made opaque to X-rays with iodoxyl or similar substances. It is an important part of any examination for kidney disease.

Pyknolepsy: is a type of epilepsy affecting young children which is not accompanied by falling or unconsciousness in the full sense of the word. The attacks begin suddenly and last a few seconds with the child looking vacant and unable to speak or move; sometimes the eyelids twitch and the eyes roll upwards. Drugs have little effect but the attacks usually cease after puberty.

Pyloric Stenosis: this is an obstruction to the outlet of the stomach which prevents the passage of food into the small intestine; it occurs in babies of 2–3 weeks old who are three times more often male than female. The immediate cause is an overdevelopment of the muscle of the pylorus which lies between the stomach exit and the duodenum. Pyloric stenosis is easily recognised by the projectile vomiting, visible movements of the stomach through the abdominal wall, and constipation. Treatment may be the administration of antispasmodic drugs such as atropine methonitrate (Eumydrin) or a relatively simple operation slitting the muscle fibres (Ramstedt's operation). The results are almost always successful.

Pylorospasm: spasm of the pyloric muscle at the exit of the stomach usually caused by a duodenal ulcer.

Pyogenic: pyogenic germs are those which give rise to the formation of pus.

Pyramidon: or amidopyrine is a drug with the same properties as aspirin which has been largely given up in this country owing to its ability to cause serious blood disease.

Pyrexia: fever.

Pyridoxine: vitamin B6.

Pyuria: pus in the urine (*see* Urine).

Quassia: a bitter-tasting wood which is used as an infusion given as an enema in cases of threadworm.

Quinidine: an alkaloid which, like quinine comes from cinchona bark and is used in the treatment of such heart diseases as auricular fibrillation.

Quinine: (*see* Malaria). In addition to its effects in killing the malaria parasite quinine is also antiseptic, reduces the temperature slightly in non-malarial diseases, stimulates the womb to contract, and to some extent dilates the peripheral bloodvessels. In large doses it causes poisoning (cinchonism) with ringing noises in the ears, deafness, and fullness in the head. Still larger doses cause death from heart and respiratory failure.

Quinsy: (see Peritonsillar abscess).

Rabies: (Hydrophobia) is a virus disease occuring in certain animals notably the dog and wolf; it is transmitted to man by bites. The incubation period following a bite is about two months but this varies considerably being sometimes as long as 8 months. The disease has been stamped out in Britain by quarantine laws but at the onset the patient is irritable and excited with painful spasms of the muscles involved in breathing and swallowing, these being brought on by the act of swallowing hence the notion that water (which is frequently offered to sick people) is feared in this disease. Patients may become maniacal with a raised temperature and later the paralytic stage appears with death in about 5 days from heart-failure. Cases are rarely cured once the symptoms have begun to show themselves but those bitten by a dog with rabies should have the wound cauterised immediately and then go to a Pasteur Institute to be inoculated with material obtained from the spinal cords of rabbits which have been infected with the disease.

Rachitis: the continental name for rickets.

Radioactive Isotopes: (*see* Isotopes).

Radium: an element which was first isolated by Mme Curie in 1898 from pitchblende which, obtained largely in Czechoslovakia, is still its main source. Radium disintegrates spontaneously in a way that cannot be controlled by any chemical or physical agency save bombardment of the nucleus with neutrons or charged atomic particles and the products of its disintegration are (1) the alpha rays which are positively charged helium nuclei, (2) the beta rays which are negatively charged electrons, and (3) the gamma rays which are similar to short X-rays. It is the latter which are employed in medicine, radium and deep X-ray therapy being to some extent interchangeable and the same unit of dosage (the Röntgen) is used for both. The chief use of radiotherapy is for malignant disease but it is also used in some skin diseases. Good results are obtained with cancers which are slow-growing, e.g. those of the face, lip, mouth, breast, bladder, and uterus or womb but surgery remains the treatment of choice in cancers of the stomach and intestines although both may be used in combination.

Radius: the outer of the two bones of the forearm.

Ranula: a small swelling which occasionally develops beneath the tongue as the result of a blocked salivary duct.

Rat-Bite Fever: (Cat-bite fever) is caused by the bite of a rat, ferret or cat infected by the spirillum minus usually in India or Japan. The bite generally heals but after a week or more breaks down with enlargement of the neighbouring glands and fever. The Wassermann reaction is positive and, like most spirochaetal diseases, rat-bite fever is cured by neoarsphenamine, about three or four injections being necessary.

Rauwolfia: a drug obtained from the root of the rauwolfia serpentina, a plant found widely in south-east Asia. It is employed in the treatment of high blood-pressure and as a tranquilliser (proprietary names Hypertane, Hypertensan, Rauwiloid, Raudixin).

Raynaud's Disease: in this condition there are attacks when the fingers and toes suddenly become pale and dead, especially in cold weather; in more severe cases they go blue or black and there is severe pain. There may be a tendency to gangrene and when this happens the pain is very severe indeed. Occasionally the ears and nose are affected. Various drugs are used in treatment but in the more serious forms the nerves on which the calibre of the blood-vessels depend may have to be cut. This is known as sympathectomy.

Rectum: the last 9 inches of the intestinal canal which passes straight down the back of the pelvis lying against the sacrum; the last part is the anal canal, one inch long, which opens to the exterior at the anus. It is this last inch or two which is more susceptible to disease than almost any other part of the body – a fact not unconnected with the almost fanatical attention and significance some people devote to their bowel motions (see Constipation). Amongst these diseases are piles or haemorrhoids (q.v.), fissure, fistula, polypi, and itching. In the rectum itself cancer is fairly common, this being one of the most usual sites of the disease. *Fissures* are slit-like ulcers in the skin of the anus which give rise to great pain on attempting to move the bowels; they are treated by cutting out and dividing the circular muscle of the sphincter in order to rest the area. A *fistula* is an abnormal communication between the inside of the rectum and the skin around the anus being the end-result of an infection which has tunnelled its way out from the rectal or anal wall to the outside. The symptoms are those of a recurrent 'boil' which comes and goes discharging pus and then healing for a brief period. Operation is necessary since these areas never heal of themselves and after surgery recurrence is rare. *Polypi* may first show themselves by more or less severe haemorrhage from the bowels or, after a bowel motion, a mass from the size of a pea to that of a golf ball may make its appearance at the exterior of the anus. These are removed by cutting or cauterisation even when they occasion little trouble since cancer may arise from such a site. Itching or *pruritis* is common around the anus and may happen from many local causes or none at all. Occasionally it is due to worms, haemorrhoids, general diseases such as cirrhosis of the liver, colitis, and very often it appears to be largely a neurotic manifestation. The primary cause, if it can be found must be eliminated, otherwise various drugs taken internally and the application of benzocaine, anti-histamine creams, or hydrocortisone externally will help (*see* also Prolapse).

Cancer of the rectum and sigmoid colon is a disease of later life which shows itself by alternating attacks of diarrhoea and constipation increasing thinness and weakness, and blood or blood-stained discharge which, however, is not usually large in amount as in the case of a polypus. The treatment is obviously surgical and must be carried out as soon as possible. On the whole the results of surgery are good.

Reflex Action: (*see* Nervous System).

Regional Ileitis: (*see* Ileitis).

Relapsing Fever: this is a disease caused by a spirochaete, the *treponeme recurrentis*, conveyed to man by body and head lice; by the *treponeme duttoni* conveyed by a tick; and by several other varieties of spirochaetes. The incubation period is 2–10 days and the onset sudden with a rigor, headache, pains in the eyes and limbs, vomiting, and abdominal pain. The spleen is enlarged and after a week the temperature falls only to recur in a further week for a period of two days. In the prevention of this tropical disease lice and ticks must be destroyed but it is cured by a single injection of neoarsphenamine.

Renal Calculus: or stone in the kidney may arise from numerous predisposing factors, e.g. urinary infections, disorders of calcium or protein metabolism, vitamin deficiencies, gouty tendencies, or partial obstruction at the outlet of the kidney.

Once a stone or stones has formed it may remain in the kidney without producing symptoms; remain and cause attacks of pain, infection, or bleeding; remain and cause destruction of the whole kidney; or leave the kidney and pass down the ureter (the tube leading to the bladder) causing attacks of renal colic. During these there is great pain in the small of the back which radiates down towards the groin and is intermittent in type. Stones in the kidney will be dealt with according to circumstances but when a stone is small enough to enter the ureter it will in about 80–90% of cases be passed either spontaneously or with the help of catheters passed up the tube through a cystoscope. The remaining 10% of stones which get stuck in the ureter require operation if the function of the kidney is not damaged. Recovery takes place in a week or ten days.

Reserpine: the active principle of rauwolfia (q.v.).

Reticulocytes: are newly-formed red blood cells.

Reticulo-endothelial System: the cells of the bone-marrow, spleen, lymph glands, and liver which destroy foreign particles and bacteria, break down old red blood cells, and transform haemoglobin into bile pigment.

Retinitis: inflammation of the retina at the back of the eye which may result from diabetes, nephritis, leukaemia, etc. (also Retinopathy).

Retrobulbar Neuritis: inflammation of the optic nerve at the back of the eye.

Retroflexion: a displacement backwards as in a retroflexed uterus.

Rheumatism: this word describes a group of diseases which on the whole seem to have very little to do with each other and have almost nothing in common save that they predominantly affect muscles and joints and even this is untrue of the allegedly rheumatic disease of chorea. The rheumatic diseases as ordinarily classified include rheumatic fever which is related in some as yet not understood way to streptococcal infections; rheumatoid arthritis the cause of which is completely unknown; osteoarthritis, which is due to the degenerative changes of old age aided sometimes by injury; chorea, or St Vitus' dance, which is a disease of the nervous system; gout, which is generally a disease of high living, and fibrositis, lumbago, and so on which are frequently symptoms of some other condition. Fibrositis in particular may have a very considerable psychological element and it is quite wrong to attribute every ache and pain to 'rheumatism.' Rheumatic fever or acute rheumatism is a disease of temperate climates, poor housing, and overcrowding; its increasing rarity must be related in some way to better social conditions but there is no evidence that it, or any other form of 'rheumatism,' has any direct connection with cold or damp. Here the evidence is quite clear that the streptococcus is to blame and a sore throat invariably precedes the disease. There is sweating with fever and pain and swelling develops in one or more joints. Recovery is slow and the heart tends to be affected; before modern treatment it was common to find children and young adults (who are most usually attacked) with a history of two or more episodes of rheumatic fever. Treatment involves the use of the salicylates or aspirin but penicillin is now the main standby and, indeed, aborts the attack if given early. Chorea is described under that heading as are the other conditions. Rheumatoid arthritis often starts without evident cause in early adult life (although a history of emotional shock is common) and affects the small joints of the fingers and toes. No infective process has been discovered, yet the disease tends to be chronic, sometimes better, sometimes worse. It is a disease commoner in temperate climates and in women and can be seriously disabling before it finally burns itself out. Rheumatoid arthritis may very well be a stress reaction in which the secretion of cortisone by the suprarenal glands is inadequate to protect the body from responding too strongly to injury. Cortisone, although less useful than at one time appeared to be the case, is used in treatment along with many other drugs and forms of physiotherapy. *Osteoarthritis*, as mentioned above, is a disease of old, prematurely old, or sometimes injured people where the bone of the larger joints has overgrown, e.g. in the hip, knee, shoulders, or spine, making movement painful and difficult. There is no specific treatment but physiotherapy and pain-killing drugs may help in many cases. *Gout*, on the other hand, is a metabolic disease described elsewhere and is the only condition in which the 'crystals' dear to the heart of patent medicine advertisers could truthfully be said to exist. The cases of 'muscular rheumatism' are of such varied origin that it serves very little purpose to discuss them together as a group; the pain may arise from muscular strain, from a slipped disc, from neuritis, possibly from toxins of bacteria in various septic foci in the body (although the thesis of focal sepsis is not so popular as it once was), and a very large number are the result of spasm resulting from emotional stress, e.g. the typical 'pain in the neck' associated with resentment. Treatment for these conditions is varied and familiar depending mainly upon the application of counter-irritation by heat; but it seems highly improbable to say the least of it that mineral salts taken by mouth have the slightest physiological effect. That they frequently relieve is an indication more of their psychological power and the often psychological nature of the complaint than of any direct action. *Sciatica*, of course, is a form of neuritis and there is no reason to suppose that it has any necessary connection with 'rheumatism' whatever.

Rheumatoid Arthritis: (*see* Rheumatism).

Rh Factor: (*see* Icterus Neonatorum Gravis).

Rhinitis: inflammation of the lining of the nose.

Rhonchi: the harsh whistling sounds of varying pitch heard through the stethoscope in cases of bronchitis.

Rhubarb: rhubarb root from *Rheum palmatum* once popular as a purgative especially for children with diarrhoea. It is also allegedly effective as a cholagogue stimulating the flow of bile.

Riboflavine: is vitamin B2.

Rickets: formerly known as the English disease probably because of the part lack of sunlight plays in its genesis, sunlight preventing rickets by elaboration of vitamin D from the ergosterol of the body. The disease, due to the deficiency of vitamin D found mainly in fats, is now uncommon in its fully-developed state as the result of better feeding and cod-liver oil supplements but at one time it was a common cause of bony deformities such as pigeon chest, bow legs, and curvature of the spine.

Rickettsia: a group of organisms spread to man by the bites of lice, fleas, ticks, and mites, and responsible for such diseases as typhus Q fever, Rocky Mountain spotted fever and Japanese River fever.

Rigor: the shivering attack which accompanies a sharp rise in temperature.

Ringworm: a contagious skin disease due to infection with the fungi *microsporon audouini* or *trichophyton*. It causes little disability but is socially a nuisance through its infectivity in such places as schools, swimming-baths, etc. The main forms are tinea (ringworm) of the scalp, tinea of the beard, tinea of the groin, tinea of the body, and tinea of the nails. Scalp infections are much less frequent than at one time but the condition is a very infectious one which, since the fungus is within the hair itself, usually has to be treated by epilation, i.e. removal of all the hair by X-rays or thallium acetate by mouth. The hair grows again in a few weeks. On the body as on the scalp the typical rings are seen, in the latter as round patches of dry and broken hairs, in the former as reddish discs which become pale in the centre while advancing around the edges. There may be a good deal of itching. Ringworm of the groin is the so-called Dhobie Itch of the East where it was believed to be spread by the dhobie or laundryman, and ringworm of the foot is the so-called 'athlete's foot' where a sodden and whitish appearance develops between the last two spaces between the toes or on the sole of the foot. Ringworm of the skin responds to various substances such as Whitfield's ointment and Castellani's paint, but today the most commonly used is powder or ointment containing undecylenic acid. A most important point is to avoid reinfection from the clothes, boots, or shoes, and socks which must be sterilised, the boots and shoes by dusting inside with fungicidal powder, the clothes by boiling. Ringworm of the nails, once resistant to treatment can now be dealt with by an oral antibiotic.

Rocky Mountain Spotted Fever: a fever of the typhus group first discovered in the area indicated by its name but later in many other parts of the United States. The disease is a serious one but the new antibiotics give excellent results, notably chloromycetin (chloramphenicol). The fever is spread by a tick and its most striking feature is the rash.

Rodent Ulcer: a chronic ulcer found in the region of the eye and nose in elderly people. It is a slow-growing cancerous condition but in most cases responds satisfactorily to X-rays or radium which cause it to heal completely.

Rombergism: unsteadiness in standing with the eyes closed found, e.g. in locomotor ataxia (q.v.)

Rorschach Test: the 'ink-blot' test devised for discovering personality traits either in normal or abnormal people.

Rosacea: (*see* Acne Rosacea).

Roundworms: (*see* Parasites, Worms).

Rubella: German Measles.

Rubeola: measles.

Rupture: (*see* Hernia).

Sacrum: the triangular bone composed of five vertebrae fused together which lies between the haunch bones at the lower end of the spinal column. It forms the back wall of the pelvis.

Sadism: a sexual perversion in which pleasure is gained by inflicting cruelty on others.

Safe Period: a method of contraception based on the assumption that a woman is only fertile and capable of becoming pregnant on certain days of the menstrual cycle. Ovulation taking place about 15 days before the next period, and allowing for five days on either side of this, it follows that the fertile period is from the 8th to the 18th day of the ordinary 28 day cycle. Any time outside this is said to be safe. The drawback is that only those with very regular menstruation can use the method and even so it seems probable that emotional and other influences can change the date of ovulation.

St Vitus Dance: (*see* Chorea).

Salicylates: the salts of salicylic acid which is derived from oil of wintergreen, sweet birch, and many other plants. The main one is sodium salicylate which has much the same effects as aspirin in relieving pain and reducing temperature; it is used as a specific in acute rheumatism.

Salpingitis: the commonest cause of salpingitis or inflammation of the Fallopian tubes is gonorrhoea, but other germs such as the streptococcus, staphylococcus, pneumococcus, and tuberculosis bacillus can also invade the tubes. In acute salpingitis there is severe pain in the lower abdomen, tenderness on pressure over the tubes, and fever. Today treatment with the antibiotics has superseded surgical treatment unless there is actual abscess formation.

Salvarsan: or arsphenamine was the original anti-syphilitic drug which has been largly replaced by Neosalvarsan (neo-arsphenamine). These substances are useful in the treatment of many diseases due to protozoa and spirochaetes.

Sand-Fly Fever: phlebotomus or three-day fever was common in the Middle East during the last war and is a mild virus infection spread by the sandfly. As its alternative name indicates, its influenzal-like symptoms rarely last for more than three days. Prophylaxis is as for mosquitoes, treatment is as for influenza, i.e. aspirin.

Santonin: a yellow drug used in the treatment of roundworms.

Saphenous Vein: refers usually to the internal saphenous vein which is a superficial vein in the leg which can be seen running up the inside of the limb all the way from the ankle to the groin. It is important as the usual site of varicose veins. The external vein is shorter and runs up the outside and back of the leg only as far as the back of the knee.

Scabies: (*see* Parasites).

Scapula: the shoulder-blade.

Scarlet Fever: the disease is due to a streptococcus which produces the toxin responsible for the rash, sore throat and red tongue with which scarlet fever begins. The onset is usually sudden with sore throat, headache, shivering, and vomiting, the temperature rising to about 102 degrees. The rash appears on the second day on the neck, front of chest, trunk, limbs, and especially in the flexures. It consists of tiny red dots which ultimately run together forming an almost uniform red. Typically there is an area of pallor (circumoral pallor) around the mouth. There is a 'white strawberry' tongue on the second day and a 'red strawberry' tongue on the fourth. On the fifth day the temperature begins to fall. Complications are nephritis, middle ear disease, valvular heart disease, and pericarditis. The incubation period is 1–8 days and isolation is usually maintained for four weeks although with the advent of penicillin treatment it is likely that any infectious discharge from the nose or elsewhere will have cleared up before then. The young children who are generally affected probably catch the infecion from droplets coughed or sneezed by sufferers, by infected milk, or by contact with infected clothes, etc.

Schistosomiasis: (*see* Bilharzia).

Schizophrenia: (*see* Mental Illness).

Sciatica: this may be a form of neuritis due to focal sepsis, 'rheumatism,' diabetes, alcoholism, etc., or simply come on for no apparent cause. Or it may be a symptom of disease elsewhere, the nerve being compressed by some inflammatory process such as fibrositis, a spinal cord tumour or a tumour in the pelvis, and possibly a slipped disc. In some cases the pain is referred from osteoarthritis of the hip or sacro-iliac strain. There is numbness and tingling in the heel, leg, or back of the thigh along the course of the nerve (i.e. right down the back of the leg from the buttocks to the heel) and later very severe pain often associated, if the condition lasts long, with wasting of the muscles of the back of the leg. It is first of all necessary to discover whether the pain is a symptom of some process or other going on in the pelvis or spine and, when these have been eliminated, rest will be recommended in severe cases with various forms of physiotherapy, pain-killing drugs, and possibly vitamin B complex. In a few cases injection of the nerve is necessary or surgical stretching.

Scoliosis: one of the most important conditions affecting the spine; it is a curvature of the spine in the vertical plane with rotation and may be idiopathic or secondary to poliomyelitis. The idiopathic type (i.e. of unknown origin) occurs in actively-growing adolescents especially girls but it has nothing to do with posture as has so often been thought in the past. That secondary to poliomyelitis occurs when one side of the body has been paralysed whilst the other remains healthy so that the strong muscles work against the flaccid ones to pull the spine out of alignment. Sometimes a similar result happens from one-sided diseases of the chest as in chronic tuberculosis. Prolonged treatment and observation is usually necessary but in most cases dealt with early only a slight scoliosis is left. In more serious cases spinal fusion operations are carried out; these fuse together one third of the spinal column and a plaster jacket must be worn for some time.

Scopolamine: (*see* Hyoscydmus).

Scurvy: this condition is due to a deficiency of vitamin C in the diet either in infants being fed on boiled milk or some other unsuitable milk substitute or in adults in war-time who lack fresh foods. Formerly scurvy was rife amongst sailors on long sea voyages and the English got their name of 'Limeys' from their use of lime juice to prevent scurvy. There are haemorrhages from the gums and the nose, bruising of the skin, and in children bleeding under the periosteum (the delicate covering of the bones) may give the appearance of paralysis owing to pain of movement. In adults the teeth soon fall out. Scurvy, even in minor degrees, is rare since the regular administration to children of orange juice. The treatment is of course to supply the missing vitamin; this may be given either in suitable foods or in the form of ascorbic acid tablets.

Sea-sickness: is one form of travel sickness, although possibly the most violent so that those who cannot tolerate sea travel would be well advised to go by some other means of transport. Recent effective drugs for the prevention of the condition are Avomine, Benacine (Benadryl with hyoscine hydrobromide), Cyclizine Hydrochloride, Dramamine (dimenhydrinate), Marzine, and Stelazine.

Seborrhoea: a condition of the sebaceous or oil-secreting glands of the skin which leads to dandruff of the scalp and a greasy eruption with yellow scales on the face, neck, back and chest. The latter are probably infected from the scalp and the rash must be treated by reduction of the oily secretion. The scalp should be washed several times a week with a non-oily and preferably a detergent shampoo and one of the various sulphur lotions applied to the rash elsewhere. It is best to use lotions rather than ointments although non-greasy creams are quite suitable.

Sedimentation Rate: the measurement of the rate at which the red blood cells in a specimen sink to the bottom. In active infections the rate of sinking is increased and this is therefore a test of the activity of a disease process .

Senna: is one of the safest purgatives to use if purgatives are actually necessary. It is standardised in the form of Senokot granules or tablets (*see* Constipation).

Septicaemia: (*see* Blood-poisoning).

Sequestrum: a fragment of dead bone separated off from the living part during the process of necrosis (*see* Bone).

Sex and Sexual Problems: it was for long the custom to think of sex as an impulse arising at puberty and dying out in women at the change of life and in men a little later. This totally false belief caused many to feel that any manifestations of sex before or after these ages must be abnormal but it is now realised that the impulse is present in various forms from the earliest months until the end of life. Infants (quite apart from the Freudian theory that sucking and defaecation are both forms of sexuality in the widest sense) evince interest in their sexual organs and their interest is carried on throughout childhood with the special characteristic that this stage is *autoerotic*, i.e. the main interest is centred on the child's own body. Masturbation is a feature of this stage and an almost universal one which causes no physical or mental harm in spite of dread warnings dating from Victorian times. On the other hand it is necessary to note that masturbation carried on to excess may well be a *sign* of something wrong, usually indicating extreme anxiety rather than overdeveloped sexuality. Just before puberty there is a brief *homosexual stage* which may or may not be marked by physical manifestations of interest in the same sex. Ordinarily this is the time when schoolgirls develop 'crushes' for older girls or schoolteachers, and schoolboys similarly have their heroes. There are few people who have not at one time or another manifested homosexual tendencies and there is nothing necessarily abnormal about this since the natural development of sex is from the self, through the similar, to the quite different, i.e. the other sex.

Puberty is the stage when the interest becomes *heterosexual* or directed towards the other sex and at the same time the body matures so that parenthood becomes possible, the menstrual periods beginning in girls and seminal emissions in boys. Such emissions are normal and it is wrong to believe – as indeed a little thought quite apart from theoretical knowledge would make obvious – that emissions are weakening. Clearly they are no more so than sexual intercourse in adults. The periods need equally be no cause for distress in girls who have been properly educated and it is worth while noting that a great deal of dysmenorrhea (pain with the periods) is related to faulty teaching which associates them with guilt or shame (*see* Menstruation). The proper way to educate children in sex matters is (1) to answer from the earliest days every question the child asks about sex and to answer truthfully; (2) to answer only what has been asked without elaborating or giving long lectures; (3) to ensure that lectures are given at the proper time and place, i.e. in school as a part of biology lessons. Parents who fail to do this are living in a fool's paradise since nearly all children learn the 'facts of life' in a garbled form from their comrades and the choice is not between some information or none but between accurate and inaccurate information. Faulty upbringing has also much to do with later difficulties in sexual relations during married life which in nearly all cases are difficulties of personal relationships showing themselves in sexual guise. Thus although *impotence* in men is occasionally the result of a general disease such as serious diabetes or Addison's disease, it is much more usually the expression of unconscious or conscious conflicts such as fear of failure or lack of genuine interest in the partner. *Frigidity* in women ranges from total frigidity to the very common inability to reach orgasm which in our own civilisation is perhaps more often the rule than the exception. Both these disabilities, if they trouble the individual, should be referred to a doctor who deals with such problems. *Sterility*, the inability to have children, is often mistakenly thought to be the fault of the woman although a large number of the cases concern the man; problems of sterility should be discussed with the family doctor who will probably arrange a consultation and treatment at the Fertility Clinic of the local hospital. Problems associated with the menopause are discussed under that heading.

Sexual perversions are cases of failure to develop beyond a certain level of childish sexuality or the replacement of normal sexual feeling by tendencies which, although not necessarily abnormal in themselves are abnormal when they became the whole aim of the act. *Homosexuality* as mentioned above is a normal stage of development through which everyone passes but becomes abnormal when it is retained into adult life. The cause of homosexuality is always psychological and frequently related in the male to a dominating mother. The outlook for treatment in a confirmed case is not good since few homosexuals have any desire to be cured. *Sadism* and *masochism*, the obtaining of sexual pleasure from hurting and being hurt respectively are examples of a normal component of sex which has got out of hand and become the main aim as is *fetishism* which is sexual satisfaction associated with inanimate objects such as shoes, brassieres, and hair. Here again it is not abnormal to feel attraction to articles associated with the beloved but quite abnormal to make them the sole object of sex. Such perversions require psychological treatment and the outlook is reasonably good in cases where there is a real desire to achieve normality; in

491

other cases where treatment seems unlikely to be successful and the impulse is a threat to others or to the individual himself it is possible to produce 'pharmacological castration' by administering stilboestrol, the female sex hormone. This, of course, is not irreversible (*see* Impotence, Orgasm).

Shaking Palsy: paralysis agitans or Parkinsonism (q.v.).

Shell Shock: the name given to war-neurosis during the First World War under the false impression that it was caused by the physical effect of shell explosions rather than emotional stress.

Shingles: Herpes Zoster (q.v.).

Shock: two kinds of shock are ordinarily described: nervous shock and surgical shock. The former simply means great mental distress caused by some distressing event and necessitates treatment with sedatives, the latter refers to a state of the body following severe injury or haemorrhage and it is with this we are concerned here. Although there are still various problems involved as to the exact nature and cause of surgical shock there is fairly general agreement that its main feature is a diminution in the fluid content of the blood caused by the effect of a substance known as histamine which is released by the injured tissues. Histamine causes the small blood-vessels to dilate and the fluid part of the blood to seep through the walls into the surrounding tissues. The patient with shock is severely prostrated and pale with skin which is often beaded with perspiration. The pulse is feeble and rapid, the respirations sighing and irregular, the temperature often below normal, and there is great thirst. The patient feels cold and clammy. As is well known, the first-aid treatment of shock is to keep the patient warm (but not too warm), give hot sweet liquids, e.g. tea (provided there is no sign of abdominal injury), relieve pain with morphia, and keep the feet higher than the head. Since the blood is too concentrated, the doctor may given transfusions of blood plasma as an early measure.

Siderosis: (*see* Pneumoconiosis).

Silver: in general silver is used externally only in medicine either in the form of silver nitrate (lunar caustic) which is used in sticks for cauterising warts and in very weak solutions for conjunctivitis of the eyes, or as silver proteinate (argyrol, protargol, etc.), for the eyes, nose, and throat, and urethra.

Simmond's Disease: (pituitary cachexia) a disorder caused by destruction of the anterior lobe of the pituitary gland. There is premature senility, wasting, loss of hair, and impotence.

Sinusitis: is an inflammation of the mucous membrane lining of one or more sinuses, the spaces in the bones of the skull which open into the nose. Sinusitis is usually secondary to an infection of the nose although the maxillary sinus in the upper jaw can be infected from a tooth in this area. Swimming and diving may drive infection from the nose into the sinuses and various nasal deformities or polyp formation within the nose predispose to it. The symptoms vary with the sinus affected: in addition to the maxillary sinuses of the upper jaw, there are the frontal sinuses above and between the eyebrows the ethmoidal sinuses on either side of the root of the nose, and the sphenoid sinus deep behind the same area. There is pain over the affected part, fever, a blocked nose with some discharge, and headache. The diagnosis is made from a history of a 'cold' which has persisted for more than a week, from the presence of the above symptoms, from the evidence of X-rays or *transillumination of the sinuses* when a light is shone through the part in a dark room (e.g. in the case of the maxillary sinuses the light would be in the mouth) and opacity is revealed in the infected sinus. Most of these cases clear up with rest in bed, inhalations to shrink the swollen lining of the nose and let the pus escape from the sinuses through the canals which connect each with the inside of the nose, nasal sprays or drops for the same purpose, and antibiotics. In only a few cases is operation necessary, its aim being to allow drainage from the infected sinus. Apart from the frontal sinus, the others can be approached through the inside of the nose, the maxillary sinuses often being dealt with by pushing a large hollow needle through the thin wall on the lateral aspect of the nasal cavity.

Skin: the skin has two layers, the epidermis or cuticle and the true skin, cutis vera, or dermis which lies underneath the other. The epidermis is bloodless and consists of layers of epithelial cells the outermost of which are dead scales, the lower actively multiplying to replace those worn or washed away, and being nourished by lymph. The thickness of the epidermis varies greatly throughout the body and is thickest on the palms of the hands and the soles of the feet; nails and hairs are outgrowths of the epidermis. The true skin or dermis is a layer of fibrous tissue which merges gradually into the loose subcutaneous tissue beneath; at its surface it rises into rows of conical *papillae* containing loops of blood capillaries and in some papillae there are nerve endings or *tactile corpuscles*. The hairs and hair follicles with their *erector pili* muscle fibres which cause 'goose-flesh' and make the hair 'stand on end' arise from the dermis and both layers of skin are traversed by the ducts of the sweat glands. Here, too, the pigment granules are found within the cells which are more numerous in certain races. The skin is constantly renewed from its deeper layers and on the palms and soles the rows of papillae form continuous ridges with intervening grooves; these remain constant throughout life and are typical of the individual being the basis of finger-printing for identification.

The skin is an excretory organ aiding to some extent the kidneys (q.v.) and taking over some of their function when they are damaged by disease. It is respiratory carrying on to a rather small degree the work of the lungs (although in some animals such as frogs respiration through the skin is much more important). It regulates the temperature of the body and is the main channel for loss of heat; but when the surrounding air is cold the sweat glands close, the skin becomes pale, and the phenomenon of shivering occurs which is nature's way of raising the temperature. The skin can also absorb, not only drugs (some of which were given in this way by inunction (q.v.) to supply the whole body) but also water since thirst is partly relieved by immersion, and another very important function is the exclusion of germs from the body (which is why we cover up cuts when the skin is broken). Sebaceous glands situated in the dermis give out a greasy secretion known as sebum into the hair follicles thus lubricating the hair and keeping it healthy whilst the sweat glands in the same area separate the sweat out from the lymph bathing them, sweat playing a large part in the process of losing heat as well as excretion. The glands are provided with special regulating nerves.

A healthy skin is obviously important but it is as well to realise that the health of the skin depends upon the health of the body and that therefore, whatever the cosmetic advertisements may say, applications on the surface of the skin have only a limited usefulness except in the case of disease. Thus one may supply grease to a dry skin to replace the normal secretion but it is extremely doubtful whether it makes much sense to talk of 'feeding' the skin because the skin is fed only from within. Feeding the hair is even more absurd because hair is a dead structure so all hair tonics might as well be poured down the drain so far as their 'tonic' effect is concerned. Nor, in spite of the mystique attached to the subject, is any one soap (provided the quality is reasonably good) better than another. Consumer's Research for example showed that a cheap toilet soap made by Boots was in no important respect different from one costing nearly six times as much. Furthermore, since *all* soaps are antiseptic by their very nature, it is doubtful whether 'antiseptic soaps' are any more so. Regular washing is especially important for those with greasy skins, although honesty compels one to admit that some of the most attractive women in primitive societies rarely wash at all and never with soap. The significance of washing and bathing is partly social (since we would smell offensively if we did not) and partly important for removing the dead cells and secretions of the epidermis. Skin diseases are dealt with under their appropriate headings. For skin grafting *see* Graft.

Skull Fractures: (*see* Concussion).

Sleep, Disorders of: *dreams* as is well-known can be stimulated by many factors: an uncomfortable or unfamiliar bed, a heavy or indigestible meal, a worrying day just past or a possibly worrying one to come, but these are not the origin of dreams which are disguised forms of our own personal problems. In some cases they are an attempted solution to such problems, but for the individual the main issue is whether they are pleasant or unpleasant. Unpleasant dreams are what we describe as nightmares in which primitive impulses from the unconscious seem about to break into awareness and if these are frequent, especially in children, it is best to see a psychiatrist or child psychologist. In children these often take the form of *night terrors* where the child wakes in a state of fear and may not be pacified or capable of recognising his surroundings for some minutes after waking. *Somnambulism* or sleep-walking has a similar origin and if at all frequent is best handled by a child psychologist. Probably due

495

to a lag in the awakening of different parts of the brain is 'paralysed wakefulness' where the individual wakes up intellectually but finds himself unable to move for some minutes or seconds after attaining full consciousness. This, if unpleasant, is of no serious significance. Insomnia is dealt with under that heading.

Sleeping Sicknss: or trypanosomiasis is a tropical disease caused by a trypanosome spread by the tsetse fly and must not be confused with *sleepy sickness* which is *encephalitis lethargica* (q.v.). Trypanosomiasis is found in West and East Africa, the Congo and Rhodesia, trypanosoma gambiense being spread by the fly *glossina palpalis* and trypanosoma rhodesiense by *glossina morsitans*. The most characteristic feature of the disease is its long latent period, the early stage of periodic rises in temperature, swelling of the spleen and lymph glands, and oedema (swelling) of the legs lasting up to three years before the next stage of tremors, vacant expression, and slow speech. Later, the patient becomes increasingly sluggish and weak and sleeps or dozes during the day; there is wasting, apathy, and a subnormal temperature and he becomes comatose and bedridden before death. Treatment is with Suramin (Bayer 205) in early cases where the trypanosome has been found in the blood; later, tryparsamide gives good results.

Slimming: (*see* Obesity).

Slipped Disc: (prolapsed disc) the intervertebral discs are made of spongy but firm elastic tissue and act as shock-absorbers to the spinal column being held in place by a strong ring of fibrous tissue (the annulus fibrosus) which surrounds the vertebra. When this wears out at the back of the vertebra, the disc is able to slip out and cause pressure upon one or other of the spinal nerve roots causing very severe pain. Slipped disc is one of the commonest causes of pain in the back and, usually occurring in the lumbar region, it involves the nerves going to the buttocks, thighs, calves, and feet; hence the initial diagnosis is often sciatica. Diagnosis is made by X-ray by the use of *myelogram* where a radio-opaque substance is injected into the spinal canal prior to filming. The usual treatment is rest in bed, but even with traction (stretching) and other measures full recovery may take three to six months. In about 20% of cases recovery does not follow conservative treatment and it is necessary to carry out a *laminectomy*. In this operation a portion of the arch of the vertebra is removed and the herniated part of the disc cut away. With this treatment it is possible to get out of bed a few days after the operation and to go home in about two weeks.

Smallpox: (variola) an acute infectious fever once prevalent in Britain but rarely seen since the introduction of vaccination; it attacks people of all ages and is equally prevalent in males and females. Infection is spread by contact, by articles handled by the infected person, by third persons, and probably by flies and air, the virus being inhaled. The cause is a filterable virus which gives rise to the so-called Paschen bodies found in the fluid of the pocks, and the incubation period is 10–14 days. The onset is usually sudden with headache, vomiting, backache, and a rigor as the temperature rises to 103 degrees; often there is a 'prodromal' reddish rash rather like scarlet fever before the true one makes its appearance on the third day. When the true rash appears the temperature falls to normal, and initially the rash takes the form of spots and papules which turn into blisters on the fifth day and pustules on the ninth. During the pustular stage the temperature begins to rise again and the pustules burst about the twelfth day forming crusts on the sixteenth. When the crusts separate in 2–3 weeks depressed scars are left behind. The rash makes its first appearance on the peripheral parts of the body, slowly moving towards the trunk, i.e. it is likely to arise on the forehead and scalp, the legs, and the back of the wrists before spreading inwards. (This is the opposite of chickenpox where the rash begins on the trunk and moves outwards.) Three types of the disease are usually described. (1) discrete, the ordinary type where the pustules remain more or less separated from each other and the outlook is fairly good; (2) confluent, where there are many pustules which coalesce sometimes forming superficial abscesses and usually there is great prostration and delirium with a correspondingly grave prognosis; (3) haemorrhagic, where there is bleeding into the pustules and haemorrhages from the mucous membranes and into the conjunctivae. Haemorrhagic smallpox is the most fatal type. There is no specific treatment but the patient must be in bed, the hair cut short, and the skin bathed with 1% potassium permanganate solution; it is important to protect the eyes and face as much as possible and the eyes should be frequently bathed. Prophylactic treatment is to vaccinate in infancy, at the age of 7, 14, and 21 years, and again if there is an epidemic. Contacts should be vaccinated and observed for 16 days. The patient must be isolated for six weeks and until all the scabs have separated.

Smoking: the term generally refers to the smoking of tobacco and it is in this sense that it will be employed here although many other substances can also be smoked, e.g. various herbs sold in herbalists' shops, opium, and stramonium which some use in the form of cigarettes in the treatment of asthma.

Tobacco was in use by the American Indians from the remotest antiquity and was introduced into Europe by Francisco Hernandez de Toledo, a physician to Philip II of Spain, in 1559. It reached the French court in the following year through the medium of an ambassador Jean Nicot (who thus gave his name to the botanical term for the plant which is Nicotiana, and to the alkaloid nicotine which is found in tobacco). Sailors returning from the Americas first introduced smoking to England about 1565 and Sir Walter Raleigh brought it to court circles. Initally, tobacco was thought to be of great medicinal value and, indeed, almost a cure-all, but at a later date laws supported by heavy punishments and even the threat of excommunication by the Church were introduced to exterminate the practice; these had as little success as the modern propaganda of today. Cigarette-smoking was brought to this country by soldiers after the Crimean War. Tobacco, of course, is not only smoked but also chewed or taken in the form of snuff.

Enough has been said about the dangers of lung cancer under the heading of Lung Diseases, and, whilst it is probably true that most of the heavy smokers we have known did not develop cancer, the fact is that these belong to the lucky seven out of eight and perhaps we did not meet the eighth, the unlucky man who died of it. What concerns us here are the other real or alleged consequences of smoking, and what can be done by those who wish to give up the habit which will bring us to consider what makes people smoke in the first place. Perhaps it is best to begin with those conditions which are *known for certain* to be either caused or worsened by smoking, and here it is necessary to remember that the death-rate of middle-aged people who smoke more than twenty cigarettes a day is more than twice that of non-smokers *taking all diseases into account*, i.e. not necessarily from lung cancer. Although rather rare now, tobacco used to be a common cause of cancer of the lips and tongue in poor people who smoked broken clay pipes, the jagged edge of the stem causing a sore which became cancerous when the hot tobacco smoke incessantly came into contact with it. Buerger's disease or thromboangiitis obliterans, a disease in which the arteries of the leg become narrowed and thickened is believed by many authorities to be a form of allergic response to tobacco and, at any rate, is always associated with heavy cigarette-smoking. The well-known 'smoker's cough' is usually of local origin, being a form of pharyngitis or laryngitis brought on by irritation, and bronchitis, if there is little ground for supposing that it is caused by smoking, is certainly worsened by it. Patients with a peptic ulcer are usually advised not to smoke (or at least not to smoke on an empty stomach) because nicotine stimulates the gastric juices which is the last thing one wants to do in this condition. Nicotine also stimulates the heart which beasts faster (although this effect is much less noticeable in those who smoke habitually) and by some is believed to be a cause of tachycardia or palpitation; the bowels are stimulated, too, and the smoker often finds that his first pipe or cigarette of the day brings on the desire to defaecate. Whether, as some believe, coronary thrombosis is linked with smoking is a more dubious matter – and so, in the view of the writer, is the idea implicit in the statement already made that twice as many heavy smokers die in their middle years from all causes as non-smokers. The fact is indubitable, but the inference that smoking in itself is the cause of this mortality is not at all certain. In spite of a few doubters, most doctors feel that we have virtually *proved* the direct connection between smoking and lung cancer, but such a claim cannot yet be made of coronary disease or the high death-rate from other diseases of heavy smokers. What is obvious is that the heavy smoker is likely to be a certain sort of person: he is tense and nervous, possibly drives himself too hard, and very likely eats and drinks alcohol to excess just as he smokes to excess. Now this is often the coronary type, and the type who is liable to have a stroke or a duodenal ulcer, and his eating, drinking, and working habits are quite adequate to account for his liability to death in middle-age without bringing in smoking, even if this plays a part. As pointed out in the section on lung diseases, proof of correlation between two events does not demonstrate for certain that they are related in terms of cause and effect.

Smoking cures come under three, or perhaps four, general headings: (1) the use of a mouth-wash containing e.g. a dilute solution of silver nitrate which makes smoking taste so unpleasant that it is supposed to turn the smoker against the habit; as with most aversion treatments, the 'cure' is more likely to be given up than the habit. (2) The use of a dummy cigarette which may contain something to give it a taste such as menthol; whether this helps or not one would not be prepared to say but there is some evidence that menthol itself can occasionally produce unpleasant symptoms or illness. (3) Simply stopping smoking abruptly which is probably the only effective way, or turning to one of the herbal mixtures already mentioned; the trouble about the latter method is (a) that the smoker will probably become a social outcast, and (b) that in all probability some other clever individual will come along sooner or later to prove that they, too, are carcinogenic. (4) The use of one of the new drugs containing lobeline or one of its derivatives. Lobeline is an alkaloid (q.v.) which produces effects on the body when taken by mouth similar to those produced by nicotine and the theory is that it can be used to tide the smoker over the initial stages of deprivation. Now whether this works or not depends upon whether one regards smoking as an addiction (in the correct sense of the word rather than the pejorative one employed by the lunatic fringe to signify its disapproval of smoking as such) or as largely a social habit. What this means is described under the heading of Drug Addiction, but, broadly speaking, a drug of addiction is one which causes unpleasant physical symptoms when it is withdrawn. If smoking comes into this caterory, then quite possibly lobeline derivatives will help withdrawal; if it does not, then any effects produced by the tablets are due to faith alone. The writer's own opinion (and it is only an opinion) is (a) that the smoker carries on with his habit because he likes the taste of tobacco and not at all because he likes its physical effects which, in the first place, are only prominent in the novice, and in the second place are wholly unpleasant (consisting of palpitation, nausea, coughing, and excessive salivation); this is not the case with the drug addict who takes something not particularly pleasant in itself – even the alcoholic often loathes the taste of spirits – in order to produce certain physical and mental states, (b) the withdrawal of tobacco produces in some a vague irritability and in all the desire for a smoke, but it cannot be said to produce symptoms as does the withdrawal of alchohol or cocaine in the addict, (c) apart from the pleasant taste, the most fundamental reason for smoking is social; it begins as a prestige symbol in the youth who regards it as manly, and later there is something calming about the whole ritual involved in lighting a pipe or a cigarette (tobacco in itself does not calm the nerves) and introductions or uneasy breaks in a conversation are facilitated. There is something about most human beings which makes them want to play around with an object in their hands, especially in company, and Moslem men, for example, carry a string of beads which they play about with when alone and thinking or with others whilst talking. It is this that mainly troubles the individual who has ceased to smoke – what to do with his hands. Shall he keep them embedded in his pockets, clasped before him or behind his neck, or tap them on the edge of the chair? This, perhaps, is why the smoker wants to retain his habit rather than addiction to a drug, and there is the additional calming effect of the pleasant smell and the sight of the smoke curling lazily upwards. It is not without significance that many heavy smokers feel no desire to smoke when they have a heavy cold and that, as is well-known, those who become blind often give up the habit spontaneously. Still, it is a dangerous habit, and the best solution is not to begin. If one has already started then we can only say that, having come to the realisation that he is taking a calculated risk (as we have to do in many other spheres of life) he must decide, according to his own temperament, to stop altogether or to continue. Recent work shows that drug treatments are useless.

Soap: (*see* Skin).

Sodium: only the salts of the metal sodium are used in medicine, the main ones being sodium bicarbonate or baking soda used as an antacid (sodium carbonate is washing soda), sodium chloride or common salt which was given in large doses in Addison's disease and is a very effective expectorant and emetic, and sodium citrate and acetate which are both diuretics.

Soft Sore: (Chancroid so called because the initial sore resembles the chancre of syphilis except in being soft rather than hard. Chancroid is a venereal disease due to the Haemophilus ducreyi with other organisms and is a local condition which does not spread beyond the glands of the groin which may break down and ulcerate in untreated cases. The incubation period is very short and the condition rapidly responds to the sulpha drugs or, in more resistant cases, to aureomycin or streptomycin.

Sore Throat: (*see* Throat).

Spanish Fly: (*see* Cantharides).

Spastic: any condition where spasm is present as in a spastic gait caused by damage to the upper part of the nervous system connected with movement (upper motor neurone). This causes the lower parts to get out of control, instead of being totally paralysed as in the case of the flaccid paralysis of a lower motor neurone lesion.

Spectacles: there are four types of refractive errors which require the use of glasses: myopia (short-sightedness), hypermetropia (long-sightedness), astigmatism, and presbyopia. Short-sightedness is due to the refractive power of the eye being too strong so that the image is brought to a focus in front of the retina producing blurred vision. This is often a problem in children who consequently are unable to see objects at a distance such as the blackboard at school and it is important that suitable glasses should be supplied as early as possible. Long-sight is the reverse condition in which the refractive power of the eye is reduced and the image of near objects is brought to a focus behind the retina; whereas in myopia a concave lens is used for viewing distant objects, in hypermetropia convex lenses are used for near work and distant vision is not affected. In astigmatism the curvature of the cornea is not symmetrical so that the rays of light in one plane cannot be focused at the same time as those in the plane at right angles to it. There is distortion of both near and distant vision so that a circle is seen as an ellipse and is blurred at two points opposite each other. The lens for this type of defect must be cylindrical, i.e. flat in one plane and curved in the one at right angles to it. Astigmatism may occur in long or short-sighted people or mixed astigmatism may exist in which the eye is longsighted in one meridian and short-sighted in the other. In presbyopia the changes due to age cause the lens to lose its ability to accommodate for near vision and glasses become necessary; this is the case with most people after 45 and nearly all after 50. Dark glasses, although fashionable from time to time, are very rarely a medical necessity – rather are they a sign of exhibitionism, the desire to conceal one's thoughts from others, or a status symbol.

Speech Disorders: (*see* Stammering and Stuttering).

Sphincter: a ring of muscle surrounding and controlling the exit from an organ, e.g. the bladder or rectum.

Sphygmomanometer: an instrument for measuring the blood-pressure by means of an inflatable band around the upper arm attached to a tube of mercury which measures the pressure necessary to obliterate the pulse.

Spinal Column: the bones or vertebrae of the spinal column are 33 in number in the child, but in adult life the lowest 4 unite to form the coccyx and the 5 above that unite to form the sacrum leaving only 26. These are arranged as follows: 7 cervical vertebrae in the neck, 12 thoracic vertebrae with attached ribs in the region of the chest, and 5 lumbar vertebrae in the region of the loins, the remaining being the sacrum and coccyx in the pelvis. Diseases of the spine and spinal cord are dealt with under their own names.

Spirochaetosis Icterohaemorrhagica: also known as Weil's disease, leptospiral jaundice, and spirochaetal jaundice, is an infection caused by the Leptospira icterohaemorrhagiae which is transmitted to man by rats which excrete it in their urine. Infection may be due to taking contaminated food or water, or the germ may enter through the skin, eyes, nose, or mouth. The disease is liable to occur amongst workers in places infested by rats, e.g. sewers, mines, barges, fish markets, slaughter-houses and piggeries. The incubation period is 6–10 days after which there is a sudden onset with high fever, headache, pains in the muscles, and vomiting. Later there is jaundice (appearing on the second or third day in 60% of cases), enlargement of the liver and spleen, nephritis, and bleeding from the nose. Occasionally a rash may be present.

The disease can occur in any country and is particularly common amongst workers in the paddy-fields of Japan where the water, which is another factor in the spread of the condition, is often infected. The *preventive* treatment is to destroy all rats, pumping out water (e.g. in mines) whenever possible, removing all waste material such as offal, prophylactic immunisation, testing each man in places where the disease is endemic for immunity, and insisting on personal cleanliness such as washing the hands before meals. In *curative* treatment the specific antiserum together with penicillin must be used as soon as possible; for unless it is started within the first four days, the outlook is serious.

Spleen: the spleen lies behind the stomach high up on the left side of the abdomen and is attached by two ligaments of peritoneum one going to the stomach the other to the left kidney. It is through the latter ligament that the blood vessels supplying the organ pass to its hilum or root. Inside the spleen consists of a network of fibrous tissue which supports the pulp whence blood from the splenic artery passes to be distributed and later collected by the splenic vein which subsequently joins the portal vein. The functions of the spleen are not fully understood but it appears that it plays some part in forming the white corpuscles of the blood and it may be that, like the liver, it also destroys the used red ones. Since the operation of splenectomy for removal of the spleen is not uncommon and the general health does not appear to suffer afterwards it may safely be assumed that the spleen carries out no function which cannot be duplicated elsewhere in the body. Thus removal is followed by an increase in size of the lymph glands in the body.

Splenectomy: (*see* above).

Splenic Anaemia: the term refers to two conditions: splenic anaemia of children or Von Jaksch's anaemia and splenic anaemia of adults or Banti's disease. The former occurs in young children from 1–4 years and there is progressive anaemia with enlargement of the spleen although most cases recover with iron treatment within a year. The latter is a rather confused title for what may be a group of ill-defined diseases such as acholuric jaundice or cirrhosis of the liver with enlargement of the spleen; typically the patient is a young adult with cirrhosis of the liver, jaundice, enlargement of the spleen, and bleeding from the nose or by vomiting (haematemesis) which may cause death. The treatment is splenectomy.

Splenomegaly: enlargement of the spleen which may be due to a great many causes among them infections by protozoa such as malaria, bacterial infections such as typhoid, blood diseases such as pernicious anaemia and leukaemia, rickets, obstruction of the portal vein in cirrhosis of the liver, syphilis, hydatid cysts, abscesses and tumour formation.

Spondylitis: is inflammation of the vertebrae of the spine which may occur at any age. *Ankylosing spondylitis* is a disease of young males from 20–40 which unless treated early is likely to lead to complete fixation of the spine. The treatment is deep X-ray therapy and the use of the drug phenylbutazone (Butazolidin).

Spondylolisthesis: this is the name of a condition in which one vertebra slips out of line and slides forward over the vertebra immediately below. It most commonly affects the last (5th) lumbar vertebra which slides forward over the first sacral one. There is discomfort which ranges from a chronic ache to severe and acute pain and treatment is usually with a back brace and change to less strenuous work. In other patients an operation bringing about fusion of the affected vertebrae gives good results in a majority of cases.

Sprains: (*see* Joints, Disease of).

Sprue: a group of diseases characterised by diarrhoea with the passage of large, pale, and offensive motions; sore tongue; anaemia, and loss of weight. Sprue was at one time thought to be an exclusively tropical disease, but it is evident that coeliac disease in infants and adults (non-tropical sprue) is unrelated to geography or climate. The condition in infants and adults appears to be the result of an inborn error of metabolism which causes the intestines to be unable to absorb fats; this is followed by malabsorption of other food substances such as carbohydrates, minerals, and vitamins. The bulky pale motions are due to the failure to absorb fat, the sore tongue and anaemia to poor absorption of minerals and vitamins. In coeliac disease of infants girls are mainly affected and the infant fails to gain weight, is backward in walking, has a poor appetite, and loose bowels. The abdomen is protuberant and tetany (from lack of calcium) sometimes develops.

Treatment is dependent on finding a diet containing as much fat as can be absorbed and giving iron and vitamin supplements. Good results are obtained from the giving of over-ripe bananas, two to three a day and vitamins A and D are especially important. Coeliac disease in adults or non-tropical sprue is probably a prolongation of the same process since most of the patients are women and many give a history of diarrhoea and rickets in infancy. The treatment is similar. In tropical sprue, the onset is insidious with looseness of the bowels in the early part of the day, soreness of the tongue and mouth, and loss of weight. There is hypochlorhydria (q.v.) and the stools are bulky, pale and frothy; the blood shows changes similar to those in pernicious anaemia. Tropical sprue, first described in 1879 by Sir Patrick Manson, is found in South-East Africa, the West Indies, and South America, but it is not known what bearing this distribution has upon the disease. In treatment a milk diet or the substance known as Sprulac should be given together with lightly cooked minced steak and such other foods as strawberries, bananas, apples, and pounded fish. Iron and liver extract is given for the anaemia, vitamins A and D with calcium lactate for calcium deficiency.

Squint: a condition in which the two eyes do not look in the same direction at one time; it results from over or underaction of one or more of the muscles which move the eyeball and may have a number of different causes. *Long-sightedness* in childhood may cause an inward squint especially on looking at objects close at hand and if the refractive error in one eye is greater than that in the other the good eye alone is used resulting in a greater or lesser degree of blindness in the other. Similarly *short-sightedness* may produce an outward squint when it has not been compensated for by proper glasses, and *defective vision in one eye* is a less frequent cause. Squint appearing in later life is usually the result of *paralysis of the nerves* supplying the eye muscles (four straight and two oblique) or disease in the brain which affects these nerves. Thus paralysis of the abducent nerve gives rise to a strong inward squint in one eye.

Treatment must begin as early as possible in life with the wearing of suitable glasses which may or may not have one dark lens to stop the child using the good eye. This prevents the bad one from becoming worse. Orthoptic exercises to train the child to use its eye muscles correctly must be given at a later stage, and in more severe cases operation may be necessary to strengthen a poorly acting eye muscle or weaken an overacting one.

Stammering and Stuttering: these are common forms of speech disorder due to incoordination of the muscles around the larynx. In stammering there is hesitation in the pronunciation of a syllable, in stuttering a machine-gun-like repetition of the initial letters. Stammering may arise in childhood or make its first appearance in adolescence or later life and it is generally believed that the former type is predominantly physiogical in origin, resulting from something wrong with the organisation of the neuromuscular apparatus concerned with speech whilst the latter type is psychological. This is not to say that emotional factors may not exacerbate the first condition, but it is common to find a family history of stammering together with a history of left-handedness which has given rise to the theory that the basic cause is an incomplete dominance of the leading hemisphere of the brain. Indeed it is frequently found that electroencephalogram recordings show that the two hemispheres of the brain give rise to alpha waves which are out of phase (*see* Electroencephalogram). Treatment of this type of stammer takes the form of training in breath control and speech therapy coupled with psychological treatment to remove any emotional problems which may exacerbate the stammer or have arisen because of it. Some types of childhood stammer are mainly psychogenic and in Freudian terminology centre around conflicts of a deep-seated nature associated with the oral (mouth) region. The later-developing stammers are all psychogenic and essentially of a hysterical nature; they readily respond to treatment of the underlying anxiety state but are in any case not usually of long duration.

Status Lymphaticus: a condition characterised by the overgrowth of lymphatic tissues throughout the body and persistence and enlargement of the thymus gland in the neck. It is a common cause of death under anaesthetic – or has conventionally been said to be so.

Sterility: (*see* Sex).

Stilboestrol: is a synthetic oestrogen active by mouth and with an action closely resembling that of the natural ovarian hormone. It is used in many gynaecological conditions and in men to slow down the the growth of cancer in the prostrate gland. In psychiatry it is given to men with psychopathic sexual tendencies to reduce the drive by inducing 'pharmacological castration'; this state, of course, is not irreversible.

Stokes-Adams Syndrome: a condition in which attacks of unconsciousness are associated with an abnormally slow pulse. The cause is heart-block (*see* Heart Surgery).

Stomach Diseases: the main stomach diseases are acute and chronic gastritis, stomach ulcer, and cancer of the stomach. Gastritis is inflammation of the stomach lining and the acute type is caused by an unsuitable meal or too much alcohol although irritant poisons also cause gastritis. The symptoms are those of a 'hangover,' i.e. headache, loss of appetite, depression, and in the words of P. G. Wodehouse, 'a feeling that you're going to die in about five minutes.' The treatment is to avoid irritating the stomach further, bland food, and a drink of alkaline effervescent salts. In chronic gastritis the common causes are persistent indulgence in irritant foods or drinks such as over-stewed tea or strong alcohol (chronic gastritis is almost an invariable accompaniment of chronic alcoholism), but it may also arise as a complication of kidney, lung, heart, or blood diseases and in severe diabetes. Its treatment is a medical problem.

Peptic ulcer is a name covering two separate conditions: gastric ulcer (i.e. stomach ulcer) and duodenal ulcer. The immediate cause of ulceration is that the digestive juices have digested away part of the mucous lining of the stomach or duodenum and the following facts are relevant to the understanding of this very common condition:

(1) About 10% of all adults have had at one time or another an ulcer of the stomach or duodenum.

(2) Nearly 90% of these ulcers clear up solely with medical treatment.

(3) Most people who believe themselves to have a 'stomach ulcer' are in fact suffering from an ulcer in the duodenum since the latter outnumbers the former in the ratio of 12 to 1.

(4) The indications for operation are in general: (*a*) when the ulcer is chronic and medical treatment has failed; (*b*)

when there is severe bleeding from the ulcer; (c) when, as somtimes happens, the ulcer forms scar tissue which contracts and obstructs the passage of food; (d) when the ulcer perforates.

A perforated ulcer is one which has eaten through the stomach wall and in these circumstances an emergency operation is necessary if peritonitis is to be avoided.

Typically, ulcer pain is in the upper abdomen and comes on from half an hour to two hours after meals depending upon its site; it is relieved by alkalies or taking more food. The medical treatment consists of dieting on easily digested foods taken little and often so that the stomach is 'never empty, never full.' Alkalies are prescribed by the doctor for taking after or between meals and these may be combined with an antispasmodic drug such as atropine or propantheline bromide (Pro-Banthine) and a sedative or tranquilliser in view of the relationship between mental stress and peptic ulcer. It cannot be too strongly emphasised that symptoms persisting any length of time should be referred to the doctor and that self-treatment is risky. Surgical treatment is designed to reduce the hyperacidity which causes the trouble. The two main operations performed are *gastrojejunostomy* in which part of the jejunum is stitched to the stomach so that the alkaline juices of the small intestine can enter and neutralise the excess acid, and, much more frequently nowadays, *partial gastrectomy*. In this operaton the part of the stomach which bears the acid-secreting glands is completely removed, the stump of the duodenum closed, and the remaining quarter of the stomach stitched to the small intestine. Following this operation only about 1% of cases have any further trouble. *Vagotomy*, the cutting of the vagus nerve through which the impulses that stimulate acid production pass, is sometimes performed.

Duodenal ulcer is a disease caused by stress, more common in industrial communities than in agricultural ones, more frequent in those who worry about their work or who work under pressure. There is no reason to suppose that irregular meals or the other dietary reasons usually given have any connection with the condition – and, in fact, some eminent authorities do not believe that diet plays any great part in its treatment and have given their ulcer patients in hospital beds the same diet as the others. Certainly the old diets of milk and slops with large amounts of alkali can hardly have been good for the general health whatever they may have done for the ulcer. Duodenal ulcer (q.v. is common in the fairly young and otherwise fit, whilst gastric ulcer occurs predominantly in the old and poorly. The former almost never become malignant but about 10% of stomach ulcers do even when there has been no previous history of serious dyspepsia. *Cancer of the Stomach* is found most frequently in men between 45 and 60. The pain in cancer tends to be constant and nagging rather than periodic, and there is increasing loss of weight and anaemia. Operation is necessary but the outlook is quite good if the condition is discovered in time. There would be much less chance of cancer getting beyond the stage when operation is likely to be successful if people with 'indigestion' in this age-group would put themselves immediately under medical care with periodic check-ups. A curious feature of cancer of the stomach is that hydrochloric acid is totally absent. For functional dyspepsia and gastric neuroses *see* Dyspepsia.

Strabismus: Squint (q.v.).

Streptomycin: an antibiotic obtained from the soil mould *actinomyces griseus* and discovered in 1944 by Waksman in the United States. It is active against certain Gram-negative organisms that are unaffected by penicillin in ordinary concentrations and, most important of all, it is effective against the germ of tuberculosis the treatment of which has been revolutionised by the discovery. Similarly valuable is its close relative dihydrostreptomycin. The main drawbacks of these drugs are their liability to create resistant strains of the organism and their production of certain toxic symptoms such as giddiness. The former disadvantage can be partly overcome by combining streptomycin with P.A.S. (para-aminosalicylic acid) or isoniazid.

Stricture: the narrowing of a natural passage as the urethra, bowel, or oesophagus.

Stroke: (*see* Apoplexy).

Strophanthin: the active principle of an African plant which is used in the treatment of heart disease having an action almost identical with that of digitalis (q.v.).

Strychnine: the alkaloid of nux vomica, seed of an East Indian tree. It is a nervous stimulant which increases muscle tone and has been used widely in tonics and as a bitter in dyspepsia although it is much less used for these purposes now. Poisoning leads to convulsions very similar to those of tetanus and is liable to be fatal. Barbiturates are given by injection as antidotes.

Stuttering: (*see* Stammering).

Subarachnoid Haemorrhage: a haemorrhage into the subarachnoid space usually from a congenital aneurism in the vessels surrounding the area where the brain and spinal cord meet.

Subinvolution: the failure of the womb to return to its normal size following childbirth.

Succinylsulphathiazole: a sulpha drug used in intestinal infections. The proprietary name is Sulfasuxidine.

Sugars: are classified as *monasaccharides* such as glucose (dextrose), fructose (laevulose), and galactose' with the general formula ($C_6H_{12}O_6$ and *disaccharides* such as sucrose (cane sugar), lactose (milk sugar), and maltose (malt sugar) with the general formula C12H22O11. The *polysaccharides* are starches such as ordinary starch and glycogen or animal starch. Disaccharides and polysaccharides are broken down in the process of digestion into monosaccharides.

Suicide: statistics show that cases of suicide or attempted suicide are on the increase; in part this shows a real increase, but it must also be remembered that a more enlightened public attitude which has removed much of its stigma and realises the need for treatment in cases of attempted suicide has helped to bring to light many instances which formerly would have been concealed.

Paradoxically, suicide is a phenomenon of the prosperous countries. Wherever one looks, it becomes apparent that it is in the technically-advanced and wealthy parts of the world (or even of cities) where the suicide-rate is highest – in Sweden and Switzerland rather than Greece or Bulgaria, in well-to-do Hampstead rather than the poorer parts of London. In so-called backward lands, it is so rare that few people know what the word means or can even picture the idea of a person killing himself. Why this should be so nobody knows for certain although, in view of what facts are available, it is fair to put forward some hypotheses. The first thing to point out is that the Industrial Revolution brought about a change in the structure of the family; for, whereas in an agricultural society every member of the large family plays a useful part –

the grandparents looking after the young whilst the parents work in the fields and the children being social and economic assets from a very early age – this pattern was rudely reversed by the advent of heavy industry. Today children no longer represent riches who, even as toddlers could help on the land, but have become economic liabilities until they leave school at the age of 15 or possibly much later, and as for the old they become a nuisance in our small houses, so, once the man has retired and his family gone elsewhere, the couple are liable to feel (and with justice) cast-off, useless, and doomed to live a lonely life in the otherwise deserted house, or, worse still, in an 'old people's home.' As for the new towns, they are mostly for the young, and the married daughter no longer has her mother just along the street to give advice, chat to, or look after the baby whilst she goes shopping or to the cinema. There is a higher rate of suicide amongst the elderly, and the writer remembers how, in what was left of the old East End after the young had left for the new towns, each Christmastime the number of suicides he was called to see tragically increased amongst the lonely old inhabitants. It was at this time that they felt their position most keenly.

Loneliness at all ages is another important factor in suicide, and this again is related to the high geographical and social mobility rate of the modern society. The single man who has to move from one place to another to get a job, the student (perhaps from a foreign country) alone in his bed-sitter are high amongst the number of those who kill themselves. There is a close correlation between the number of single bed-sitters in an area and its suicide rate. Again, to take another aspect of industrial society, it is obvious that the more importance we attach to success and the greater the stigma we attach to failure, the worse we make things for even the relative failure. In this field, it is not the poor and downtrodden or those who really have something to worry about without a penny in their pockets who commit suicide, but the wealthy man who has lost a large portion of his fortune whilst still retaining ample to live on comfortably for the rest of his life. The sayings 'the further you rise the harder you fall' with its corollary 'those who are down need fear no fall' are substantially true; for the former is liable to suicide whilst the other is not. Finally, amongst the other phoney values of our, in many respects, unpleasant world-picture is that of the over-dramatisation and stimulation by the mass media of the concept of early romantic love amongst the young and romance as a continuing essential in marriage. This plays a very large part in cases of attempted suicide amongst adolescents and married women whose absurdly sentimentalised attitudes towards love-affairs or marriage have been shattered by hard realities. Suicide and suicidal attempts, then, are commonest in these groups: the elderly and old, the lonely, the unmarried, widowers and widows, the wealthy business man who thinks he has lost everything when he still has plenty by ordinary standards, and adolescents and married people amongst whom attempted suicide is most frequent.

Suicide and attempted suicide are not at all the same thing. Suicide successfully accomplished is largely a male preserve. Out of every four men who make the gesture, three succeed; but out of every four women, only one. Attempted suicide is more typical of the younger age groups (from disappointed love) and in married women for much the same reason. Thus, unlike accomplished suicide in which social isolation is a common feature, attempted suicide almost always occurs in a social setting because basically it is an appeal to others, a threat, or even a thinly disguised form of spiritual blackmail. In effect, the individual is saying: 'Look what you've made me do – and I'll do it again if you don't give me more attention!' But it would be a mistake to suppose that those who threaten to commit suicide, whatever their motive, are unlikely to carry out their threat. In one group of cases of death from suicide, investigation showed that more than two-thirds had told someone of their intention beforehand. Nor is it true, as is so often believed, that anyone who fails the first time is unlikely to succeed later. Those who merely attempt suicide to gain some end are quite often dead before help is available. Again, times have altered the methods used by suicides and in a series of 211 admitted to the Royal Infirmary in Edinburgh, 78% had taken overdoses of drugs (all but 32 from doctors' prescriptions); this is a change from the old pattern of throat-cutting, wrist-slashing, gassing, or jumping from heights.

What can the ordinary individual do to prevent these deaths or unpleasant occurrences? In the first place, every threat of suicide should be taken seriously, reported to a doctor who should be encouraged to obtain a psychiatric opinion, and no suicidal attempt hushed-up. Secondly, it should be realised that anyone who shows depression to an abnormal degree, especially without adequate external reason for it, should be similarly reported; so should the persistent hypochondriac who keeps on complaining about bodily (especially abdominal) symptoms and refuses to accept the reassurances of his doctor, that no physical disease exists. Lastly, it is sensible to remember that alcoholism is not only a condition requiring treatment, but is, after depression, the commonest cause of suicide. What for his part the doctor should learn is the danger of giving large amounts of dangerous drugs which are often kept lying around the patient's house for years as a constant temptation to suicide and a serious risk of accidental poisoning.

Sulphacetamide: a sulpha drug used mainly in the treatment of urinary infections. The preparation Albucid (soluble sulphacetamide) is used in the eyes and nose.

Sulphadiazine: a sulpha drug which is relatively non-toxic being used largely in infections caused by the pneumococcus, meningococcus, and gonococcus.

Sulphadimidine: is sulphamezathine, a very safe sulpha drug for general use.

Sulphaguanidine: a sulpha drug used in the treatment of intestinal infections and notably of bacillary dysentery.

Sulphamerazine: with the same range as sulphadiazine, sulphamerazine is a slowly excreted drug which maintains high concentrations in the blood over a long period.

Sulphanilamide: one of the earliest sulpha drugs which is still widely used for general purposes.

Sulpharsphenamine: (sulpharsenol) an arsenical drug used in the treatment of syphilis.

Sulphathiazole: one of the earlier sulpha drugs which has the advantage for some diseases of being rapidly excreted in the urine. Hence its use in urinary infections. It is, however, somewhat more toxic than later sulpha drugs. Sulphathiazole is also used for local application to wounds.

Sulphonal: a relatively rarely used hypnotic which is dangerous because it is so slowly excreted and its effect is therefore carried over into the following day – an undesirable quality in a sleeping potion.

Sulphonamides: the collective name for the sulpha drugs discovered in the form of prontosil by Domagk in 1935. It was found that prontosil was transformed in the body into sulphanilamide, a bacteriostatic substance. This bacteriostatic effect which interferes with the growth of bacteria whilst not killing them is typical of the sulpha group and it is believed that they work by reason of their similarity in chemical structure to p-aminobenzoic acid which is essential to the growth of organisms. The bacteria take up the sulpha drug when it is in greater concentration than p-aminobenzoic acid and this hinders their development and makes it impossible for them to reproduce themselves.

Sulphones: a group of drugs related to the sulphonamides and used in the treatment of leprosy.

Sulphur and Sulphates: these substances are widely used in medicine, sulphur mainly on the surface of the body in the form of sulphur lotions and ointment for acne and in the treatment of scabies (it was formerly popular in the treatment of constipation). Amongst sulphates, which are the salts of sulphuric acid, used in medicine are sodium, potassium, and magnesium sulphate the saline purgatives. Sodium sulphate is Glauber's salts and magnesium sulphate Epsom salts. Copper sulphate is used externally to destroy overgrowths of new tissue.

Sunburn: the effect produced, especially upon fair-skinned people, by the ultra-violet rays of the sun. The treatment for mild degrees of sunburn is calamine lotion; more severe degrees are treated with anti-histamine applications alone or combined with calamine lotion (Caladryl) and hydrocortisone creams.

Sunstroke: (*see* Heat-Cramps, Heat Stroke).

Superfluous Hair: if at all abundant is best removed by shaving which does not, as is so often stated, cause it to grow more rapidly or to become coarser. Isolated hairs can be dealt with by electrolysis and the various depilatory creams can be used in place of shaving. Care must be taken with all of these since they are irritant to many skins and dangerous if they get in the eyes.

Suppository: cones made of oil of theobroma or glycerine jelly combined with a drug for giving by rectum.

Suprarenal Glands: triangular-shaped ductless glands situated

515

one above each kidney. Each consists of a medulla or central part and a cortex or external part, the former secreting the hormone adrenaline, the latter several hormones known as corticosteroids which include cortisone and hydrocortisone. The metabolic end-products of these are 17-ketosteroids and 11-oxysteroids and also the virilising androgen sex hormones. The activity of the cortex is under the control of the anterior lobe of the pituitary gland through the hormone A.C.T.H. (q.v.) and disease of the cortex leads to the development of Addison's disease (q.v.).

Suramin: a drug used in the treatment of trypanosomiasis or sleeping sickness. (It is also known as Germanin and Bayer 205.)

Sycosis: or 'barber's itch' is a very infectious staphylococcal infection of the hair follicles of the beard which was often transmitted by infected instruments in the barber's shop, although much less frequently than formerly. Various sulpha and antibiotic preparations are used in treatment.

Syphilis: is a serious venereal disease spread by sexual intercourse with an infected person. Other methods of infection are possible but, with the exception of kissing, extremely rare and the disease is certainly not contracted from lavatory seats as popular tradition would have us believe. Children may be born with congenital syphilis contracted from the mother. Adult syphilis begins with a sore known as a hard chancre at the point where the spirochaete has entered; this is nearly always on the sexual organs but occasionally on the lips and more rarely elsewhere. In a short time, if untreated, the chancre disappears and all may seem to be well, but this primary stage is followed by a secondary stage with sore throat, a rash, headache, and enlargement of the glands. This, if left alone, also clears up only to be followed by the tertiary stage in which a chronic infection develops in some part of the body which, presumably, is the most susceptible in that particular individual. Thus there may be chronic syphilis of the skin, bones, heart, liver, or nervous system. In the nervous system the two main diseases are locomotor ataxia or tabes dorsalis (q.v.) and general paralysis of the insane or G.P.I. (q.v.).

In congenital syphilis the child is often still-born or premature and those who survive tend to look wizened like a little old man; amongst other symptoms of the disease are eye defects, 'snuffles,' a flattened nose, and when the adult teeth appear the front ones may be notched at the biting surface (Hutchinson's teeth). Diagnosis is made by the finding of a positive Wassermann or Kahn reaction and the modern treatment of syphilis is based on the use of such arsenical preparations as neoarsphenamine (neosalvarsan) and penicillin although in the past bismuth and mercury have been used. Salvarsan was Ehrlich's 'magic bullet' which could attack the organism selectively without harming the body and was, indeed, the first of the modern specific drugs. G.P.I., once hopeless, is now dealt with by malarial therapy combined with the other preparations.

Of venereal disease in general it is important to emphasise the necessity for early treatment and the following facts are also relevant: (1) V.D. does not happen solely to moral degenerates and many are infected who are no worse morally than anyone else; (2) many people believe themselves to have V.D. when they do not since every sore or discharge in the genital area is not necessarily venereal; (3) the only way of finding out for certain is to go to a doctor immediately, remembering that to him this is not a matter for criticism but just another disease; (4) all treatment is wholly secret and confidential.

Syringomyelia: a degenerative disease of the spinal cord of unknown origin in which small cavities are present in its posterior part, usually in the lower cervical and upper thoracic region, surrounded by neuroglial tissue (i.e. the connective tissue of the nervous system) which interferes with the fibres carrying impulses of pain and temperature. Later extension may affect touch and the anterior part of the cord concerned with movement. The process begins between the ages of 10–30 when the patient begins to notice pains or weakness in the hand or arm accompanied by a loss of the sense of pain when the part is cut or burned. Later there is wasting of the small muscles of the hand and sometimes in the shoulder together with a spastic condition of the legs. The anaesthesia of the parts affected is dissociated, i.e. there is retention of the sense of touch together with loss of the senses of pain, heat, and cold. Trophic changes occur due to faulty nutrition of the areas and there may be painless disease of the shoulder or elbow joints or at the wrist and painless ulcers of the fingers

517

are common. There is no specific treatment but death may not ensue for 10–20 years.

Tabes: in the general sense not now much used the word means a wasting disease but today the term is almost exclusively applied to tabes dorsalis or locomotor ataxia (q.v.).

Tachycardia: means a rapid heart-beat which may result from exercise, emotion, fevers, chronic infections, anaemia, haemorrhage, and certain drugs. In *paroxysmal tachycardia* attacks of palpitation may last for a few minutes to a week or more. The most common cause of palpitation is anxiety neurosis in which the heart itself is not affected but only its nervous control mechanism.

Talipes: club-foot (q.v.).

Tannin: (Tannic Acid) is a pale brownish powder with an astringent taste which is used in many conditions in medicine because of its ability to coagulate proteins. Its main use is in burns although other methods are now preferred in the more serious cases because of the tendency of tannic acid to form contracting scars; ulcers and sores are similarly treated. Enemas of the substance have been used for ulcerative colitis and inflammation of the rectum, the ointment of galls (from which tannic acid used to be obtained) with opium is used for piles, and glycerine and tannin is a familiar application for sore throats. Small wounds can be treated with tannin to stop bleeding.

Tape-Worm: (*see* Worms).

Tarsus: the region of the heel which has seven bones: the heelbone or calcaneum, the astragalus which supports the tibia and fibula of the leg, the scaphoid, cuboid, and three cuneiform bones.

Tartar Emetic: (Antimony and Potassium Tartrate) was originally, as the name indicates, used as an emetic but this is not now recommended since it is slow of action and produces depression of the heart and breathing. It is used as an expectorant in cough medicines and is extremely important in the treatment of certain tropical diseases, notably kala-azar (Leishmaniasis), sleeping sickness (trypanosomiasis), bilharziasis, filariasis, yaws, oriental sore, and relapsing fever.

Teeth: in man there are 32 permanent teeth, 16 in each jaw, and these are divided up as follows on each side of the jaw:

two incisors, one canine, two premolars, and three molars. The incisors are used for cutting, the canine (well-developed in carnivorous animals) for tearing and piercing, and the premolars and molars for grinding. The outer layer of a tooth is made of enamel which is a hard substance composed of calcium phosphate, magnesium phosphate, calcium carbonate, and calcium fluoride whilst the rest of the tooth is composed of dentine made up of the same materials but not so hard as the enamel. In the dentine are many small channels which communicate between the enamel and the pulp in the centre of the tooth which is contained in the cavity and consists mainly of blood-vessels and nervous tissue. The root of the tooth is single in the incisors and canine and usually in the first premolar tooth, but the second premolar has two roots and the molars of the upper jaw three; the molars of the lower jaw have two roots each and the last and smallest molar is known as the 'wisdom tooth.' The 'milk teeth' which precede the permanent ones are fewer, smaller, whiter, and somewhat different in shape, the permanent teeth developing from the 5th to the 20th year.

Teething: is often given as the cause for the numerous minor complaints of infancy, probably in the majority of cases quite unjustly. However the irritation or pain caused by erupting teeth can cause loss of sleep and appetite with consequent loss of weight and fretfulness; that it can also cause skin eruptions, cough, and diarrhoea is rather more doubtful. Parents ought to be careful about giving 'teething powders' some of which are decidedly dangerous and capable of causing much more serious trouble than the original one. One may justly attribute troubles to teething when the child rubs its gums and salivates profusely. The best treatment is to give it rusks to chew which will aid in the process. *Dental caries* is essentially a disease of civilisation caused in large measure by eating 'civilised' foods which are too soft and too sweet. These weaken the gums and jaws and the carbohydrates cause bacteria to multiply which produce lactic acid to disintegrate the enamel and subsequent infection attacks the dentine breaking down the whole tooth and destroying the pulp. One of the symptoms of this is *toothache* which may also be caused by a dental abscess or *gumboil*. The treatment of the pain in toothache (which will afterwards require the dentist's attention) is to wash the mouth out with an alkali such as baking soda, give aspirin, and if a cavity exists it should be plugged with a piece of cotton-wool soaked in oil of cloves. Lack of dental care or infections of the mouth are the cause of *gingivitis* or inflammation of the gums in which during the acute stage the gums are swollen, red, and bleed easily on being brushed. A soft toothbrush should be used gently in cleaning, the gums should be massaged daily, and penicillin lozenges or an antiseptic mouth-wash may help. *Pyorrhoea alveolaris* or *paradontal disease* differs from gingivitis in that pockets of pus are formed around the junction of the teeth and gums. In both conditions the teeth tend to become loose in their sockets and the gums shrink exposing the necks of the teeth. The ultimate treatment of gingivitis and pyorrhoea should be left to the dentist.

The teeth should be brushed up and down and to and fro in the morning and at night and after each meal if possible and those who wish to keep their mouths healthy would be well advised to discourage in themselves and others the use of excessive amounts of sweets, carbohydrate foods, and sweet drinks. The effect of dental health upon the health of the body is a matter of controversy. Obviously in very severe cases of pyorrhoea it is undesirable to be constantly swallowing the pus produced around the gums but very few doctors nowadays believe that dental decay has the dread results it was once supposed to have. Thirty years ago or more it used to be thought that 'focal sepsis' could cause a multitude of diseases from rheumatoid arthritis to insanity – indeed, every disease which had no other known cause was attributed to focal sepsis and unfortunate schizophrenics and sufferers from rheumatism had their teeth ruthlessly drawn in the hope of betterment of their condition. This, of course, was rubbish and there is also no reason to suppose that gastric diseases have any close relationship to dental disorders; for the obvious fact is that certain types of people are likely to get ulcers no matter what they do, or do not, eat, whilst others who may have no teeth at all eat (or at any rate swallow) any kind of food, chewed or unchewed, with impunity. A more moderate attitude is that dental disease is largely confined to the mouth but is nevertheless unpleasant, unaesthetic, and painful and few normal people would wish to be wearing dentures if a little attention to their teeth from the early years could prevent it. The prevention of decay in the teeth by adding fluorine to drinking water is mentioned under the heading of Fluorine.

Temperature: (*see* Fever).

Tendon: the cord attaching the end of a muscle to its bone.

Tennis Elbow: (*see* Elbow).

Teratoma: a tumour composed of embryonic tissues, sometimes containing hair or teeth, and usually arising from the ovary or testicle.

Terramycin: (*see* Oxytetracycline).

Testicle: the testicles, epididymides, and spermatic cords lie within the scrotum, the loose bag beneath the penis. The spermatic cord contains the blood-vessels supplying the testicle and epididymis which is a system of coiled tubes through which the spermatozoa manufactured in the testicle pass by way of another tube known as the vas deferens to the seminal vesicles and prostate gland. The semen, which is the combined secretion of the prostate and the spermatozoa from the testicle, is stored in the seminal vesicles until required. Amongst the commoner conditions affecting this area are infection, injury, hydrocele, and varicocele. Cancer of the scrotum used to be very common amongst chimney sweeps and cotton spinners but this is rarely seen now although tumours of the testicle, also rare, are very malignant. Dermatitis of the scrotum is fairly frequent and often difficult to treat.

Infection of the testicle (orchitis) can arise from any condition affecting the urethra, urinary tract, or the prostate gland; sometimes tuberculosis attacks the epididymis which usually has to be removed leaving the testicle in place, but the commonest type of infection used to be gonorrhea although this is less often seen since the introduction of antibiotics. *Injuries* are not often serious ones except in war or industrial cases where the testicle may be so badly damaged as to have to be removed; removal of one testicle does not affect the individual in any way. However, even slight blows to the gland are liable to cause great pain and shock. *Hydrocele* is dealt with under that heading. *Varicocele* is a condition of varicose veins in the spermatic cord occurring nearly always on the left side of the scrotum which when examined feels like a bag of worms. The condition is not serious nor need it give rise to any symptoms although some feel a dragging sensation in the groin. If it is necessary to operate this can be done quite simply and there is no later disturbance of testicular function.

Testosterone: the hormone produced by the testicles which can replace their function in cases of eunuchoidism. Testosterone is also an anabolic substance which aids in the utilisation of proteins and is sometimes used to improve nutrition in wasting diseases; it also diminishes the pain in angina pectoris. The hormone is of no use whatever in cases of impotence due to psychological causes nor is it usually helpful in sterility. In women it is given for a number of disorders such as certain types of excessive uterine bleeding and in cases of cystic mastitis (lumps in the breast caused by multiple cysts).

Tetanus: is an infectious disease characterised by violent muscular contractions and caused by the tetanus bacterium *Clostridium tetani* through a wound contaminated with soil containing spores, or at one time by catgut or wool used for dressings. The incubation period is about 12 days but varies considerably on either side. The patient notices muscular stiffness in the jaw (lockjaw), neck, or arms and legs and this is followed in a few hours by painful cramps. Epileptiform spasms then occur affecting the whole body, and if the period between the onset of the first symptoms and the onset of the first generalised spasm is less than two days the outlook is very grave. Although opisthotonus may occur when the spasm is so great as to cause the patient to be bent like a bow with only the heels and back of the head touching the bed and the patient suffers terrible pain, his mind remains clear. The only other condition resembling this is strychnine poisoning (q.v.). The risk of tetanus has been very much reduced since the introduction of tetanus antitoxin and toxoid, the latter providing protection against the disease. Antitoxin is given immediately after a wound has been received which may be contaminated. After the symptoms have started it is necessary to clean the wound and, although it is less helpful at this stage, antitoxin is injected around the area and into the spinal canal. Curare and other muscle relaxants are given together with sedatives such as paraldehyde or the barbiturates whilst the patient is kept quiet in a dark room. An onset within a week of wounding has a mortality rate of 60% whereas if it delayed to a month or more the mortality rate is 15%. Immunisation with toxoid is given to all soldiers and many believe that those

522

living in parts of the country where soil is much contaminated with organic matter should be immunised also. The organism of tetanus was discovered in 1889 by the Japanese scientist Kitasato.

Tetany: a disorder manifesting itself in muscular spasms of the hands and feet, the larynx, and in severe cases the whole body. The hands assume the so-called accoucheur position (i.e. tips of fingers and thumb together in a cone), the arms are held close to the body, the knees are bent and the feet turned up and inwards with the sole concave. The cause is deficient calcium or alkalosis which may result from: parathyroid deficiency; deficient absorption of calcium as in rickets, osteomalacia, coeliac disease, etc.; alkalosis as in pyloric stenosis in infants, prolonged vomiting, and overdosage of alkalies in the treatment of peptic ulcer; overbreathing in hysteria, and during pregnancy and lactation loss of calcium may bring about attacks. Spasm of the larynx (laryngismus stridulus) may cause death in infants. In adults generalised spasms may resemble epilepsy but there is great pain and no loss of consciousness in tetany. The treatment must include dealing with the causative condition together with administration of parathormone and calcium either by mouth or injection.

Theobromine and Theophylline: two alkaloids, the former found in cocoa, the latter in small amounts in tea or prepared synthetically and both used as diuretics.

Thiourea: a drug which has the power to interfere with the synthesis of thyroxine in the thyroid gland and has therefore been used in the treatment of toxic goitre. It was later replaced by *thiouracil* and this in turn has been replaced by propyl-thiouracil, methylthiouracil, and tapazole, all derivatives of the original substance. They are given (*a*) to prepare a thyroid patient for operation, (*b*) in patients who are mild cases or poor operative risks as the main form of treatment. In the latter case younger patients may remain cured after stopping the drug but about half the older ones relapse.

Thoracic Duct: the large lymph vessel which collects the lymph from the legs, abdomen and left side of the chest, neck, and head. It passes into the large veins at the left side of the neck (*see* Glands).

Thoracoplasty: the operation of removing a number of ribs in

523

order to collapse the lung in cases of pulmonary tuberculosis or bronchiectasis.

Thorax: the chest.

Thread-worm: (*see* Worms).

Throat Diseases: the main diseases considered here are acute and chronic laryngitis, pharyngitis, and carcinoma of the oesophagus. *Acute laryngitis* often follows the common cold or accompanies one of the infectious fevers such as measles, scarlet fever, and diphtheria; on the other hand it may be due to excessive or wrong use of the voice. The symptoms are well-known: slight fever and malaise, a burning sensation in the throat, cough at first dry and later moist, and a voice which may be hoarse or disappear altogether. The treatment is rest in bed, gargles, inhalations of Friar's balsam, and aspirin but in more severe cases the antibiotics or sulpha drugs may have to be used. *Chronic laryngitis* may be the result of many attacks of the acute form or be secondary to infection in the nose and throat, tuberculosis of the lungs, or syphilis. In many cases the people affected are those who use their voice a great deal, e.g. 'clergyman's sore throat.' However, hoarseness which persists beyond a fortnight should always be referred to a doctor and if necessary to a specialist since the risk of cancer of the larynx especially in males over 40 is considerable. *Pharyngitis* is inflammation of the throat proper – the ordinary 'sore throat.' The symptoms are very much the same as in laryngitis with cough, etc., but the back of the throat is painful and red on examination. Gargles, inhalations and sulpha drugs or antibiotics in bad cases may be given. The oesophagus or gullet is the site of several disorders usually characterised by pain or difficulty in swallowing. *Oesophagitis* or inflammation may result from drinking irritant or too hot liquids and difficulty in swallowing may also be due to disorders of nervous control. But the most important disease affecting this area is *cancer of the oesophagus*. This is responsible for about 1% of all cancer deaths and usually occurs in men over the age of 50, the main symptoms being difficulty in swallowing and loss of weight. Until recently the outlook in this condition was absolutely hopeless and relatives had to stand by helplessly whilst the patient literally starved before their eyes as swallowing became more and more difficult. But now advances in chest surgery make it possible for an operation to be carried out in which the diseased area is removed and the stomach brought up into the chest and stitched to the remainder of the gullet. Still more recently the whole oesophagus has been removed and replaced by a plastic tube; this, of course, is only possible if the disease is diagnosed at an early stage.

In many cases difficulty in swallowing or a feeling of choking has a purely emotional cause, this being known as *globus hystericus* which must be treated psychologically. Often it is symptomatic of an intolerable situation facing the patient and is the body's way of saying 'I can't swallow that,' i.e. 'I can't stand this situation' in organ jargon. Lastly, there may occur the bulging in the wall of the oesophagus known as a *diverticulum.* This does not necessarily cause trouble but the larger ones do in that they collect food which periodically comes back into the mouth and the putrefying contents are liable to cause lung disease or pressure on surrounding parts. In this case the only treatment is surgical removal, a major operation but one after which recovery is the general rule.

Thromboangiitis Obliterans: (Buerger's disease) is a rare condition occurring more commonly in men between 40 and 50 and allegedly often Jews and heavy smokers. There is progressive thickening of the medium-sized arteries and veins notably in the legs which soon leads to the symptom of intermittent claudication, i.e. cramps brought on by walking and relieved by rest. The feet are cold and there is loss of pulsation in the artery at the ankle; gangrene of the toes may occur. The treatment is usually surgical, the sympathetic ganglia which lead to spasm being removed.

Thrombosis: the formation of a clot within the blood vessels or heart (*see* Coronary Thrombosis).

Thrush: this is a fungus infection characterised by the presence of white patches in the mouth usually in infants whose bottle-feeding has not been as hygienically carried out as is necessary. The fungus is the *oidium albicans* and the usual treatment is painting with glycerine or borax and sodium sulphite; potassium chlorate is given externally and internally.

Thymol: an antiseptic derived from oil of thyme; it is used in the treatment of hookworm infestations.

Thymoleptic Drugs: drugs used in psychiatry which alter the patient's mood and are usually employed in cases of depression (*see* Mental Illness). Amongst the most generally employed are phenelzine, iproniazid, and nialamide (proprietary names Nardil, Marsilid, Niamid).

Thymus Gland: this lies in the upper part of the chest and lower part of the neck having two lobes composed of a central medulla and an external cortex. The gland decreases in size after puberty and its true function is unknown although it probably has some connection with the changes taking place at that time. Enlargement of the thymus is found in some cases of myasthenia gravis and in the condition known as status lymphaticus (q.v.). Removal of the gland in the treatment of myasthenia gravis is known as thymectomy.

Thyroid Gland: the thyroid gland consists of two lateral lobes conical in shape and joined by a narrow isthmus lying across the windpipe at the base of the neck. Structurally it consists of follicles lined with epithelium which secrete a sticky substance known as colloid and its main function is the production of the hormone thyroxin which increases the rate of metabolism. Oversecretion leads to Graves' disease or exophthalmic goitre, undersecretion to cretinism in infancy and myxoedema in later life. The activity of the thyroid is measured by taking the basal metabolic rate (B.M.R.), i.e. measuring the patient's oxygen consumption over a period of 10 minutes or so whilst he is at complete rest. A more modern test is carried out by measuring the patient's speed of iodine metabolism by means of radioactive iodine. A tracer dose is given which is detected by a special apparatus in its movements through the body. The thyroid is under the control of the anterior pituitary gland (*see* Goitre).

Tibia: the inner and larger of the two bones in the leg.

Tincture: an alcoholic solution of a drug.

Tinea: (*see* Ringworm).

Tinnitus: noises in the ears (*see* Deafness).

Tobacco: (*see* Smoking).

Tolbutamide: proprietary name Rastinon, is a sulphonamide derivative used in the treatment of diabetes in which it lowers the level of the blood sugar. It is used only in selected cases especially those which are fairly mild or in older people.

Tongue, Diseases of: *glossitis* or inflammation of the tongue may be the end-result of many causes and shows itself in some unusual appearance or sensation: redness, soreness, white or black patches, or ulcers. Sometimes the patches are in the form of a map (geographical tongue) and quite often nowadays the cause may be the excessive use of penicillin lozenges which by killing some organisms encourage the growth of others. Other causes of glossitis are irritant foods, excessive smoking, oral sepsis, or general conditions such as gastritis, pellagra, sprue, pernicious anaemia, etc. In leucoplakia the tongue is white and furrowed. All these conditions should they last any length of time must be referred to the doctor, especially if they occur in older people or if ulcers be present. Ulcers of the tongue, if often of little significance, may be very serious and a manifestation of cancer; they should always be reported immediately. Although in the conditions mentioned the appearance of the tongue is a guide to something wrong with the general health of the body few doctors now believe that a coated tongue has the sort of significance it was once thought to have and chronic tongue examiners should give up their practice.

Tonics: it is necessary to state at the outset that there is no such thing as a tonic since, broadly speaking, anybody who feels unwell is either suffering from a specific disease for which he requires the appropriate treatment or is simply psychologically upset, i.e. suffering from depression, being 'fed-up,' bored, etc. Conventional tonics are of various kinds. Thus those who have the custom of demanding such after an illness might be surprised if they knew what they were getting when they make an impossible demand of their long-suffering general practitioner. It may be a mixture of potassium bromide and nux vomica (strychnine) given on the assumption that bromides relax the nerves – as they do – and that strychnine stimulates – although it only stimulates the lower centres rather than the brain and is more likely to lead to nervousness than calm. Or it may be one of the many old-fashioned iron preparations, an 'iron tonic' such as Parrish's food or Easton's syrup, which has neither enough iron to do any good nor in any case would iron be useful unless anaemia were present. Some have great faith in vitamins in spite of the fact that, unless used for some specific disease, they are only necessary to those who lack them and it is unfortunately the case that the more overfed a nation is the more vitamin pills it consumes. In the sense of a preparation which *really* makes one more fit none of these drugs have any effect and, in fact, apart from their psychological effect, they do not even make the patient *feel* better. In recent years many substances have been developed which have the latter effect so that the patient feels better by reason of a genuine stimulating or sedating effect on the brain without actually being better in any way. Such preparations are justified in some cases to tide the individual over a difficult period whilst the body is getting well in its own good time but many have the danger of addiction. Amongst these are such drugs as the stimulants related to amphetamine with or without a sedative which cheer the patient up whilst relaxing him at the same time, the tranquillisers, and other newer drugs which speed up the metabolism. If the doctor advises these then he knows what he is about but in general the tonic habit is a bad one although there is no harm in giving children a vitamin preparation after a feverish illness which has exhausted their resources.

Tonsillitis, Tonsils and Adenoids: the tonsils lie one on each side at the back of the mouth where they can clearly be seen when it is opened wide; the adenoids, on the other hand are not so readily visible being situated in the pharynx behind the inner openings of the nose. Tonsillitis may be a disease on its own or an accompaniment of most of the acute fevers because this area is the point of entry of many infections. In the former case the onset is usually sudden with vomiting and a high fever, the infecting organism being the streptococcus, and the chief danger is that it is prone to lead to a number of dangerous conditions such as rheumatic diseases, damage to the heart, and nephritis when the kidneys are affected. The tonsils on examination are large and swollen, sometimes almost meeting across the mid-line and points of pus may be visible on their surfaces. Chronic tonsillitis occurs as the result of previous acute attacks and is more likely to occur in children who are run-down or who live in poor surroundings; it is nearly always associated with adenoids and the sufferer usually gives a history of many sore throats, colds, or sinus trouble since infection in the throat can spread directly to any part of the nose, sinuses, and (by way of the Eustacian tube) to the ears. If the adenoids are grossly enlarged a typical facial expression develops with the child looking dull and listless and breathing through the mouth which is fishlike and constantly open; the speech sounds as if it had a permanent cold in the head. However this only occurs in the severe cases and is much less common today; for although most children have some trouble with their tonsils and adenoids the tissues tend to shrink after the tenth year and difficulties after that time are infrequent. Antibiotics and the sulpha drugs quickly cure acute tonsillitis, but removal of tonsils and adenoids is required when the tissues are so enlarged as to make breathing difficult, when there are recurrent attacks of tonsillitis, or when the condition does not respond to medical treatment and a chronic infection exists.

Toxaemia: a state of poisoning due (*a*) to the absorption of bacterial toxins from a localised infection such as an abscess, or (*b*) to interference with excretion as in kidney disease leading to uraemia. (For toxaemia of pregnancy *see* Eclampsia.)

Tracheitis: inflammation of the trachea which is usually part of a general infection of the breathing tubes associated with bronchitis.

Tracheotomy: a minor operation for making an opening through the neck into the windpipe which is performed (*a*) to save life when the larynx is obstructed or (*b*) as a preliminary to the operation of removal of the larynx. A tube is inserted in the opening and the patient breathes through this. When the tube is no longer necessary it is removed and the opening allowed to heal up of itself.

Trade Diseases: (*see* Occupational Diseases).

Tranquillisers: the name given to a group of drugs which make the individual feel more calm without making him sleepy as do the ordinary sedatives. There are many of these mostly introduced by drug firms and they include such substances as Atarax (hydroxyzine hydrochloride), Suavitil (benactyzine hydrochloride), Largactil (chlorpromazine hydrochloride), Equanil and Miltown (meprobamate), Pacatal (pecazine hydrochloride), Serpasil (reserpine), Librium, Sparine (promazine hydrochloride), etc. Whereas the barbiturates and ordinary sedatives given in sufficient dosage produce predictable effects, the effect of most tranquillisers is rather variable leading to apparently magical results in some cases and to none at all or unpleasant ones in others. Tranquillisers should never be taken without medical advice since some have very unpleasant side-effects such as giddiness, depression, heaviness in the legs, extreme drowsiness in individual cases, and even severe liver disease. Used properly they are a great advance in medicine.

Transillumination: (*see* Sinusitis).

Transvestism: a sexual perversion in which the individual chooses to wear the clothes of the opposite sex.

Travel Sickness: (*see* Sea-Sickness).

Trephining: the operation of making a hole in the skull either in order to relieve pressure inside or as a preliminary to brain surgery.

Trichiasis: a disease of the eyelids in which the eyelashes grow towards the surface of the eye causing great irritation.

Trichlorethylene: (Trilene) a rapid and safe anaesthetic used in childbirth, when it may be self-administered, and in dentistry for brief anaesthesia.

Trichomonas Vaginalis: a protozoon frequently present in the vagina which may give rise to no symptoms at all or multiply to the point of causing discharge. The infection can be spread to men causing urethral discharge. The condition is fairly easily treated but must be referred to a doctor as it can only be diagnosed for certain by the microscope.

Trigeminal Nerve: the 5th cranial nerve which consists of three divisions: the ophthalmic nerve supplying sensation to the forehead; the superior maxillary nerve supplying sensation to the forehead; the superior maxillary nerve supplying sensation to the cheeks, upper jaw and teeth, and the lining of the mouth and throat; the inferior maxillary nerve supplying sensation to the lower jaw and teeth and the tongue. The latter is also a motor nerve supplying the muscles concerned with chewing (*see* Neuralgia).

Trypanosomiasis: (*see* Sleeping Sickness).

Tryparsamide: an arsenical preparation used in the treatment of sleeping sickness and neuro-syphilis.

Tsetse Fly: (*see* Sleeping Sickness).

Tubal Pregnancy: (*see* Ectopic Gestation).

Tuberculosis: this is caused by the *myobacterium tuberculosis* and in adults the organisms are usually of the human type whereas the glandular tuberculosis of children is most often due to bovine bacilli. The disease may attack almost any part of the body, e.g. the lungs in pulmonary tuberculosis, the intestinal tract (tabes mesenterica), the lymph glands, the bones and joints, the skin (lupus), or the meninges covering the brain (tuberculous meningitis), and the basic lesion is the tubercle. In this the point attacked by the bacillus breaks down to form thick cheesy pus which may subsequently calcify and, surrounded by fibrous tissue, heal. Over 90% of adults in this country have these healed tuberculous lesions in the lungs. On the other hand the tubercle may not calcify but, surrounded by varying amounts of fibrous tissue, remain latent to break down under any circumstances which weaken the body defences; or, finally, it may not become circumscribed at all but eat its way gradually through the surrounding tissues when if not halted it may soon lead to death. Sometimes a balance is struck between the processes of attack and defence, the disease becoming chronic and more or less static, and the tuberculous lesion may burst into a bronchus or on to the surface of the skin forming a persistent discharging sinus. If a lesion bursts into the blood-stream the result may be miliary tuberculosis in which the infection spreads rapidly throughout the body resulting formerly in inevitable death in 2–3 months. The onset of acute pulmonary tuberculosis is characterised by haemoptysis (spitting blood), the spontaneous collapse of a lung, or the signs of pneumonia or bronchopneumonia, the diagnosis being confirmed by finding T.B. germs in the sputum and the results of an X-ray. The signs in the more insidious type are cough, tiredness, loss of weight, stopping of the periods in women, and other rather vague symptoms which, again, require to be confirmed by radiological and bacteriological tests.

The three common types of tubercle bacillus are the human, the bovine, and the avian (occurring in birds), but only the first two types occur in man. In England 99% of pulmonary tuberculosis and 75% of non-pulmonary are due to the human type; the remaining 25% of bovine tuberculosis, as mentioned above, occurs mainly in children whose bones and glands are affected. The main sources of infection are other human beings with T.B. or infected cattle; in the former case the infection is spread by coughing or direct contact and, since the germ is very resistant in the dried state, infected dust may be a source of danger for many months. In the latter case the infection is spread to human beings by infected milk and meat. However, there can be no doubt that infection depends almost as much on the soil as on the seed and everyone who is exposed to T.B. does not necessarily contact it. Bad social and environmental conditions were, therefore, a major point for attack in trying to eradicate the disease and treatment by prevention has been a basic principle. Its striking success is illustrated by the figures: the death-rate of T.B. in 1900 was about 150 per 100,000, in 1950 it was 50, and in 1954 only 17 per 100,000. Apart from improving social and nutritional standards, measures have been taken to weed out infected cattle. Tuberculin testing of herds is widespread and T.T. milk is readily available, whilst the pasteurisation of milk is nearly universal. As a result of this the bovine infections of the bones, glands, and intestines have become much less common. In the human infections early diagnosis by means of mass X-rays with reference to chest clinics and observation of contacts, and vaccination with B.C.G. have played an important part. There seems little doubt that B.C.G. has a considerable effect in preventing tuberculosis when administered to young children. The main principles of treatment have been rest, fresh air, and a rich diet with plenty of vitamins A and D together with such surgical measures in suitable cases as artificial pneumothorax, phrenic crush, and thoracoplasty all of which are designed to collapse the lung and allow it to heal. More recently, pneumonectomy or complete or partial removal of the affected lung has been successful, but the major advance is in the field of chemotherapy since Waksman and his colleagues in the U.S.A. demonstrated the effectiveness of the new antibiotic streptomycin in tuberculosis. Two other drugs isoniazid (I.N.H. and para-aminosalicylic acid (P.A.S.) have a similar effect and all have a profound effect on tuberculous infections especially in younger people. In older and more chronic cases they are capable of making the sputum negative so that today tuberculosis tends to become a chronic rather than an acute disease. Cases of military tuberculosis and tuberculous meningitis which were invariably fatal prior to the discovery of streptomycin can now be saved. Although the new drugs have greatly reduced the mortality of the disease they have not as yet reduced the number of notifications of new cases to the same degree since the mass radiography campaigns have discovered many cases and very often symptomless ones which are therefore in need of early treatment. Lupus and Tuberculous

Meningitis are discussed elsewhere, the latter under the heading of Meningitis.

Tuberose Sclerosis: a condition found in infants obviously mentally defective from birth where there are sebaceous swellings about the face and internally congenital tumours in the heart and kidneys whilst nodules of neuroglia (q.v.) of varying sizes are found embedded in the brain. Most of such cases also suffer from epilepsy and nothing can be done for them to alter the situation for the better.

Tularaemia: a disease spread from rabbits or other rodents to man, the infecting organism being the bacterium tularense named after the county in California (Tulare) where it was first found. The disease occurs both in North America and Europe outside Britain and is characterised by low fever lasting several weeks, exhaustion and depression, with considerable emaciation in the later stages, but streptomycin has proved successful in its treatment.

Tumour: in medical parlance simply means any swelling whatever whether it be benign or malignant. Thus to say that swollen glands create a tumour in the groin simply means that they create a swelling. Malignant tumours are discussed under the heading of Cancer.

Twilight Sleep: the administration of morphine and scopolamine either prior to surgical operations or in childbirth where it is given hourly during the course of labour. It is very effective in producing freedom from pain but has the disadvantages of weakening the force of the contractions of the womb and sometimes causing difficulty with the breathing of the child after birth.

Typhoid Fever: (Enteric) is caused by the *bacillus typhosus* and spread by those sick with the disease, carriers who are infected but not sick, contaminated food such as milk, shellfish, ice-cream, water-cress and other uncooked stuffs, water, and flies. Epidemics are usually due to carriers contaminating food or to sewage contamination of water. Typhoid is a disease of both temperate and tropical countries and occurs mainly in the autumn months, the patients being predominantly young (between 15–25 years). The incubation period is 7–21 days and the onset usually insidious with headache, constipation, and nose-bleeds; during the first week the temperature rises in a stepladder fashion to be maintained at about 101–103 degrees during the second week and gradually falling to normal during the third. The pulse is relatively slow compared with the temperature and the spleen is enlarged with abdominal pains and bowel motions which may be loose or costive. About the 7th day a rash of small pink spots (rose spots) appears on the abdomen and chest and typhoid bacilli appear in the blood in the first week, showing themselves in the urine and faeces (which are therefore highly infectious) during the second and third weeks. The Widal reaction (q.v.) is positive after the 10th day. Amongst complications are deafness, intestinal haemorrhage and perforation during the third week, relapses which may occur on or after the fourth week, and thrombosis, neuritis, pneumonia, and acute cholecystitis may also occur. Of mental symptoms delirium of a low muttering type is sometimes present and memory is often impaired in the early stages. The paratyphoid fevers have similiar symptoms but the duration of the illness is shorter.

The outlook in typhoid has been dramatically changed since the introduction of chloramphenicol (q.v.) and nursing is no longer so much of a problem as formerly. It is still necessary, however, to keep the patient in bed for three weeks on a bland and nutritious diet if complications are to be avoided. Those who are travelling to countries where typhoid is endemic such as India should have T.A.B. injections before leaving.

Typhus Fever: a group of diseases of world-wide distribution caused by organisms of the Rickettsia type which are intermediate between bacteria and viruses in their properties and spread by lice, ticks, fleas, and mites according to the particular form of typhus. The classical form is caused by the Rickettsia prowazeki which is carried by lice and therefore predisposed to by the sort of conditions with which lice are likely to be associated: undernutrition, famine, dirt and overcrowding. The incubation period is 5–21 days and the onset sudden with headache, pains in the back and limbs, and rigors. The rash, known as a 'mulberry rash,' appears on the fourth day and consists of rose-pink spots with larger papules and a mottled appearance under the skin; it appears first on the body and then spreads to the limbs, disappearing on the second week. The temperature rises to 103 degrees and falls by crisis (i.e. suddenly, as in lobar pneumonia) from the 10th to the 14th day. Typhus is a disease which causes great prostration and delirium is a common feature as the name (which means mist or smoke) indicates, the mind being almost invariably clouded whilst the fever lasts. Prior to the advent of modern methods of treatment almost all patients over the age of 50 died. The prophylactic treatment depends, of course, upon the control of lice and fleas and the rats carrying the fleas and this process has been revolutionised by the introduction of D.D.T. which undoubtedly saved Europe in the period following the last war from the epidemics which were so terrible a sequel to the 1914–18 war in Eastern Europe. Curative treatment has changed from being wholly symptomatic to wholly specific by the use of the antibiotics chloramphenicol, chlortetracycline (aureomycin), and oxytetracycline (terramycin). These alter the outlook very considerably. The other types of typhus are Flea typhus (murine), Tick typhus, Rocky Mountain Spotted Fever (q.v.), Mite Fever (Japanese river fever, Tsutsugamushi), and Tick-bite fever.

Ulcer: there are numerous different types of ulcer arising from many different causes but, broadly speaking, all are likely to result from the interplay of two factors, the one internal, the other external. Thus duodenal ulcer is the result of digestion of the mucous membrane by the juices which are normally present and ordinarily do not affect it and this happens because the mucosa has already become devitalised in some way. In bed-sores the internal factor is devitalisation of the tissues in the old or weak, the external one pressure from lying in bed, and in the commonest type of ulcer which accompanies varicose veins (q.v.) the basic factor is poor nutrition of the legs resulting from stagnating blood whilst the external one which decides where the ulcer will occur is very often (although not necessarily) a blow or other minor injury. The treatment of ulcers depends upon their cause which must in all cases be dealt with and inevitably varies greatly, but in those on the surface of the skin such as varicose ulcers the basic principle so far as the local treatment is concerned is to improve the circulation to the part. In the latter case this involves keeping the legs raised as much as possible. If sepsis is present antiseptics or antibiotics such as sulphathiazol powder may be used, but it is important to realise that prolonged use of

535

antiseptics can do nothing but harm and delays or even wholly prevents healing so it is advisable to use bland applications as soon as possible although this depends upon the judgement of the doctor.

Ulna: the inner of the two bones of the forearm which is narrow in the lower portion and thicker at the upper end which forms the olecranon process of the elbow. Fractures may occur from falling on the closed hand at the lower third and falls upon the elbow sometimes result in a chip being broken off from the olecranon process.

Ultra-violet Rays: (*see* Light).

Umbilicus: the navel.

Unconsciousness: this, of course, is ultimately the result of some process occurring in the brain which may be temporary lack of blood-supply as in fainting, injury, compression, as in tumours and abscesses, haemorrhage as in apoplexy or stroke, epilepsy, poisoning by narcotic and other drugs and anaesthetics, diabetic coma and the coma of uraemia in serious kidney disease, the two last being the result of internal poisons accumulating in the body until they affect the brain. In cases of unconsciousness it is important to be able to recognise these various causes so that the appropriate treatment may be applied. Fainting is usually easily diagnosed when the patient suddenly collapses after a brief period of uneasiness with a pale clammy skin and a faint and rapid pulse, whilst in the case of stroke the face is usually congested and the breathing stertorous, traces of paralysis being found on one or other side (*see* Apoplexy). It is necessary to distinguish this from narcotic poisoning; for whilst a case of stroke must be allowed to rest, poisoning requires immediate and active treatment with emetics and stimulants. Epilepsy is not difficult to diagnose when the unconsciousness is preceded by convulsions and later recovery is rapid. In diabetic coma the breath may smell sweet from acetone and the diagnosis will be confirmed by a urinary test whilst uraemia also requires that the urine should be tested to make certain of the cause. Hypoglycaemic coma from an overdose of insulin can also occur and requires the opposite treatment from diabetic coma, sugar being administered in place of insulin.

Undecylenic Acid: a substance used in the treatment of tinea (*see* Ringworm).

Undulant Fever: (*see* Malta Fever).

Uraemia: results from the failure of the kidneys to excrete waste products as a terminal stage in chronic nephritis. The condition is divided into acute and chronic uraemia. In the former type the onset may be with twitchings and drowsiness, headache with a furred tongue and foul breath, gradually deepening into coma; or the state may begin with convulsions and a high fever, and sometimes with great breathlessness. Chronic uraemia manifests itself in many ways, e.g. with gastro-intestinal symptoms of persistent vomiting and diarrhoea or hiccough and cramps, with nervous symptoms such as headache, insomnia, mental symptoms, or transient blindness and signs of stroke although no actual lesion in the brain exists. In latent uraemia there are few initial symptoms except irritability, loss of appetite, a dry tongue, and small pupils, but the condition ends in acute uraemia. The main purpose of treatment is to get the bowels and skin to carry on the functions of the failing kidneys by means of hot packs, etc., to induce sweating and strong purgatives to cause excretion of fluid by the bowels. This, of course, has to be done in hospital.

Urea: is the chief waste product excreted from the body by the kidneys being formed in the liver and transported to the kidneys in the blood. Urea arises mainly from the breakdown of proteins and was the first organic substance to be synthesised. It is used as a test of kidney efficiency and is occasionally given as diuretic.

Ureter: the tubes leading from the kidneys to the bladder (*see* kidneys).

Urethra: the tube passing from the bladder to the exterior. Inflammation of the urethra is known as urethritis and may accompany or cause cystitis or inflammation of the bladder. The two most common causes are infection which is most frequently from gonorrhoea but may be due to other organisms, and irritant substances in the urine as in gout, crystals in the urine, and the taking of various drugs such as cantharides or even alcohol in those liable to the condition. The treatment depends upon the cause, the sulpha drugs and penicillin being used in gonorrhoea (q.v.). Stricture may be the result of a temporary spasm or due to the contraction of a scar causing progressive narrowing of the tube. In the latter case the danger is that the increasing difficulty in passing urine may lead to urinary infection in the bladder and subsequently spread to the kidneys causing death. The stricture may be dilated with bougies or divided by an instrument passed along the urethra (internal urethrotomy) or from outside (external urethrotomy). Injuries to the urethra follow from severe crushing injuries to the pelvis or from injuries sustained by falling astride some object. The diagnosis is made by the presence of blood in the urine or complete stoppage following such an accident.

Uric Acid: (*see* Urine).

Urine: the fluid secreted by the kidneys which is 96% water and the remainder solids resulting from the waste-products of metabolism. The kidneys extract these substances from the blood and pass the resulting urine down the ureters to be stored in the bladder until excreted through the urethra. Normally urine is straw-coloured but this varies with the degree of concentration; the reaction is usually acid but after a meal it may become alkaline when, if it is allowed to stand, a cloud of phosphates may form which are of no pathological significance. The most important constituents of urine are urea (which is formed from the amino-acids resulting from the digestion of proteins), uric acid, and creatinine. Uric acid in the urine is increased after large meat meals, in gout, in leukaemia: it has no connection whatever with rheumatism other than gout in spite of what the patent medicine advertisements say. A normal man passes about 2½ pints of urine in 24 hours but this varies greatly with the fluid intake and the weather, the amount of urine being in inverse relationship to the amount of sweat. Thus in hot weather when much fluid is lost by sweating less urine is passed, whilst in cold weather when there is little sweating the flow is increased.

The flow of urine is increased in certain disease conditions, notably certain types of chronic nephritis and diabetes; it is diminished in acute nephritis and in fevers or heart disease. Complete stoppage is of two types: *suppression* when the urine is not in fact being manufactured by the kidneys, and *retention* when it is manufactured but unable to escape as in inflammation of the prostate or stones in the ureters or urethra when the cause may also be a stricture. The colour of the urine, as mentioned above, may be pale when it is dilute or of a deeper colour when it is concentrated; it is orange or red after taking certain drugs such as senna, when blood is present, or in the presence of urates which often appear in the urine following violent exertion or during fevers; a smoky opaque appearance is typical of small amounts of blood; a greenish-yellow tinge appears when bile is present as in jaundice and black in a few conditions as when (at one time) carbolic dressings were used or when creosote has been taken. The odour of urine also varies being ammonical when it has begun to decompose, fishy when bacillus coli infections exist, like new-mown hay in the presence of diabetes, and smelling of violets when aromatic drugs have been taken or, allegedly, if passed by a saint. Sir Thomas More who was canonised in 1935 claimed to have manifested this form of the odour of sanctity. Abnormal substances found in the urine are albumen (*see* Albuminuria), sugar (*see* Diabetes), blood, pus, and in the more severe cases of diabetes acetone and diacetic acid.

Urology: the branch of medicine dealing with disorders of the urinary tract.

Urticaria: (*see* Nettle-rash).

Uterus: the womb which is a small pear-shaped organ in the non-pregnant state slung by ligaments within the pelvis with the bladder in front and the rectum behind. It is 3 inches long, 2 inches wide at the widest point, and 1 inch thick from before backwards. The Fallopian tubes enter the upper corners lying close to the ovaries at their other ends. At its narrow lower end the uterus projects into the vagina as the cervix with its opening or os uteri. Amongst the more common conditions affecting the uterus are displacements, inflammation, and tumours. The womb normally points upwards and forwards but sometimes the organ may bend further forward producing a kink in itself (anteflexion) or tilt forward as a whole (anteversion); backward bending and tilting are known as retroflexion and retroversion respectively. Anteflexion may be congenital or due to chronic inflammation of the ligaments; the former type may cause painful periods, scanty menstruation, and sterility and is relieved by dilating the cervix. Retroversion and retroflexion may also be congenital when they do not necessarily lead to any symptoms, or acquired when they are usually associated with prolapse and result from relaxed ligaments, lying in bed too long after childbirth, or a tumour which drags the womb backwards. There are no symptoms unless some degree of prolapse is also present when there will be backache, dysmenorrhea, excessive bleeding at the periods, and discharge in between due to to associated endometritis. The condition is dealt with either by inserting a pessary to keep the uterus in position or surgically by tightening the supporting ligaments. In prolapse the womb is displaced downwards and in bad cases may appear outside the vulva. There is a feeling of 'something coming down,' frequency in passing water, vaginal discharge, and backache. Here, too, the treatment is either by pessary or surgical operation. Acute inflammation of the lining of the womb is known as endometritis and usually follows labour or miscarriage whilst chronic endometritis results from infections by streptococci, staphylococci, gonococci, etc., in similar circumstances or may be caused by retroversion or fibroids. Curettage or radium treatment may be necessary or the condition may clear up with drugs. Fibroids are dealt with under that heading and cancer, the other form of tumour, may affect either the body of the uterus or the cervix, the latter type being 30 times more common than the former and occurring usually in women who have borne children. Cancer of the body is more common in those who have never been pregnant, but both types occur between the ages of 40–45. The early symptoms include blood-stained discharge and it is therefore important that any woman over 40 who has excessive loss at the periods or irregular bleeding should see her doctor at once since cure either by radium or surgery depends for its success in cases of cancer upon early diagnosis. Such symptoms of course do not necessarily indicate that cancer is present but it is as well to make sure.

Uvula: the prolongation of the soft palate which hangs down in the middle.

Vaccination: vaccinia is a disease of the cow (cow-pox) which, when inoculated into man produces local pocks at the site of inoculation and slight general symptoms thus affording protection, as Jenner discovered in 1796, against smallpox. The exact nature of the condition produced by vaccination is not known for certain but the two possible theories are (1) that it is small-pox modified by passing through the calf, and (2) that it is quite a separate disease. Most authorities believe that vaccinia (cow-pox) and variola (small-pox) are really the same disease and that the difference between them results from the suscepti-bilities of the animal in which they occur.

Vaccination should be performed on infants at the age of six weeks and every seven years thereafter, the material used being glycerinated sterilised calf lymph. The duration of the immunity conferred is about 12–15 years and this diminishes the liability to contract smallpox and, even if the disease occurs, it is much milder and less likely to be fatal. Compli-cations of vaccination are now very rare, those described being (1) generalised vaccinia, (2) cellulitis from secondary infection by other germs entering the arm at or after the time of vaccination, (3) encephalitis which is the rarest complica-tion of all. Whatever its critics may say there is no doubt that vaccination has caused a great decrease in the mortality of the disease since 1880; thus in Sweden which made vaccination compulsory in 1816 and practised it widely from 1801 there were 2,049 deaths per million population in 1800, 623 per million yearly between 1802–11, and in the years 1890–99 only 1 death per million. Of course the word vaccination can be applied to the giving of any vaccine, the most recent of which is the quadruple one protecting simultaneously against polio, whooping-cough, diphtheria, and tetanus.

Vaccine: a preparation of dead or attenuated infectious material injected into the body with the purpose of increasing its power to resist or to get rid of a disease.

Vaccinia: cow-pox (*see* Vaccination).

Vagina: the female genital passage. Vaginal discharge may arise in the vagina itself or come from the cervix, uterus, Fal-lopian tubes, and other pelvic organs. It may be due to vari-ous germs, to trichomonas vaginalis (q.v.) or the yeast monilia or be non-infective. Some discharge is normal and is more plentiful in some women than others or during pregnancy but any discoloured or offensive discharge should be referred to the doctor. Vaginal discharge is also known as leucorrhoea or 'the whites.'

Vaginismus: spasm of the vagina on attempted intercourse which often makes it impossible. In a few cases this is due to pain from some local condition but the vast majority of cases are wholly psychological.

Vagus: the 10th cranial nerve which supplies branches to the organs in the chest and abdomen having an opposite action to the fibres of the sympathetic nervous system, e.g. the heart is slowed, the intestines stimulated.

Valerian: the root of valerian a common European plant which is, or was, much used in the treatment of neurosis and particularly hysteria. There is no evidence that it has any pharmacological effect at all and there can be little doubt that its main effect was psychological since its unpleasant smell doubtless hastened recovery in those cases who were appalled at the thought of continuing to take it indefinitely.

Valgus: a bending inwards at the knees (knock-knee) or at the ankles as in flat-foot (q.v.).

Valvular Disease of the Heart: (endocarditis) the main enemies of the heart are rheumatic fever and streptococcol infections generally, e.g. tonsillitis and scarlet fever, together with diphtheria and chronic syphilis. All of these can attack the valves of the heart which are the pulmonary, the tricuspid, the mitral, and the aortic each of which may be damaged in one or other of two ways – by narrowing so that the blood cannot easily be pushed through, or by leaking so that the blood pushed through slips back again. The first condition is known as stenosis, the second as regurgitation or incompetence and when one or more valves are damaged the heart attempts to compensate. Thus in incompetence of the aortic valve which lies between the left ventricle and the aorta the blood is pumped out but because the valve cannot close properly much of it returns to the ventricle which, in order to deal with it, becomes greatly enlarged and thickened. But if this does not happen the increased pressure in a chamber which is unable to empty itself completely is passed back through the rest of the circulation; the left auricle overfills, the lungs become congested, and finally the right side of the heart is affected leading ultimately to varying degrees of heart failure. In a great many cases the presence of a murmur heard through the stethoscope, although it does indicate some degree of damage to a valve, is of little serious significance; in mitral incompetence, for example, there need be no symptoms or disability whatever if compensation is perfect but aortic incompetence and mitral stenosis are always serious conditions. The former can be caused by rheumatic fever but syphilis used to be by far the commonest cause in middle-aged men and in elderly people arteriosclerosis is frequently to blame. As explained above, there is great enlargement of the left ventricle and later the signs of a failing heart when compensation fails. The early symptoms of this are headache, giddiness, unpleasant throbbing in the arteries, and occasionally pain in the region of the heart which may spread up the neck and down the arm. Aortic stenosis seldom occurs alone but is usually accompanied by regurgitation. In mitral stenosis the left auricle and the right ventricle are dilated and the lungs, liver, and other viscera are congested. The symptoms are a bluish tinge of the face often accompanied by a high colour over the cheek-bones, a tendency to bronchitis, and haemoptysis (spitting of blood) may occur. The fingers are often clubbed at the tips and there is shortness of breath on slight exertion. Although mitral stenosis is one of the most unpleasant forms of valvular disease the defect may be perfectly compensated for many years and indeed it may be quite unsuspected. Pulmonary stenosis is nearly always congenital (*see* Heart Disease, Congenital).

Since rheumatic fever is much less common and diphtheria and chronic syphilis equally infrequent the most usual sequence of events preceding valvular disease of the heart is as follows: a child or young adult develops a streptococcal sore throat which may clear up with little trouble as it does in the vast majority of cases, but in others the infection is followed within about ten days by pains moving from one joint to another and this too clears up within a short time. A similar episode follows at a later date and later still it may be found that these relatively trivial events have damaged the heart; the damage may be discovered by accident during a routine medical examination or because the patient has begun to complain of breathlessness or one or other of the symptoms mentioned above. When symptomless valvular disease is found no treatment is necessary except that the patient should take ordinary precautions to lead a quiet and well-regulated life and drugs are only necessary when, with the appearance of symptoms, it is evident that compensation is beginning to fail. In such cases the drugs digitalis and its derivatives or strophanthus are used and these in many cases enable the patient to lead a busy, useful, and reasonably long life. Mitral stenosis can now be treated by surgical operation in which

543

the narrowed valve is slit thus transforming the condition into the much less serious mitral incompetence.

Varicella: chicken-pox (q.v.).

Varicocele: (*see* Testicle, Diseases of).

Varicose Veins: these occur in about one out of every two women and one of every four men over the age of 40 years although they may also make their appearance in much younger people. In large measure varicose veins are the penalty man has to endure for adopting the upright position since only then does the problem arise of returning the blood to the heart against the pull of gravity; normally this is done by the contraction of the leg muscles which massages the blood upwards and by the periodic expansion and contraction of the lungs during breathing which, by creating an alternate positive and negative pressure in the chest causes the blood to be sucked up towards the heart. But both these processes are dependent on the valves in the veins of the leg which by their one-way action keep the blood once it has moved up from falling backwards. When the valves fail the veins swell and the blood stagnates within them and this is the condition described as varicose veins. The damage may be caused by pregnancy in women, by constipation, or other causes which partially block the veins in the pelvis, and jobs which involve a great deal of standing without much movement, e.g. dentists, barbers, etc., are prone to lead to breakdown. Phlebitis is both a cause and the result of varicose veins. The veins affected are not the deep ones embedded in the muscles but the superficial ones in the saphenous system (q.v.) which can be seen beneath the skin and the result of the failure of their valves is a heavy tired feeling in the legs, swelling of the ankles, and frequently skin rashes, ulcers, and phlebitis. The great danger of phlebitis (or thrombophlebitis) which is inflammation of a vein with clot formation is that the clot which sometimes contains bacteria may break loose and lodge in other vessels at some distant part of the body perhaps causing a fatal embolism or abscesses which can lead to blood-poisoning. Phlebitis is particularly likely to occur in sufferers from varicose veins and the initial cause that starts it off may be an injury, extension of infection from a nearby site, pregnancy, or an operation when the patient gets up after being in bed for some time. There are three main forms of surgical treatment for varicose veins: injection, cutting and ligation, ligation and stripping. In injection a sclerosing solution is injected into the vein forming a clot which causes the blood to change its course and travel through the unaffected deep veins; this gives relief in mild cases but in a large number of cases the veins recur. Cutting and ligation is much more effective and here the main saphenous vein and its branches are tied and divided at the groin; in addition incisions have to be made along the course of the veins in order to deal with the branches connecting superficial and deep veins. Stripping means threading a long wire through the vein from the groin to the ankle, the vein then being tied securely to the wire in the groin and pulled out from above down by turning it inside out. This is an effective but more risky operation.

Vena Cava: the superior and inferior venae cavae are the two large veins which open into the right auricle of the heart.

Venereal Disease as a Social Problem: the main venereal diseases (gonorrhoea, syphilis, and chancroid or soft sore which is the least common) have already been discussed under these headings. But since throughout this book an attempt has been made to deal not only with individual problems but with social ones, it seems important to say something about the rather serious problem presented by these diseases in Britain – and elsewhere – today. Nobody was surprised when the number of V.D. cases reached an all-time peak during the war and the subsequent two years and then slumped, but there was ground for concern when, after about 1951, a further dramatic rise began, especially in the incidence of gonorrhoea, and is still continuing. An investigation carried out by the World Health Organisation showed (a) that during the years 1957–60, out of seventy-two countries, thirty stated that gonorrhoea was on the increase and thirty-one recorded an increase in syphilis; (b) that these increases were unrelated to high or low standards of hygiene or health services; and (c) that the greatest increase was amongst teenagers.

Gonorrhoea cases in Britain have increased in the last ten years from less than 20,000 per year in 1951 to over 30,000 a year today, but in the years 1957–60 there was a national increase of nearly 70% among boys of 15–19 and 65% for girls of the same age. The increase was also high amongst young men of 20–24 where it was 56% and amongst young women of the same age-group where it was 60%. In the older age-groups the national increase for men was 33% and for women only 18%. Syphilis which constitutes only about 10% of the cases of V.D. in Britain has apparently not increased to any great extent, but it is of interest to note that a large number of syphilitic cases are homosexuals – in one London clinic the proportion was 60%. Syphilis is, of course, a killer, which can spread to any part of the body; gonorrhoea, on the other hand, tends (although by no means always) to be localised. Both are easy to diagnose in a man who can hardly fail to notice the hard sore of the former on his penis, or the thick pus exuding from his urethra in the latter. Unfortunately, although easily diagnosed by a doctor, the symptoms of both diseases are much less obvious to a woman who may therefore go on infecting others unknowingly and the fact that about one female attends a V.D. clinic for every four males suggests that many women are unaware of their condition and that the incidence of V.D. is higher than even the figures already given would suggest. As pointed out in connection with the individual diseases, the end-results of syphilis (both for the individual and the next generation) are very serious indeed, and gonorrhoea, if less serious in most cases, can also have very unpleasant consequences. Neither is as infectious as was formerly believed, and certainly cannot be contracted by the means often mentioned in the past – from cups, towels, or lavatory seats – sexual intercourse and, rarely, kissing someone with an actual sore on the lip are almost the only source of infection. Cure is relatively simple and in the earlier stages of syphilis penicillin is almost invariably successful, whilst a single penicillin injection usually suffices for gonorrhoea.

Nevertheless, the figures are disquieting and obviously it is necessary to explain them before deciding what practical measures to take. Most authorities are agreed that there are two minor and one major cause for the explosive increase in V.D. The two minor ones are that nowadays, when less social stigma is attached to these diseases, fewer cases are concealed and that therefore part of the increase is more apparent than real; another is the greater social mobility of people in the modern world which makes it possible for an infected person to infect others in widely separated areas. Emigrants form a small part of the problem; for – although they are no more immoral than anybody else – it is obvious that, as happened during the war, the existence of a large number of men without women is bound to lead to promiscuity. The major cause, however, as is evidenced by the increases in the younger age-groups, is the increasing sexual activity of the adolescent. This, in its turn, is due to the undoubted fact that children mature earlier, and to the breakdown of old moral standards.

What can be done about it? Propaganda, except in so far as it is informative, is of little use. Information performs a really useful function but those responsible for public health propaganda have yet to learn that terror campaigns have been proved beyond doubt by psychological research to be not only useless but to bring about exactly the opposite results from those desired. You cannot terrify people out of smoking or sexual promiscuity – but you can often terrify them into it. Nor can we by moral dictate control peoples' sexual activities as so many churchmen and politicians seem to suppose. In fact the only feasible solution is more and better sex education both by parents and teachers. This should be objective and based on discussion rather than preaching. Many of those adolescents who became infected with V.D. are doubtless children with delinquent tendencies, but the great bulk are ordinary children who would not run the risks of pregnancy and disease had they been better informed and treated with greater understanding. It is not only imperious sexual desire that causes juvenile promiscuity – many children fornicate for the same reason that they smoke: to prove their adulthood and because grown-ups threaten them and tell them that these are things they must not do. Their behaviour is in the nature of a 'dare' or challenge. Thus the headmaster of a school where smoking was rife, called his pupils together and gave them a factual, truthful, and unemotional talk about the risk attached to the habit following up his talk with a statement that all those who wished to do so could smoke in a small room in the school during the last half-hour of the lunch break, but at no other time. So far from increasing, smoking practically ceased altogether, because (a) those who went to the room to smoke were caused to feel rather silly and cut off from the rest of their school-mates, and (b) the daring aspect of the habit had been removed. We are not suggesting that exactly the same procedure should be carried out in relation to V.D., but it is suggested that those who lead public opinion should learn from psychological research; that there should be a far wider spread of cold, factual, information; and that thundering from the pulpit or parliamentary bench is likely to spread the very evil it is trying to curb.

Venesection: the removal of blood by opening a vein.

Ventriculography: the process of taking an X-ray of the ventricles of the brain after the cerebrospinal fluid has been replaced by air. This enables any bulging into the ventricles, e.g. from a tumour to be observed.

Verruca: a wart (q.v.).

Vertigo: or giddiness with a sense of lack of balance has numerous causes which can best be classified as those connected with the inner ear such as Ménière's disease (q.v.), those connected with the eyes such as refractive errors, those caused by injury or disease in the brain as in arteriosclerosis and tumours, diseases of the nerves, gastric causes such as gastritis and stomach upsets, and many minor conditions such as neurosis, too large intake of tobacco or alcohol, migraine, and bloodlessness of the brain produced by fainting or disease of the heart. Treatment depends upon the cause but many cases respond well to prochlorperazine maleate (Stemetil).

Vesical: connected with the urinary bladder.

Vesicle: a little blister.

Vincent's Angina: a form of sore throat characterised by a membranous and ulcerative condition of the tonsils rather similar to that of diphtheria and caused by a spirillum and a fusiform bacillus. It is frequently associated with pyorrhoea of the gums and a generally run-down state of health. There is only slight fever and little pain but the glands in the neck are swollen. The condition clears up on painting the throat with salvarsan.

Virilism: the appearance of masculine characteristics in the female usually the result of disease of the suprarenal glands, e.g. over-action or a tumour of the cortex.

Virus: (*see* Infection).

Visceroptosis: a general dropping of the abdominal organs due to laxity of the peritoneal ligaments and weakness of the abdominal muscles. The symptoms vary but there is often a considerable neurotic element in those who are aware of the existence of this condition.

Vitamins: the following is a list of the known vitamins, their sources and diseases associated with their absence:

Vitamin A: fat-soluble, found in fish-liver oils, milk, and green vegetables. Absence causes xerophthalmia and night-blindness.

Vitamin B complex:

(a) Vitamin B1 (aneurin, thiamin) found, like the others, in yeast and liver. Absence causes beri-beri.

(b) Vitamin B2 (riboflavine). Absence causes cheilosis.

(c) Nicotinamide. Absence causes pellagra.

(d) Vitamin B6 (pyridoxin, pyridoxal, pyridoxamine).

(e) Pantothenic acid.

(f) p-aminobenzoic acid.

(g) Inosotol.

(h) Choline.

(i) Vitamin H (biotin).

(j) Folic acid.

(k) Anti-pernicious anaemia factor (vitamin B12).

Vitamin C: water-soluble (ascorbic acid) found in fresh fruit and vegetables, raw meat. Absence causes scurvy.

Vitamin D: fat-soluble (calciferol) found in liver oils, herrings, dairy produce, and formed by the influence of sunlight on the skin. Diseases caused by its absence rickets, osteomalacia.

Vitamin E: fat-soluble (alpha-tocopherol), found in wheat-germ oil and lettuce. Absence causes habitual miscarriage and sterility.

Vitamin K: (alpha-phylloquinone, menaphthone). Absence exists in haemorrhagic disease of the new-born, obstructive jaundice, and chilblains. Its action is anti-haemorrhagic.

Vitamin P: exists in association with vitamin C (citrin, hesperidin) and diminishes the permeability of capillary walls. It is given in purpura. (*See* Tonics).

Vitiligo: a skin disease characterised by light coloured patches in the skin and hair.

Volvulus: an obstruction of the intestine caused by the twisting of a loop of bowel on itself.

Vomiting: this has many causes both physical and psychological all of which act through the vomiting centre on the floor of the fourth ventricle of the brain. Many acute fevers, especially in children, begin with vomiting and any form of gastric irritation whether from disease or irritant substances taken into the body has the same effect. Other abdominal conditions not connected with the stomach such as intestinal obstruction, peritonitis, pregnancy, renal and biliary colic, and brain diseases such as tumour, abscess, injury, and meningitis are associated with vomiting and retching Certain drugs such as apomorphine have the same effect, and perhaps one of the commonest causes is the vomiting associated with giddiness (Ménière's syndrome, travel sickness) or with psychological causes in connection with the emotions of fear or disgust.

Vulva: the external female genitals.

Warts: or verrucae are extremely common both in childhood and later life. They are usually considered to be a virus infection and are certainly capable of spread. Freezing with carbon dioxide snow is the best treatment since it leaves no scar but in mild cases glacial acetic acid applied on a stick wrapped in cotton-wool or the use of silver nitrate will cure the condition. Extensive infection with warts can be dealt with by the application of X-rays. Plantar warts, unlike the common type, are painful, appearing on the soles of the feet and usually contracted in swimming-baths, etc; they may occur in epidemics in schools and are treated by incision, scraping out, and cauterisation. Care should be taken against infecting others.

Wassermann Reaction: the complement fixation test used in the diagnosis of syphilis. It is accurate in at least 90% of cases and, although positive in certain other diseases, these are not such as could easily be confused with syphilis clinically.

Waterbrush: the bringing-up into the mouth of sour-tasting fluid from the stomach which is associated with excessive acidity of the stomach contents and sometimes with duodenal ulcer.

Weil's Disease: (*see* Spirochaetosis Icterohaemorrhagica).

Weir-Mitchell Treatment: a treatment consisting of absolute rest and a nourishing and easily-digested diet formerly used in the treatment of neurosis. The patients probably got well out of sheer boredom.

Wens: cystic tumours sometimes reaching a large size and occurring on the face and scalp as the result of blockage of a sebaceous gland. They are harmless but unsightly and require to be surgically removed.

Whites: a popular name for leucorrhoea (*see* Vagina).

Whitlow: a popular term for any inflammation and infection of the fingers, generally on the finger tip in the pulp or at the base of the nail.

Whooping-cough: (pertussis) this disease is caused by the *haemophilus pertussis* and spread by droplet infection. The patient is usually a child who, after an incubation period of 6–17 days, develops a fever, running nose, and cough. The attacks of whooping begin about a week later with an explosive cough leading up to a long-drawn-out crowing inspiration which may be followed by vomiting. The whites of the eyes become congested and the face swollen until the whoop disappears in about six weeks. Complications include bronchitis, middle ear disease, bronchopneumonia, and convulsions and quite often there are haemorrhages from the nose, in the sputum, and into the eyes. Cases should be isolated and given as much fresh air as possible consistent with keeping warm. Antispasmodic drugs such as belladonna and bromide are given for the cough and the sulpha drugs and penicillin are given to reduce the risk of complications. Chloramphenicol and the tetracyclines seem to attack the organism directly but are not used as a routine being reserved for very young children and cases with complications. A prophylactic vaccine is available which seems to prevent the disease or modify its course when given early enough.

Windpipe: the trachea (q.v.).

Womb: (*see* Uterus).

Worms: numerous types of worm infest the human body and some of these have been described elsewhere. The common worms in this country are the tape-worm, the round-worm, and the thread-worm. Tape-worms are spread by infested food, *taenia solium* by pork, *taenia mediocanellata* by beef, and *dibothriocephalus latus* by fish mainly in the Baltic countries. The length ranges from 6–12 feet for the pork tape-worm to 25–30 feet for the fish tape-worm, each worm having a small head with suckers and, in the case of taenia solium, hooks, the rest of the body being composed of a varying number of segments or proglottides (from 500–1,000). Rather different is the *taenia echinococcus* which is only ¼ inch long and with four segments; this type inhabits the intestines of the dog and, on entering the human intestines perforates the wall and reaches various parts of the body to produce hydatid cysts which can only be treated surgically. The first three forms of tapeworm inhabit the flesh of animals but are localised solely in the human intestine where they produce, contrary to general belief, no symptoms although the knowledge that a tapeworm is present is liable to lead to various neurotic symptoms after the fact has been discovered. Treatment must be under medical care and usually involves the giving of male fern extract which can only be counted successful when the head is expelled.

Ascaris lumbricoides, the round-worm, inhabits the upper parts of the small intestine and is about the size of a large earth-worm. There is no intermediate host and infestation is probably through drinking infected water. Round-worms are treated by santonin. Occasionally irritability, a 'run-down' appearance, and convulsions occur in children. Thread-worms or *oxyuris vermicularis* are very common and range from ¼–½ inch in length. Localised in the rectum and colon, they give rise to itching around the anus and are very infectious from one child to another and it is important to keep the child from scratching and to keep the hands clean and the nails short. The usual treatment is thymol, but Benadryl, gentian violet, piperazine, and diphenan are probably more effective. Anthiphen (dichlorophen) and chloroquine sulphate or phosphate are more modern remedies for tape-worm.

Wounds: these are classified as incised, contused, punctured, and lacerated. An incised wound is one that is clean-cut as with a knife; the opening tends to gape and, depending upon its size, to bleed a good deal. Treatment in this case is to clean thoroughly with antiseptic and, when necessary, stitch the edges of the wound together to allow it to heal by 'first intention,' i.e. the two surfaces become joined by a film of lymph which is later replaced by connective tissue. The point of entry of a punctured wound caused by a pointed instrument is often quite small but the obvious danger is that internal organs have been damaged and that internal bleeding may be going on. This can only be diagnosed by careful observation of the patient's general condition, internal bleeding being indicated by pallor, rapid weak pulse, and falling blood-pressure. A watch must also be kept for signs of sepsis which may have been introduced into the wound by the instrument. Contused wounds result from a fall or a blow with a blunt instrument; here, too, there is usually little bleeding but considerable bruising and injury to bones, etc., must be looked for. Because of the bruising such wounds often take some time to heal but, on the other hand, there is less risk of sepsis. Lacerated wounds are those in which the tissues are torn as in some types of industrial or road accidents; here there is considerable risk of sepsis and shock is likely to result if the injury is at all extensive. Cleaning is very important and anti-tetanus serum is even more important than in the other cases where it may be unnecessary if there is no suspicion that dirt has got into the wound; repairs to the injured tissues may have to be carried out by the surgeon before leaving the wound to heal. This type of injury usually heals by 'second intention,' i.e. a film of lymph forms over the area and new granulation tissue grows which later turns into a more or less extensive scar. In bad cases skin grafts may be necessary. Penicillin and sulphonamides are much used both locally and otherwise when wounds are infected but thorough cleaning and arrest of bleeding are always the first steps.

Wrist: this region lies between the end of the forearm which consists of the ends of the radius and ulna and the metacarpal bones of the hand; it contains eight small carpal bones and the radius and the triangular cartilage at the end of the ulna articulate with three of these – the cuneiform, scaphoid, and lunar bones. Dislocations of the wrist are rare but sprains are quite common and the tendons in front of the joint are liable to tenosynovitis or inflammation. A ganglion (q.v.) is not uncommon in this area.

Writer's Cramp: (see Cramp).

Wry-neck: a twisting of the head to one side as the result either of the contraction of a scar or spasm of the muscles which may be psychological in origin.

X-rays: these are electromagnetic waves of the same type as wireless or light waves but much shorter, a property which gives them the ability to penetrate bodies opaque to ordinary light. The absorption of X-rays depends upon the nature of the atoms of the body concerned, so that the heavier the atoms the greater the absorption. Thus a thin sheet of lead will absorb much of a beam of hard X-rays that would easily penetrate several feet of wood. A beam of X-rays passing through the body is less easily absorbed by the flesh than by the bone and so if a fluorescent screen be placed behind the body the bones will be revealed by the shadows they cast. Other parts of the body can be made opaque to X-rays by injecting or giving the patient appropriate substances to swallow, e.g. the barium meal to outline the intestines, special substances given to outline the gall-bladder and kidneys, the arteries of the brain or its ventricles. Permanent X-ray records are obtained by replacing the fluorescent screen by a photographic plate which is sensitive to X-rays. The other function of X-rays in medicine is in treatment. They are used in dealing with many types of cancer because malignant cells are more readily destroyed by X-rays than are normal ones. They are also used for certain skin diseases. Radioactive substances such as radium are also used for radiotherapy and the action of some of them depends on the gamma-rays or very hard X-rays that they emit (*see* Radium).

Xeroderma: a disorder of the skin characterised by the formation of scales on a rough dry surface.

Xerophthalmia: a dry thickened state of the conjunctiva of the eyes together with chronic conjunctivitis caused by lack of vitamin A.

Yaws: (*see* Framboesia).

Yeast: a soft light-brown cheese-like material consisting of a mass of minute single-celled organisms (saccharomyces) belonging to the group of fungi. They are rich sources of the B vitamins and of ergosterol, a source of vitamin D, and are used in medicine because of this characteristic. However it must be remembered (*a*) that when vitamin B complex is really needed it is much more conveniently available in tablet form which also has the advantage that the dose is standardised, and (*b*) that yeast has no effect at all, least of all a 'tonic' one in those whose diet is not lacking in the vitamin. Yeast has not the slightest effect on a neurosis although it is commonly advertised for 'nerves.'

Yellow Fever: this is a virus infection spread by a mosquito, the Aëdes aegypti, and found mainly in central America and east and west Africa. Jungle yellow fever occurs in Brazil but it is not known how man is infected in this type, although monkeys and other animals probably act as reservoirs of infection for all types. The incubation period is 3–6 days and the onset sudden with a rigor, the initial fever lasting about three days when jaundice appears and there is vomiting in which the vomit contains bile and perhaps blood. There is then a period of remission for a further three days and the temperature falls; this may be the beginning of convalescence but more often a stage of secondary fever follws when the temperature rises again but the pulse remains slow. There is black vomit at this stage due to the bringing up of altered blood and the urine is dark and scanty due to red blood cells, haemoglobin, and bile. Rashes and bleeding from the nose are common. In severe cases the patient has a high fever, vomits blood, and the urine is totally suppressed leading to death. The preventive treatment is directed to mosquito destruction, the use of mosquito nets, and the giving of yellow fever vaccine which affords complete protection. People coming from an infected area should be kept in quarantine for 10 days. There is as yet no specific treatment for the fever and good nursing is the main necessity with measures to deal with stoppage of urine should this occur.

Zymotic Diseases: a term formerly used to apply to the acute infectious fevers, e.g. scarlet fever, measles, diphtheria, typhus and typhoid, cholera, etc.

A Selection of Biography from Sphere

A Selection of History and Archaeology Titles from Sphere

Titles in the Beginners Guide Series from Sphere

All these titles are illustrated